FUNDAMENTALS OF
Orthopaedics

FUNDAMENTALS OF
Orthopaedics

Mark R. Brinker, MD
Director of Acute and Reconstructive Trauma
Director, The Center for Musculoskeletal Research
  and Outcomes Studies
Fondren Orthopaedic Group LLP
Texas Orthopaedic Hospital
Houston, Texas
Clinical Associate Professor of Orthopaedic Surgery
Associate Director of Orthopaedic Resident
  Education
Tulane University School of Medicine
New Orleans, Louisiana
Adjunct Associate Professor of Orthopaedic Surgery
Director of Orthopaedic Basic Science Education
Adjunct Associate Professor, School of Public
  Health,
University of Texas at Houston Medical School
Houston, Texas

Mark D. Miller, MD
Chief of Sports Medicine
Director of Resident Research
Deputy Chairman, Orthopaedic Surgery
Wilford Hall USAF Medical Center
Lackland Air Force Base
San Antonio, Texas
Clinical Associate Professor
Uniformed Services University of the Health
  Sciences
Bethesda, Maryland
Clinical Associate Professor of Orthopaedic Surgery
University of Texas Health Sciences Center
San Antonio, Texas

W.B. SAUNDERS COMPANY
A Division of Harcourt Brace & Company
Philadelphia London Toronto Sydney

W.B. SAUNDERS COMPANY
A Division of Harcourt Brace & Company

The Curtis Center
Independence Square West
Philadelphia, Pennsylvania 19106

Library of Congress Cataloging-in-Publication Data

Brinker, Mark R.

Fundamentals of orthopaedics / Mark R. Brinker, Mark D. Miller.

p.   cm.

ISBN 0–7216–6698–1

1. Orthopedics.   I. Miller, Mark D.   II. Title.
  [DNLM: 1. Orthopedics.   WE 168 B858f 1998]

RD731.B83 1998   616.7—dc21

DNLM/DLC   97–43313

FUNDAMENTALS OF ORTHOPAEDICS   ISBN 0–7216–6698–1

Last digit is the print number: 9   8   7   6   5   4   3   2   1

*To my parents, Allen and Carole Brinker, who gave me the ability,
and my sister, Marjorie Ivy Brinker, who taught me what to do with it.*

MARK R. BRINKER

*To my wonderful wife Brenda; my beautiful daughter Melissa; and her
three doting big brothers. With love and appreciation for all the
sacrifices that they make.*

MARK D. MILLER

Preface

In a small plane somewhere over Iowa we conceived of the idea for a basic orthopaedic textbook. We have entered an era when primary care providers have become the gatekeepers for patients' access to subspecialists. Because of this trend, there has been increasing pressure on primary care physicians to manage a vast array of musculoskeletal problems. Medical students, primary care physicians, and young orthopaedic residents now have too much to learn and find it difficult to rapidly synthesize the core information of musculoskeletal medicine.

Therefore, we planned this textbook with two goals in mind:

1. The text can be used as a reference, allowing a provider of musculoskeletal care to rapidly obtain knowledge about a patient being seen in the office. It will serve as a blueprint for treatment and a guideline for referral.
2. The text can be read cover to cover, educating the novice on the fundamentals of orthopaedic knowledge.

As we developed the idea and began writing the text, we discovered that the book would likely have a much wider appeal. When we put the finishing touches on the proofs, we envisioned primary care physicians, medical students, young orthopaedic residents, physiatrists, neurologists, radiologists, osteopaths, podiatrists, chiropractors, physical therapists, occupational therapists, physician assistants, nurses, and many many others who would benefit from this book.

The final text is in many ways a compromise between the authors, one anxious to cut to the chase and get to the bottom line, and the other insistent on making sure that every detail is clear to even the most junior student. What has resulted is a well-planned journey through orthopaedics unlike any other textbook currently available. We sincerely hope that we hit the mark and that the reader shares our enthusiasm and interest in musculoskeletal medicine. Read on!

MARK R. BRINKER
MARK D. MILLER

Acknowledgments

No project of great magnitude can be completed without the help of many individuals; this textbook is no exception. The authors are indebted to the members of Fondren Orthopedic Group and Wilford Hall Medical Center for their generous contributions of clinical cases and their support of academic excellence. Special thanks to Michele Clowers and the staff of the Joe W. King Orthopedic Institute (Rodney Baker, Lou Fincher, Jeff Russell) for their assistance in the preparation of the text and figures. We would also like to express our gratitude to the Radiology Technologists (Kathy Kroupa, Becky Atkinson, Jennifer Brammer, Becky Leggett, Vincent Lusk, Janet McGowan, Cathy Ramsey, Kelly Ryan, John Thomas, Dee Partridge-Yawn, Lila Bernal) and the Orthopedic Technologists (Jake Trivitt, Richard Blanton, Jimmie Edmonds, Robert White) of the Fondren Orthopedic Group for all of their assistance. We are grateful to Dr. Jeffrey London and Dr. Linda Nachmani for all of their efforts and to Peggy Pierce and Karen Yates, the "Great Facilitators." Also special thanks to Mrs. Annemarie Hamori, the best orthopedic librarian in the universe, for all of her valuable assistance. Thanks to the residents and staff at Wilford Hall USAF Medical Center, The Uniformed Services University, and the University of Pittsburgh; special thanks to Dr. Michael Wilson, Dr. Rich Howard, and Dr. Norman Rich. The authors appreciate all the people at W.B. Saunders who worked so hard to bring this project to completion. We are particularly grateful to our editor, Richard Lampert; our Production Managers, Linda Garber and Shelley Hampton; our copy editor, Amy Norwitz; and our illustrator, Suzanne Edmonds. Finally, we would like to express our profound gratitude to our mentors, the faculty of the departments of orthopaedic surgery at Tulane University School of Medicine, Wilford Hall USAF Medical Center, and the University of Pittsburgh.

MARK R. BRINKER
MARK D. MILLER

Contents

CHAPTER 1

Basic Sciences

BONE

HISTOLOGY OF BONE

Types of Bone (Fig. 1–1)

On a microscopic level, bone may be classified into two types—lamellar (cortical or cancellous) and woven (immature or pathologic) (Table 1–1)

Cortical bone
- Also known as compact bone
- Makes up 80% of the skeleton
- Composed of tightly packed osteons (haversian system)
- Osteons are connected by haversian canals, which contain
  - Arterioles
  - Venules
  - Capillaries
  - Nerves
  - ? Lymphatic channels
- Interstitial lamellae lie between osteons
- Cement lines define the outer border of an osteon
- Nutrition of cortical bone via intraosseous circulation
  - Haversian canal vessels
  - Canaliculi (cell processes of osteocytes) (see Fig. 1–1)

Cancellous bone
- Also known as spongy or trabecular bone
- Less dense than cortical bone
- Remodels more than cortical bone; remodeling is along lines of stress (Wolff's law)
- Higher rate of turnover than cortical bone
- More elastic than cortical bone

Table 1–1
TYPES OF BONE

Microscopic Appearance	Subtypes	Characteristics
Lamellar	Cortical	Structure is oriented along lines of stress
		Strong
	Cancellous	More elastic than cortical bone
Woven	Immature or pathologic	Not stress oriented
		Random organization
		Increased turnover
		Weak
		Flexible

Cellular Biology of Bone

Osteoblasts
- Form bone
- Produce type I collagen

Osteocytes
- Make up 90% of the cells in the mature skeleton
- Maintain bone
- Represent former osteoblasts that have been trapped in matrix
- Important for controlling the extracellular concentration of calcium and phosphorus

Osteoclasts
- Resorb bone
- Multinucleated giant cells (from monocytes)
- Possess a ruffled "brush border" to increase surface area (to increase bone resorption)
- Bone resorption occurs in depressions known as Howship's lacunae

Osteoprogenitor cells
- Become osteoblasts

Lining cells

Bone Matrix

Composed of organic and inorganic components
- Organic components make up 40% of the dry weight of bone; they include collagen, proteoglycans, noncollagenous matrix proteins, and growth factors and cytokines
  - Collagen
    - Responsible for the tensile strength of bone
    - Makes up 90% of the organic matrix
    - Mostly type I collagen (the word "bone" contains the word "one" as its terminal three letters, so it's easy to remember that bone is composed primarily of type I collagen)
    - Collagen structure is a triple helix of tropocollagen (two α_1 and one α_2 chains) (Fig. 1–2)
  - Proteoglycans
    - Responsible for the compressive strength of bone
    - Composed of glycosaminoglycan (GAG) protein complexes
  - Noncollagenous matrix proteins
    - Promote mineralization and bone formation
    - Include osteocalcin, osteonectin, osteopontin, and others
  - Growth factors and cytokines
    - Include transforming growth factor β (TGF-β), insulin-like growth factor, interleukin-1, in-

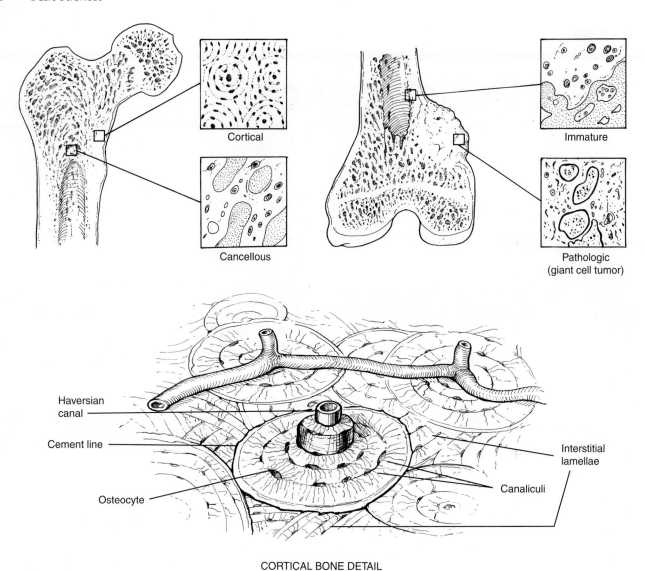

CORTICAL BONE DETAIL

FIGURE 1–1 ■ Types of bone. *Cortical* bone consists of tightly packed osteons. *Cancellous* bone consists of a meshwork of trabeculae. In *immature* bone, there is unmineralized osteoid lining the immature trabeculae. In *pathologic bone,* atypical osteoblasts and architectural disorganization are seen.

terleukin-6, and the bone morphogenic proteins (BMPs)

Inorganic (mineral) components make up 60% of the dry weight of bone

Calcium hydroxyapatite [$Ca_{10}(PO_4)_6(OH)_2$]

Also responsible for the compressive strength of bone

Responsible for matrix mineralization

Makes up the greatest portion of the mineral component

Osteocalcium phosphate (brushite)

Makes up a lesser portion of the mineral component

Bone Remodeling

General concepts of bone remodeling

Both cortical and cancellous bone are continuously being remodeled by osteoblastic and osteoclastic activity

Bone remodeling is affected by mechanical forces according to **Wolff's law**

Removal of external stress leads to bone loss

An increase in external stress leads to bone formation

Bone remodeling is also affected by piezoelectric charges

Compression side of bone is electronegative and stimulates osteoblasts and bone formation

Tension side of bone is electropositive and stimulates osteoclasts and bone resorption

Remodeling of cortical bone (Fig. 1–3)

Remodeling process of cortical bone begins with osteoclastic tunneling (cutting cones), followed by layering of osteoblasts and deposition of layers of lamellae until the size of the cutting cone tunnel has narrowed to the size of the osteonal haversian canal

The head of the cutting cone is made up of osteoclasts that bore holes through hard cortical bone

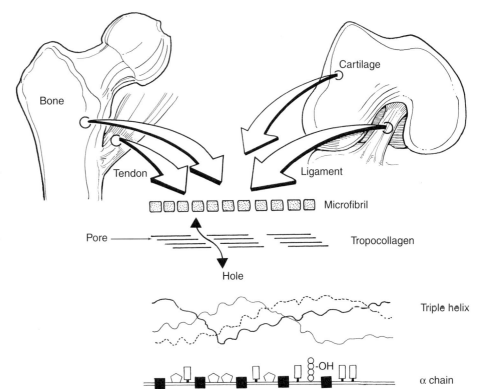

FIGURE 1–2 ■ Microstructure of collagen. Collagen is composed of microfibrils that are packed in a quarter-staggered fashion to form tropocollagen. Note hole and pore regions for mineral deposition (for calcification). Tropocollagen, in turn, is made up of a triple helix of α chains of polypeptides.

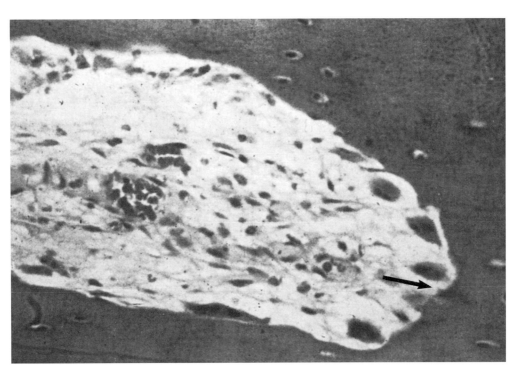

FIGURE 1–3 ■ Remodeling of cortical bone. Head of the cutting cone for osteoclastic tunneling (*arrow*). (Modified from Bogumill GP, Schwamm HA: Orthopaedic Pathology: A Synopsis with Clinical and Radiographic Correlation. Philadelphia, WB Saunders, 1984, p 34.)

Behind the osteoclastic front, osteoblasts lay down osteoid to fill the resorption cavity

Remodeling of cancellous bone

Remodeling is similar to cortical bone but is less organized

Osteoclasts resorb bone, followed by new bone deposition by osteoblasts

Bone Circulation (Fig. 1–4)

Anatomy of bone circulation

As an organ system, bone receives 5% to 10% of the cardiac output

Long bones receive blood from three sources

Nutrient artery system

Nutrient artery originates as branches from major arteries of the systemic circulation

Nutrient artery enters diaphyseal cortex through the nutrient foramen and enters the medullary canal

Nutrient artery branches into ascending and descending small arteries and arterioles within the medullary canal

Branching arterioles penetrate the endosteal cortex to supply at least the inner two thirds of mature diaphyseal cortex via vessels that traverse the haversian system (see Fig. 1–4)

Nutrient artery system is a high-pressure system

Metaphyseal-epiphyseal system

Arises from periarticular vascular plexus (e.g., genicular arteries about the knee)

Periosteal system

Composed primarily of capillaries

Supplies the outer third of mature diaphyseal cortex

Low-pressure system

Bones with a tenuous blood supply include

Scaphoid

Capitellum

Talus

Navicular

Base of the 5th metatarsal

Femoral head

Odontoid process of C2 vertebra

Physiology of bone circulation

Direction of flow

Arterial flow in mature bone is centrifugal (inside to outside), a result of the net effect of the high-pressure endosteal versus the low-pressure periosteal system

In the case of a completely displaced fracture, the endosteal system is disrupted and the periosteal system predominates (direction of flow is reversed and is centripetal [outside to inside])

Arterial flow in immature bone is centripetal (periosteum is highly vascularized and predominates)

Venous flow in mature bone is centripetal

Bone circulation and fracture healing

Bone blood flow is the major determinant of fracture healing

Blood flow is responsible for delivery of nutrients and growth factors to the site of bony injury

Tissues Surrounding Bone

Periosteum

Connective tissue membrane that covers bone

Responsible for the blood supply to the outer third of mature diaphyseal cortex

More highly developed in children

Responsible for growth in bone diameter in children

Bone marrow

Source of progenitor cells

Red marrow slowly changes to yellow marrow with aging

Yellow marrow is inactive

Enchondral Bone Formation/Mineralization

Cartilage model process

Formed from mesenchymal anlage

Vascular buds invade

Osteoprogenitor cells differentiate into osteoblasts

Formation of primary centers of ossification in the mid diaphysis

Cartilage model grows in width (appositional) and length (interstitial)

Secondary centers of ossification develop at the ends of bone, forming epiphyseal centers of ossification (growth plates)

Note: Remember, bone replaces the cartilage model; cartilage is not converted to bone

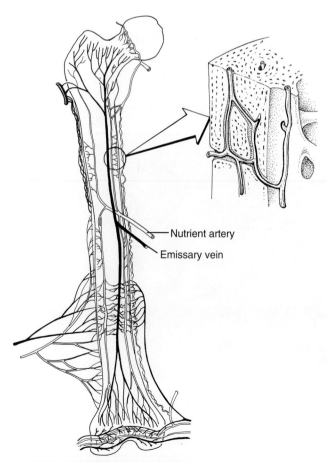

—Nutrient artery

Emissary vein

FIGURE 1–4 ■ Blood supply to bone.

Physis (growth plate) (Fig. 1–5)
  Two growth plates exist in the immature skeleton
    Horizontal growth plate (physis)
      Responsible for longitudinal growth of the long bones
    Spherical growth plate
      Allows for growth of the epiphysis
      Less organized than the horizontal growth plate
  Physeal cartilage is divided into zones based on growth and function
    Reserve zone: matrix production and storage (cells store lipids, glycogen, and proteoglycan aggregates)
    Proliferative zone: cellular proliferation and matrix production
    Hypertrophic zone: preparation of matrix for calcification that begins in the zone of provisional calcification; the hypertrophic zone is sometimes subdivided into three zones:
    Maturation
    Degeneration
    Provisional calcification

Various conditions affect one or more of the physeal zones (Table 1–2)
Metaphysis
  Adjacent to the physis
  Expands with skeletal growth
  Several conditions affect the metaphysis, including
    Osteopetrosis
    Scurvy
    Osteogenesis imperfecta
    Pyle's disease (metaphyseal dysplasia)
    Acute hematogenous osteomyelitis
    Metaphyseal chondrodysplasia
Periphery of the physis is composed of two elements
  Groove of Ranvier—supplies chondrocytes to the periphery of the growth plate for growth in width
  Perichondrial ring of La Croix—dense fibrous tissue anchors and supports the physis (see Fig. 1–5)

Intramembranous Ossification

Occurs without a cartilage model
Usually involves the flat bones and the clavicle
Provides for growth in width of the long bones

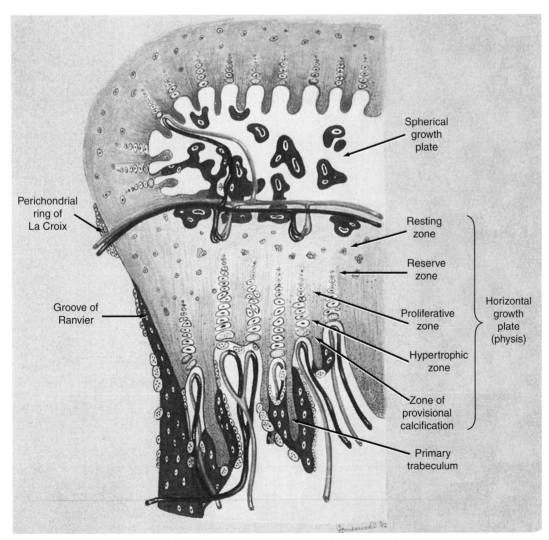

FIGURE 1–5 ■ Physeal architecture. (Modified from Bogumill GP, Schwamm HA: Orthopaedic Pathology: A Synopsis with Clinical and Radiographic Correlation. Philadelphia, WB Saunders, 1984, p 17.)

Table 1–2
CONDITIONS AFFECTING PHYSEAL ZONES

Zone	Condition	Etiology
Reserve	Lysosomal storage diseases (such as Gaucher's disease)	
	Kneist syndrome	Proteoglycan abnormality
	Diastrophic dwarfism	Type II collagen abnormality
Proliferative	Achondroplasia	Deficient chondrocyte proliferation
	Gigantism	Growth hormone causes increased proliferation of chondrocytes
Hypertrophic (sometimes divided into three zones: maturation, degeneration, and provisional calcification)	Mucopoly-saccharidoses (Hurler's, Hunter's, Sanfilippo's, and Morquio's syndromes) (affect zones of maturation and degeneration)	Lysosomal acid hydrolase abnormalities
	Rickets, osteomalacia (affect zone of provisional calcification)	Abnormal matrix calcification
	Enchondromas	
	Physeal fractures	
	Slipped capital femoral epiphysis	

BONE METABOLISM

General Concepts

Calcium and phosphate metabolism are affected by an elaborate interplay of hormones and feedback mechanisms

Peak bone mass occurs between 16 and 25 years of age

Bone mass is greater in men than in women

Bone mass is greater in African-Americans

Bone loss begins in the late 20s at a rate of 0.3% to 0.5% per year

Bone loss can reach 2% to 3% per year for untreated women in the first 10 years after menopause

Calcium

Bone is a reservoir for more than 99% of the body's calcium

Plasma calcium (<1% of total body calcium) is approximately 50% free and 50% bound (usually to albumin)

Calcium is absorbed from the gut (duodenum) by active transport (regulated by the active form of vitamin D [$1,25(OH)_2$vitamin D_3])

Calcium is also absorbed by passive diffusion (jejunum)

Calcium is 98% resorbed by the kidney

Calcium is also important for nerve and muscle function

Dietary requirement of elemental calcium is as follows:

Age and Circumstance	(mg/day)
Children	600
Adult men and women (25–65 yr)	750
Adolescents and young adults (10–25 yr)	1300
Pregnant women	1500
Postmenopausal women	1500
Patients with healing long bone fractures	1500
Lactating women	2000

Hypercalcemia leads to areflexia, confusion (stupor, coma), weakness, fatigue, anorexia, nausea, vomiting, constipation

Hypocalcemia leads to hyperreflexia, tetany (positive Chvostek's sign), lethargy, confusion

Phosphate

Bone is a reservoir for 85% of the body's phosphate

Phosphate is a key component of bone mineral

Important role in enzyme systems

Parathyroid Hormone

Synthesized in the chief cells of the parathyroid gland

PTH acts at the intestine, kidney, and bone

Increases plasma calcium by increasing intestinal absorption of calcium and increasing osteoclastic bone resorption

Enhances excretion of phosphate, thereby lowering serum phosphate

Low calcium levels in the extracellular fluid stimulate the release of PTH

Vitamin D_3

A steroid

Hydroxylated in the liver to $25(OH)$vitamin D_3 (inactive form)

Hydroxylated a second time in the **kidney** to $1,25[OH]_2$ vitamin D_3 (**active form**)

Calcitonin

Produced by the clear cells of the thyroid gland

Secretion stimulated by elevated calcium levels

Important role in lowering plasma calcium levels

Other Hormones

Estrogen

Prevents bone loss (inhibits resorption)

Supplementation is helpful in postmenopausal women, but only if started within the first 5 to 10 years of the onset of menopause

Corticosteroids

Increase bone loss (cancellous bone more affected than cortical bone)

Thyroid hormones
  Lead to osteoporosis

BONE INJURY AND REPAIR

The response of bone to injury is a continuum of processes beginning with **inflammation,** proceeding through **repair,** and ending with **remodeling**
  Inflammation
    Hematoma formation from a bleeding fracture site
    Fibrin clot provides a source for hematopoietic cells that secrete growth factors
    Fibroblasts, mesenchymal cells, and osteoprogenitor cells present at a fracture site
    Osteoblasts (from osteoprogenitor cells) proliferate at a fracture site
  Repair
    Primary callus response occurs within 2 weeks
  Remodeling
    Process begins during the middle of the repair phase
    Process continues long after the fracture is clinically healed (up to 7 years)

Bone Grafts

Properties (Table 1–3)
  Osteoconductive matrix
    Acts as a scaffold or framework into which bone growth occurs
  Osteoinductive factors
    Growth factors such as BMP and TGF-β that promote bone formation
  Osteogenic cells
    Cells that promote bone formation
  Structural integrity
  Immunogenicity
    Most types of bone graft have low immunogenicity
Types of grafts
  Autograft—from the same patient
  Xenograft (heterograft)—from another species
  Allograft—from the bone bank (cadaveric bone)
  Ceramics

Hydroxyapatite
Tricalcium phosphate
Demineralized bone matrix
Bone marrow
Composite grafts

ARTICULAR TISSUES

CARTILAGE

Types of Cartilage

Growth plate (physeal) cartilage
Fibrocartilage
  Important for tendon and ligament insertion into bone
  Important in healing of articular cartilage
Elastic cartilage
  Nose, epiglottis, auricle
Fibroelastic cartilage
  Menisci
Articular (hyaline) cartilage

Articular (Hyaline) Cartilage

Plays a critical role in joint function
Decreases joint friction
Aids in load distribution
Has no arteries, nerves, lymphatic channels
Chrondrocytes receive nutrients and oxygen via diffusion through cartilage matrix
Articular cartilage composition
  Water
    Sixty percent to 80% of the wet weight of articular cartilage
    Allows for deformation of the cartilage surface in response to stress
    Responsible for nutrition and lubrication of cartilage
    Water content *decreases* with aging
    Water content *increases* in osteoarthritis

Table 1–3
TYPES OF BONE GRAFTS AND BONE GRAFT PROPERTIES

Graft	Osteoconduction	Osteoinduction	Osteogenic Cells	Structural Integrity	Other Properties
Autograft					
Cancellous	Excellent	Good	Excellent	Poor	Rapid incorporation
Cortical	Fair	Fair	Fair	Excellent	Slow incorporation
Allograft	Fair	Fair	None	Good	**Fresh** has the highest immunogenicity
					Freeze dried is the least immunogenic but has the least structural integrity (weakest)
					Fresh frozen preserves BMP
Ceramics	Fair	None	None	Fair	
Demineralized bone matrix	Fair	Good	None	Poor	
Bone marrow	Poor	Poor	Good	Poor	

BMP, bone morphogenic protein.

Table 1–4
OVERVIEW OF COLLAGEN TYPES

Type	Location
I	Bone
	Tendon
	Meniscus
	Annulus of intervertebral disc
	Skin
II	Articular cartilage
	Nucleus pulposus of intervertebral disc
III	Skin
	Blood vessels
IV	Basement membrane
V	Articular cartilage (in small amounts)
VI	Articular cartilage (in small amounts)
VII	Basement membrane
VIII	Basement membrane
IX	Articular cartilage (in small amounts)
X	Hypertrophic cartilage
	Associated with calcification of cartilage (matrix mineralization)
XI	Articular cartilage (in small amounts)
XII	Tendon
XIII	Endothelial cells

Collagen (Table 1–4; see Fig. 1–2)
  Ten percent to 20% of the wet weight of articular cartilage (>50% of the dry weight)
  Cartilaginous framework
  Responsible for the **tensile strength** of cartilage
  Type II collagen represents 90% to 95% of the collagen content of articular cartilage
Proteoglycans (Fig. 1–6)
  Ten percent to 15% of the wet weight of articular cartilage
  Responsible for the **compressive strength** of cartilage
  Produced by chondrocytes
  Proteoglycans are protein polysaccharides
  Composed of **GAGs**; GAGs include
    Chondroitin 4-sulfate
    Chondroitin 6-sulfate
    Keratin sulfate
  GAGs are bound to a protein core by **sugar bonds** to form a **proteoglycan aggrecan molecule** (see Fig. 1–6)
  Link proteins stabilize aggrecan molecules to **hyaluronic acid** to form a **proteoglycan aggregate** (see Fig. 1–6)
Chondrocytes
  Represent trapped chondroblasts
  Active in protein synthesis
  Produce collagen, proteoglycans, and some metabolic enzymes
Articular cartilage layers (Fig. 1–7; Table 1–5)
Changes in articular cartilage with aging
  Increased stiffness
  Becomes relatively hypocellular
  Decreased water content
  Increased protein content
  Overall proteoglycan mass decreased
  Decreased content of chondroitin sulfate
Increased content of keratin sulfate
Healing of articular cartilage
  Deep lacerations (extend below the tide mark)
    Heal with fibrocartilage (less durable than hyaline cartilage)
  Superficial lacerations (do not extend below the tide mark)
  Chondrocytes proliferative
  No true healing occurs

SYNOVIUM

General Concepts

Synovium mediates the exchange of nutrients between blood and joint (synovial) fluid
Contains two main cell types
  Type A cells
    Phagocytosis
  Type B cells
    Similar to fibroblasts
    Produce synovial fluid (type **B** cells produce synovial **B**roth)

Synovial Fluid

Composed of proteinases, collagenases, hyaluronic acid, and prostaglandins
Contains no red blood cells, hemoglobin, or clotting factors
Nourishes articular cartilage via diffusion
Lubricates via hydrodynamic, boundary, weeping, and boosted mechanisms
Exhibits non-Newtonian flow characteristics
  Synovial fluid is not linearly viscous
  Coefficient of viscosity is not a constant
    Viscosity decreases as the shear rate increases
Lubricin (a glycoprotein) is the key lubricating component of synovial fluid

MENISCUS

General Concepts

Composed of fibrocartilage/fibroelastic cartilage
Functions to deepen the articular surface

Table 1–5
ARTICULAR CARTILAGE LAYERS

Layer	Orientation of Collagen Fibers	Function
Superficial (gliding)	Tangential (high concentration of collagen fibers)	Versus shear
Middle (transitional)	Oblique	Versus compression
Deep (radial)	Vertical	Versus compression
Tide mark	Tangential	Versus shear
Calcified cartilage	—	Anchor

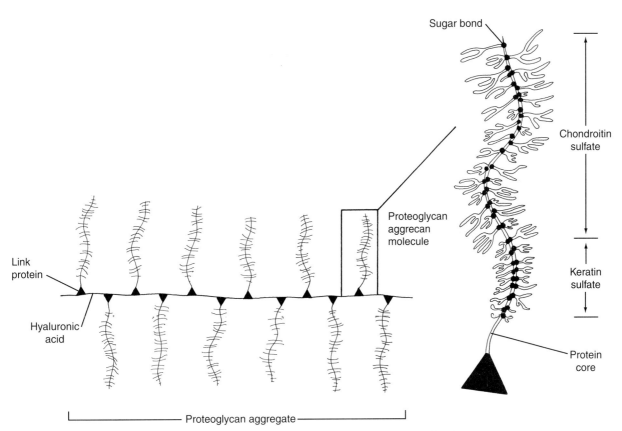

FIGURE 1–6 ■ Proteoglycan aggregate and aggrecan molecule.

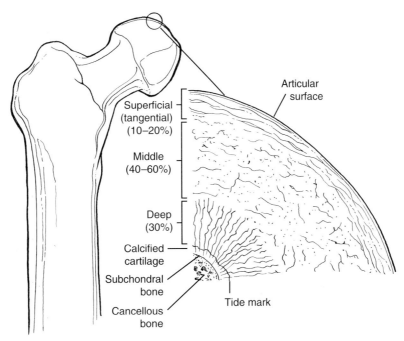

FIGURE 1–7 ■ Articular cartilage layers.

Broadens the contact area to distribute the load
Functions as a secondary joint stabilizer (assists ligaments)

Examples

Shoulder (glenoid labrum)
Wrist (triangular fibrocartilage complex)
Hip (acetabular labrum)
Knee (meniscus)

Knee Meniscus

Blood supply from genicular arteries
Peripheral 25% of the meniscus is vascular
Central 75% of the meniscus is avascular and receives its nutrition via diffusion
Peripheral meniscal tears in the vascular zone ("red zone") can heal via fibrocartilage scar
Central meniscal tears in the avascular zone ("white zone") do not typically heal

NEUROMUSCULAR AND CONNECTIVE TISSUES

SKELETAL MUSCLE

Noncontractile Elements (Fig. 1–8)

Epimysium
  Surrounds individual muscle bundles
Perimysium
  Surrounds muscle fascicles
Endomysium
  Surrounds individual muscle fibers
Myotendon junction
  The "weak link" of muscle
  Often the site of tears
Sarcoplasmic reticulum
  Stores calcium in membrane-bound channels
    T tubules
    Cisterns

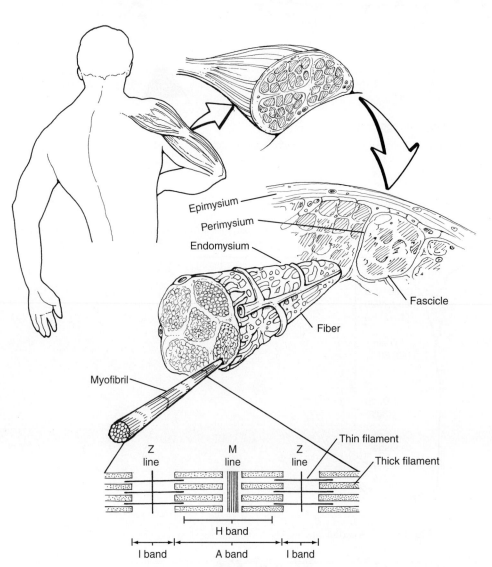

FIGURE 1–8 ■ Skeletal muscle architecture.

Epimysium
Perimysium
Endomysium
Fascicle
Fiber
Myofibril
Z line
M line
Z line
Thin filament
Thick filament
H band
I band
A band
I band

Contractile Elements (see Fig. 1–8)

Muscle
  Composed of several muscle fascicles
Muscle fascicle
  Contains several muscle fibers
Muscle fiber
  An elongated cell
  Composed of myofibrils
Myofibrils
  A collection of sarcomeres
Sarcomere (see Fig. 1–8; Table 1–6)
  Many sarcomeres per myofibril
  Composed of thick and thin filaments
    Thick filaments = myosin
    Thin filaments = actin

Action

Stimulus for muscle contraction originates in the cell body of the neuron and is carried to the neuromuscular junction via an electrical impulse propagated down the axon (from spinal cord to skeletal muscle)
Impulse reaches the motor end plate
Acetylcholine is released from presynaptic vesicles and diffuses across the synaptic cleft and binds to the receptor on the muscle membrane
Binding triggers depolarization of the sarcoplasmic reticulum, releasing calcium
Calcium binds to troponin
Actin-myosin cross-bridges form
Muscle contracts

Agents Affecting Neuromuscular Impulse Transmission (Table 1–7)

Types of Muscle Contractions

Isotonic (two types: concentric and eccentric)
  Constant tension through range of motion (ROM)
  Example: biceps curls using free weights
  Concentric
    Muscle shortens during contraction
    Tension proportional to external load
  Eccentric
    Muscle lengthens during contraction
    Greatest potential for injury
Isometric
  Tension generated in muscle
  Muscle length remains constant
  Example: pushing against an immovable object
Isokinetic (may be concentric or eccentric)
  Muscle contracts at constant speed over full ROM

Table 1–6
SARCOMERE

A band	Contains actin and myosin
I band	Contains actin only
H band	Contains myosin only
M line	Interconnecting site of the thick filaments
Z line	Anchors the thin filaments

Requires special equipment
Best for strength training
Example: Cybex machine exercises

Types of Muscle Fibers

Slow twitch (type I fibers)
  Oxidative
  Aerobic
  Endurance activities (marathon)
Fast twitch (type II fibers)
  Glycolytic (ATP–creatine phosphate [CP] system)
  Anaerobic
  Sprint

Athletics and Training

Endurance athletes have a higher percentage of slow twitch (type I) fibers
Strength-type athletes (such as sprinters) have more fast twitch (type II) fibers
  Strength training leads to hypertrophy of fast twitch fibers
Closed chain exercises
  Extremity is loaded with the most distal portion of that extremity (such as the foot) stabilized or not moving
  Safer, fewer injuries than open chain exercises (for example, decreases patellofemoral stress)
Anabolic steroids cause
  Increased muscle strength
  Testicular atrophy
  Oligospermia/azoospermia
  Gynecomastia
  Striae
  Cystic acne
  Alopecia (irreversible)
  Liver tumors
  Increased low-density lipoproteins, decreased high-density lipoproteins
  Abnormal liver enzymes
Aerobic conditioning
  Recommended 3 to 5 days per week for 20 to 60 minutes per session in healthy adults
  Training heart rate should be 60% to 90% of maximum heart rate
Female athletes (common problems)
  Amenorrhea (from decreased percentage of body fat and resultant hormonal changes)
  Osteoporosis
  Anorexia

THE NERVOUS SYSTEM

Central Nervous System (CNS)

Stroke
  Brain injury resulting from a vascular insult
  Patients may continue to improve up to 6 months after their vascular event
Traumatic brain injury
  Patients may improve up to 18 months after injury

Table 1–7
AGENTS AFFECTING NEUROMUSCULAR IMPULSE TRANSMISSION

Agent	Site of Action	Mechanism	Effect
Nondepolarizing drugs Curare, pancuronium, vecuronium	Neuromuscular junction	Competitively binds to acetylcholine receptor to block impulse transmission	Paralytic agent (long term)
Depolarizing drugs Succinylcholine	Neuromuscular junction	Binds to acetylcholine receptor to cause temporary depolarization of muscle membrane	Paralytic agent (short term)
Anticholinesterases Neostigmine, edrophonium	Autonomic ganglia	Prevents breakdown of acetylcholine to enhance its effect	Reverses effect of nondepolarizing drugs; muscarinic effects (bronchospasm, bronchorrhea, bradycardia)

Concussion (Table 1–8)
  Jarring injury to the brain
  Results in disturbances of cerebral function

Peripheral Nervous System (Fig. 1–9)

Nerve—bundle of fascicles enclosed in a connective tissue sheath
Fascicle—bundle of nerve fibers
Nerve fiber—axon plus surrounding Schwann cell sheath
  Myelinated fibers
    One Schwann cell per one axon
    Rapid conduction velocity
  Unmyelinated fibers
    One Schwann cell for many axons
    Slow conduction velocity
  Afferents
    Transmit information from sensory receptors to the CNS
    Sensory system
  Efferents
    Transmit information from the CNS to the periphery
    Motor system

Histology and Signal Generation

Neuron (see Fig. 1–9)
  Cell body—the neuron's metabolic center

Table 1–8
CONCUSSION

Severity	Characteristics	Treatment
Grade I (mild)	No loss of consciousness No retrograde amnesia	May return to play (sports) as soon as asymptomatic
Grade II (moderate)	Loss of consciousness ≤5 minutes Retrograde amnesia that lasts for minutes	First time: may return to play after 1 week Repeat episode: may return to play after 1 or more months
Grade III (severe)	Loss of consciousness >5 minutes Retrograde with or without post-traumatic amnesia that persists for more than minutes	May return to play after 1 or more months Computed tomography of the head is mandatory

Axon—conveys electrical signals via action potentials
Dendrites—thin processes that branch from the cell body to receive synaptic input
Presynaptic terminals—transmit information from one neuron to another
Glial cells
  Schwann cells—myelinate peripheral nerves
  Oligodendrocytes—form myelin for the CNS
  Astrocytes—CNS supporting structure
Resting potential of the neuron
  -50 to -80 mV
  Inside of the cell is negative relative to the external environment
Action potential
  Transmits signal via electrical impulses to other neurons or effector organs (such as muscle)
  Results from an increase in cell membrane permeability to Na^+ in response to a stimulus

Sensory System (Fig. 1–10)

Receives messages from the environment via transmission from sensory receptors
  Photoreceptors—vision
  Mechanoreceptors—hearing, balance, mechanical stimuli
  Thermoreceptors—temperature
  Chemoreceptors—taste, smell
  Nociceptors—pain
Transmission to the spinal cord is via the dorsal root ganglia

Motor System (see Fig. 1–10)

Spinal cord
  White matter
    Peripheral cord
    Fiber tracts of axons
  Gray matter
    Central cord
    Neuronal cell bodies, glial cells, dendrites, and some axons
  Spinal cord reflexes
    Stereotyped response to a specific stimulus
    Most human reflexes are polysynaptic (involve one or more interneurons)
    Pathway

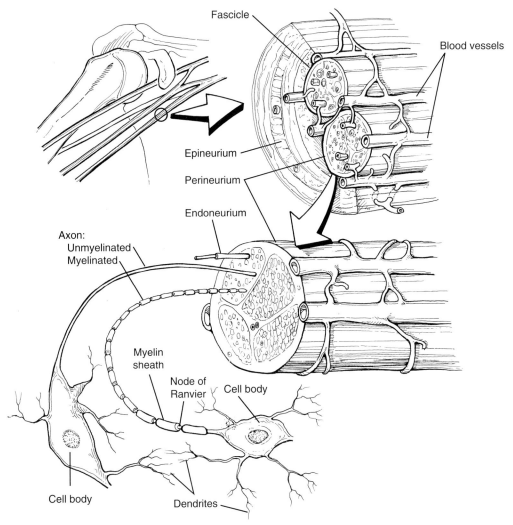

FIGURE 1–9 ■ Nerve architecture.

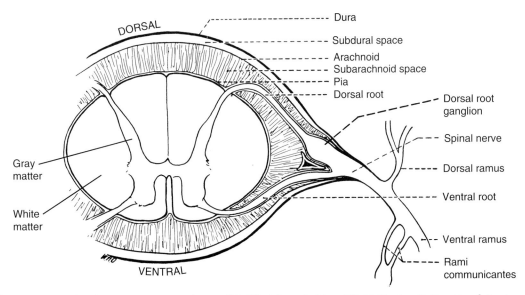

FIGURE 1–10 ■ Spinal cord and nerve root nomenclature. (Modified from Jenkins, DB: Hollinshead's Functional Anatomy of the Limbs and Back, 6th ed. Philadelphia, WB Saunders, 1991, p 205.)

Sensory organ (receptor)
Interneuron
Motoneuron
Motor unit
Alpha motoneuron and the muscle fibers it innervates
Four types
Slow, fatigue-resistant (type S)
Fast, fatigue-resistant (type FR)
Fast, fatigue-intermediate (type FI)
Fast, fatigue (type FF)
Upper and lower motoneurons
Upper motoneuron
Located in descending pathways of cortex, brain stem, spinal cord
Lower motoneuron
Located in ventral gray matter of the spinal cord
Motoneuron lesions (Table 1–9)

Peripheral Nerve (see Fig. 1–9)

Composed of nerve fibers, blood vessels, and connective tissues
Nerve fibers
Type A—heavily myelinated, rapid conduction (touch)
Type B—intermediate myelination and conduction (autonomic nervous system)
Type C—no myelination, slow conduction (pain)
Blood vessels—course through the connective tissue of peripheral nerve
Connective tissues
Endoneurium—coats axons
Perineurium—coats nerve bundles known as fascicles
Epineurium—coats peripheral nerve, which is composed of one or more fascicles
Conduction—facilitated by gaps between Schwann cells known as nodes of Ranvier
Peripheral nerve injury
Types of injuries
Neurapraxia—reversible conduction block (usually from nerve compression) characterized by local ischemia; prognosis for recovery is good
Axonotmesis—more severe injury; endoneurium remains intact; prognosis for recovery is fair

Neurotmesis—complete nerve division; endoneurium transected; prognosis for recovery is poor
Biologic response to peripheral nerve injury
Distal axons die
Wallerian degeneration (of myelin)
Proximal axonal budding (at 1 month)
Nerve regeneration (1 mm per day)
Types of operative nerve repairs
Epineural
Grouped fascicular

CONNECTIVE TISSUES

Tendon (Fig. 1–11)

Attaches muscles to bones
Composed of fascicles (groups of collagen bundles)
Enclosed within a tendon sheath (paratenon)
Composed primarily of type I collagen (see Fig. 1–2)
Inserts into bone by way of Sharpey's fibers
Tendon repair/healing
Weakest at 7 to 10 days after injury
Strong by 4 weeks after injury
Maximum strength at 6 months after injury

Ligament (see Fig. 1–11)

Attaches bone to bone
Composed primarily of type I collagen (see Fig. 1–2)
Ultrastructure similar to a tendon but a ligament has a higher elastin content
Ligament blood supply (two sources)
At its insertion site
Vincula (such as flexor tendons of the hand)
Ligament insertions (two types)
Indirect insertions
More common
Superficial fibers insert into the periosteum
Direct insertions
Deep fibers attach to bone at a 90-degree angle with transition of tissue from ligament to fibrocartilage to mineralized fibrocartilage to bone
Superficial fibers insert into the periosteum

Intervertebral Disc

Allows for motion and stability of the spine
Contains types I and II collagen
Composed of 85% water
Water content decreases with aging
Central disc (nucleus pulposus)
Hydrated gel
Responsible for compressibility of the disc
High in GAG content
Low in collagen content
Collagen is primarily type II
Peripheral disc (annulus fibrosis)
Allows for extensibility and tensile strength of the disc
Low in GAG content
High in collagen content
Collagen is primarily type I

Table 1–9
FINDINGS IN UPPER AND LOWER MOTONEURON LESIONS

Findings	Upper Motoneuron Lesions	Lower Motoneuron Lesions
Strength	Decreased	Decreased
Tone	Increased	Decreased
Deep tendon reflexes	Increased	Decreased
Superficial tendon reflexes	Decreased	Decreased
Babinski's sign	Present	Absent
Clonus	Present	Absent
Fasciculations	Absent	Present
Atrophy	Absent	Present

Adapted from Simon SR: Orthopaedic Basic Science, 2nd ed. Rosemont, IL, American Academy of Orthopaedic Surgeons, 1994, p 354.

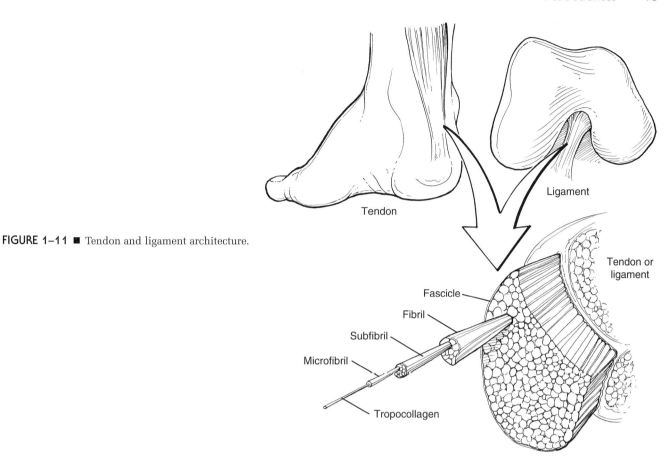

FIGURE 1–11 ■ Tendon and ligament architecture.

GENETICS OF MUSCULOSKELETAL CONDITIONS

MENDELIAN INHERITANCE

Autosomal Dominant Disorders

Typically are **structural defects**
Heterozygote state (Aa) manifests a condition
Fifty percent of offspring are affected (assuming only one parent is affected)
Normal offspring do not transmit a condition
No gender preference

	A	a
a	Aa	aa
a	Aa	aa

Examples
  Marfan syndrome
  Achondroplasia
  Cleidocranial dysostosis
  Multiple epiphyseal dysplasia (MED)
  Spondyloepiphyseal dysplasia (SED)

  Malignant hypothermia
  Kneist syndrome
  Metaphyseal chondrodysplasia
  Multiple exostoses
  Osteogenesis imperfecta (types I and IV)

Autosomal Recessive Disorders

Typically are **biochemical** or **enzymatic defects**
Homozygote state (AA) manifests a condition
Parents are unaffected
Twenty-five percent of offspring are affected (assuming both parents are heterozygotes)
No gender preference

	A	a
A	AA	Aa
a	Aa	aa

Examples
  Hurler's syndrome
  Ochronosis
  Homocystinuria
  Sanfilippo's syndrome
  Scheie's syndrome
  Maroteaux-Lamy syndrome
  Osteogenesis imperfecta (types II and III)

Gender-Linked Dominant Disorders

Heterozygote (X′X or X′Y) manifests a condition

Affected female (mating with unaffected male) transmit X-linked gene to half of daughters and half of sons

	X	Y
X′	X′X	X′Y
X	XX	XY

Affected male (mating with unaffected female) transmit X-linked gene to all daughters and no sons

	X′	Y
X	X′X	XY
X	X′X	XY

Example
  Vitamin D–resistant rickets

Gender-Linked Recessive Disorders

Heterozygote (X′Y) male is affected

Heterozygote (X′X) female is unaffected

Affected male (mating with unaffected female) transmits gene to all daughters (who are carriers) and no sons

	X′	Y
X	X′X	XY
X	X′X	XY

Carrier female (mating with unaffected male) transmits gene to half of daughters (who are carriers) and half of sons (who are affected)

	X	Y
X′	X′X	X′Y
X	XX	XY

Examples
  Duchenne's muscular dystrophy
  Hemophilia
  Hunter's syndrome
  SED

CHROMOSOMAL ABNORMALITIES

Represent an abnormality in a region of a chromosome or an abnormal number of chromosomes

Examples of Disorders Associated With Chromosomal Abnormalities

Down syndrome (trisomy 21)
Polydactyly
Vertical tali
Radioulnar synostosis

GENERAL CONCEPTS OF BIOMECHANICS AND BIOMATERIALS

BIOMECHANICS

The science of the action of forces on the living body

Newton's laws
  Inertia—a body in motion remains in motion; a body at rest remains at rest
  Acceleration—change in velocity over time
  Reactions—for every action, there is an equal and opposite reaction; allows for free body analysis

Force—an applied action that tends to accelerate or deform a body
  Force = mass × acceleration

Load—the force sustained by a body

Deformation—temporary (elastic) or permanent (plastic) change in the shape of a body

Stress—internal force generated within a body (such as bone) in response to an applied load (force per unit area)
  Stress = force/area

Strain—change in dimension of a body (deformation) that results from an applied load
  Strain = change in length/original length
    Tensile strain—a normal strain (acts perpendicular to the cross section of bone) that acts to increase the length of bone
    Compressive strain—a normal strain that acts to decrease the length of bone
    Shear strain—the production of an angular deformity caused by an externally applied load

Extrinsic factors of fracture production
  Magnitude of force
  Duration of force
  Direction of force
  Rate of bone loading

Intrinsic factors of fracture production
  Energy absorbing capacity—the more rapidly a bone is loaded, the more energy it can absorb before failure; low-energy fractures are generally loaded slowly and are linear; high-energy fractures are loaded rapidly with subsequent explosion of the bone into multiple fragments (comminuted)
  Strain energy—the energy a body is able to absorb by changing shape in response to an applied load; this is a measure of the toughness of a material
  Young's modulus of elasticity (E)—a measure of the stiffness of a material or its ability to resist deformation: E = stress/strain (Fig. 1–12)
  Yield point (proportional limit)—transition point from elastic to plastic deformation (see Fig. 1–12)

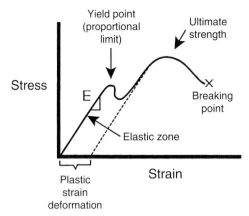

FIGURE 1–12 ■ Stress-strain curve. (Modified from Miller MD: Review of Orthopaedics, 2nd ed. Philadelphia, WB Saunders, 1996, p 102.

Breaking point—point where a material (bone) fails (fractures) (see Fig. 1–12)

Plastic deformation—change in length of a material after a load is removed (before the breaking point) in the plastic range (see Fig. 1–12)

Fatigue strength—a measure of the strength of a material under repeated or cyclical loading

Creep—time-dependent stress/strain behavior whereby there is a change in the shape of a material without actual loss of material

BIOMATERIALS

The study of the relationship between externally applied loads and the resulting internal effects and deformations on a material

Characteristics of Materials

Brittle materials—break soon after reaching the yield point
  Example: bone cement (polymethylmethacrylate [PMMA])
Ductile materials—undergo plastic deformation before failure
  Example: polyethylene
Viscoelastic materials—stress/strain behavior is time-rate dependent

Example: slow loading causes bone-ligament disruption at bone (avulsion); rapid loading results in a midsubstance ligament injury

Types of Materials in Orthopaedics

Metals
  Stainless steel (fracture fixation devices)
  Titanium (total joint arthroplasty and some fracture fixation devices)
  Cobalt-chromium-molybdenum (total joint arthroplasty)
Polyethylene (PE)
  Ultra high molecular weight (UHMW) (and high density)
    UHMWPE
    Superior wear characteristics, low friction
    Used in total joint arthroplasty (this type of polyethylene is used almost exclusively today for total joint arthroplasty)
PMMA (bone cement)
  Used for implant fixation
    Acts as a grout
    Is not a glue
  Forms mechanical interlock with bone
  Can cause systemic hypotension after insertion during surgery
Ceramics
  Composed of metallic and nonmetallic elements (ionically bonded in a highly oxidized state)
  Low tensile strength
  Superior wear characteristics with polyethylene
Biodegradable materials
  Are resorbed by the body over time
  Generally these are weaker materials
  Examples: polylactic acid, polygylcolic acid
Bone
  Strongest in compression
  Weakest in shear
  Anisotropic (mechanical properties determined by the orientation of the material to the applied force)
Ligament
  Can stretch before rupture (plastic deformation)
Tendon
  Strongest in tension
Articular cartilage
  Has viscoelastic properties

CHAPTER 2

Overview of Anatomy, the History and Physical Examination, and Diagnostic Tests

OVERVIEW OF ANATOMY

Get to bone and stay there . . . avoid cutting round structures.
Stanley Hoppenfeld, MD; Piet de Boer, MA, FRCS
In Preface, Surgical Exposures in Orthopaedics:
The Anatomic Approach, 1984

Introduction

Orthopaedic procedures are often based on reproducing normal anatomy

Bones

Contain cortical (outer) and cancellous (inner) components
206 bones in the human skeleton
80 bones in the axial skeleton (cranium, spine, and pelvis)
126 bones in the appendicular skeleton (arms and legs)
Regions of the long bones (Fig. 2–1)
  Diaphysis—located between the metaphyses of a long bone; shaft of a tubular bone
    Proximal third
    Middle third
    Distal third
  Metaphysis—located between the epiphysis and diaphysis; widened end of a tubular bone
  Epiphysis—located between the joint and the epiphyseal plate (physis) in children (or epiphyseal scar in adults)
  Physis—growth plate; the growth plate is found only in children and is responsible for longitudinal growth of the long bones

Joints

Allow motion at the ends of bones; covered with smooth articular (hyaline) cartilage

Diarthrodial joints—have hyaline cartilage, synovium, capsules, and ligaments
Nomenclature—based on planes of motion
  One plane of motion
    Example: a hinge joint (elbow)
  Two planes of motion
    Example: a saddle joint (thumb carpometacarpal [CMC] joint)
  Multiple planes of motion
    Example: a ball and socket joint (hip, shoulder)

Muscles

Provide power for movement of the extremities
Classified by arrangement of fibers: parallel, fusiform, oblique
Origin and insertion of a muscle are the key to understanding its function
Certain muscles have a dual innervation
  Brachialis (musculocutaneous nerve and radial nerve)
  Flexor carpi ulnaris (median nerve and ulnar nerve)
  Flexor digitorum profundus (ulnar nerve and anterior interosseous nerve)
  Flexor pollicis brevis (ulnar nerve and median nerve)
  Biceps femoris (peroneal and tibial divisions of the sciatic nerve)
  Adductor magnus (obturator nerve and sciatic nerve)

Nerves (Fig. 2–2)

Important for motion, sensation, and proprioception
Peripheral nerves extend from the brachial plexus or lumbosacral plexus

Vessels (see Fig. 2–2)

Bring blood to and from the extremities (and bone)
It is important to know where the vessels (and nerves)

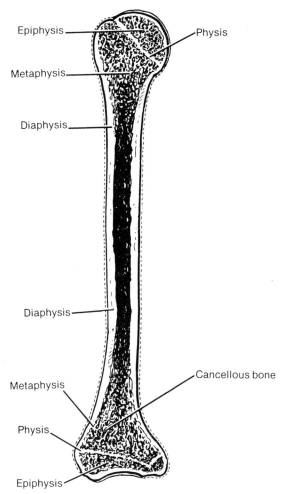

Figure 2-1 ■ Regions of the long bones. (From Gartland JJ: Fundamentals of Orthopaedics. Philadelphia, WB Saunders, 1987, p 9.)

are (and avoid injuring them) during surgical dissection

Nomenclature

Varus—bowing of the extremity with the apex away from the midline

Valgus—bowing of an extremity with the apex toward the midline; think of valgus as forming an "L"

Kyphosis—excessive forward bending (apex posterior angulation) of the spine, creating a humpback deformity

Lordosis—excessive backward bending (apex anterior angulation) of the spine, creating a swayback deformity

Recurvatum—hyperextension of a joint (most common in the knee)

Superficial—relatively close to the surface

Deep—relatively far from the surface

Superior—toward the head

Inferior—toward the feet

Anterior—toward the front of the body

Posterior—toward the back of the body

Proximal—relatively closer to the trunk (or point of origin)

Distal—relatively farther from the trunk (or point of origin)

Cephalic—upward; toward the head

Caudal—downward; toward the buttocks

Medial—closer to the midline

Lateral—farther from the midline

Planes of the body (Fig. 2–3)

Cross-Sectional Anatomy (Fig. 2–4)

Important for preoperative planning

OVERVIEW OF THE HISTORY AND PHYSICAL EXAMINATION

More mistakes are made from want of a proper examination than for any other reason.
R. J. Howard, MD

History

Age

Sex

Hand dominance (for upper-extremity problems)

Occupation

Symptoms

Mechanism of injury

Onset

Acute symptoms

Chronic symptoms

Lifestyle effects

Pain (onset, location, characteristics)

Deformity

Physical Examination

Observation—look at patients as they walk, stand, bend, and undress; look for abnormal contours, deformities, bruises, redness, etc.; look for signs of pain (limp, protected motion, grimacing, etc.)

Palpation—feel for warmth, defects, crepitus, etc.

Motion—measure in all planes

Neurovascular examination

Muscle strength testing—manual muscle strength testing should be performed on the involved anatomic area; muscle strength is graded on a scale of 5/5 to 0/5

5/5 = normal muscle strength

4/5 = some diminished strength (as compared to the contralateral normal side)

3/5 = weak but muscle is strong enough to overcome the force of gravity

2/5 = muscle can perform work but only if the force of gravity is eliminated

1/5 = fasciculations only

0/5 = no motor units fire

Sensory testing—test for sensation to fine touch and pinprick in a dermatomal distribution (Fig. 2–5)

Reflexes—an involuntary reaction to an applied stimulus (such as a knee jerk after tapping the patella tendon with a reflex hammer)

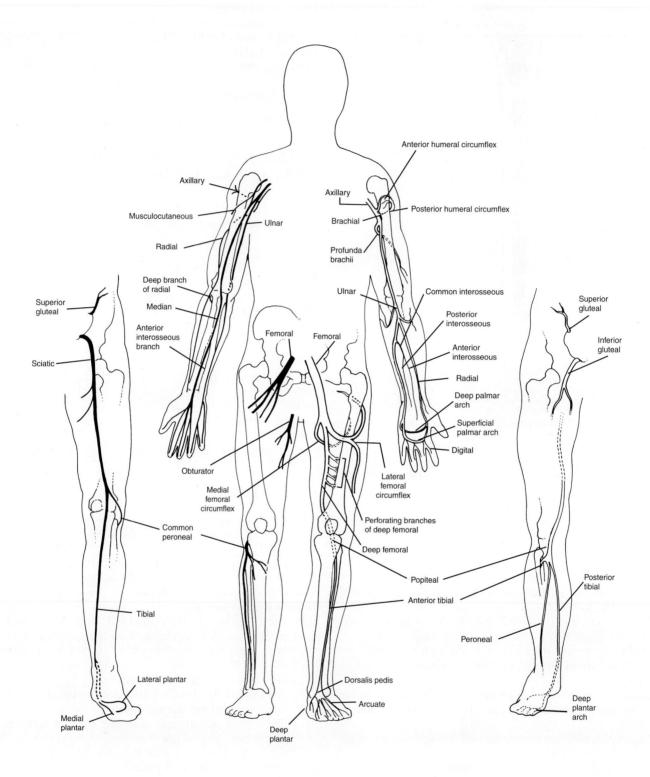

NERVES   ARTERIES

Figure 2–2 ■ Nerves and arteries.

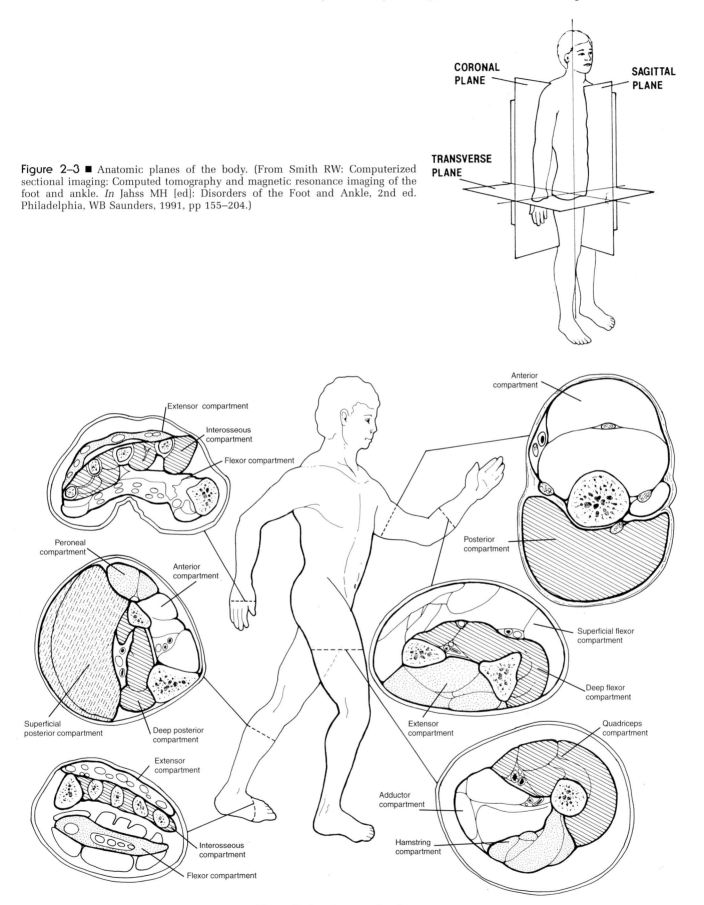

Figure 2–3 ■ Anatomic planes of the body. (From Smith RW: Computerized sectional imaging: Computed tomography and magnetic resonance imaging of the foot and ankle. *In* Jahss MH [ed]: Disorders of the Foot and Ankle, 2nd ed. Philadelphia, WB Saunders, 1991, pp 155–204.)

Figure 2–4 ■ Cross-sectional anatomy.

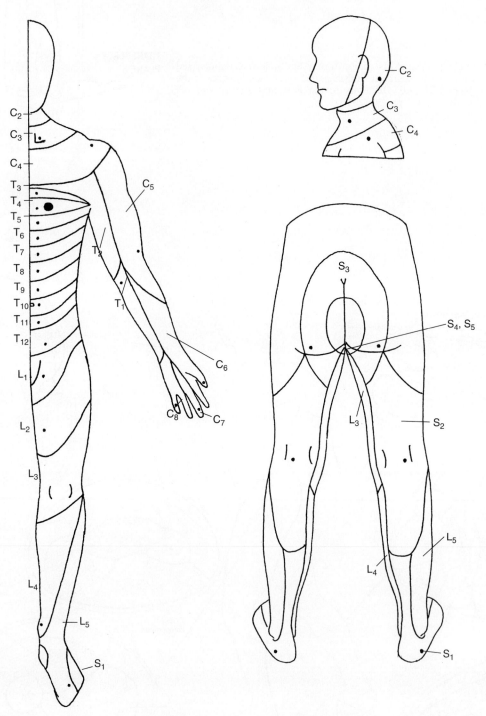

Figure 2–5 ■ Dermatomes. (From Masear VR: Primary Care Orthopaedics. Philadelphia, WB Saunders, 1996, p 53.)

Grading

    0 = absent (areflexia)

    1 = diminished (hyporeflexia)

    2 = average

    3 = exaggerated (hyperreflexia)

    4 = clonus

Pulses—important to palpate (or examine with Doppler testing) for pulses in areas of injury or disease (carotid, brachial, radial, ulnar, femoral, popliteal, posterior tibial, or dorsalis pedis)

Gait (Fig. 2–6)

Special/provocative tests

    Maneuvers that are unique for each specific anatomic area (see Chapters 8 to 22)

    Tests to rule out referred symptoms from other areas

OVERVIEW OF DIAGNOSTIC TESTS

Plain radiographs (x-rays)

    AP (anteroposterior) and lateral views are the minimum requirement for each examination of the long bones

    AP and lateral views and one oblique view are the minimum requirement for examination of all joints (or pathology near a joint)

    Special views directed at suspected pathology (by specific anatomic location)

    Be sure to study the entire film (this includes all bones and soft tissues); **you are responsible for the entire film;** look for

    Size and shape of the bone(s)

    Cortical thickness

    Trabecular pattern

    Density changes

    Lesions and their margins

    Breaks in the continuity of bone

    Periosteal changes

    Soft tissue densities

    Joint contour

    Spatial relationship between adjacent bones

    Always consider ordering a radiograph of the joint above and the joint below the area of suspected pathology

    Example: thigh pain can be referred from hip or knee pathology

Special radiographs

    Condition-specific (see Chapters 8 to 22)

Stress radiographs

    Useful for the diagnosis of ligamentous injuries

    A radiograph of the joint is taken while stress is applied to test the ligament ("check-rein" effect) in question

    Example: applying valgus stress at the knee to test the medial collateral ligament

Tomography—radiographs taken at specific depths (planes) in order to remove the overlap phenomenon seen with plain radiographs; largely being replaced by computed tomography (CT) but can help in the evaluation of certain fractures and nonunions

CT scan—helpful to define **bony anatomy;** very useful for certain fractures (distal radius, proximal tibia, spine, etc.) that are otherwise not well visualized; also useful for visualizing the bony extension of a tumor

Magnetic resonance imaging (MRI)—helpful for evaluation of the **soft tissues** (e.g., meniscus, ligaments, tendons, intervertebral discs) and marrow (e.g., determining the extension of tumor into the marrow cavity); **MRI should be used SELECTIVELY to confirm an otherwise questionable musculoskeletal diagnosis; it should not be used in place of a thorough physical examination and should not be relied upon as a routine diagnostic tool; consultation with an orthopaedic surgeon before ordering an MRI may be appropriate**

MRI terminology

    T1 = time constant of exponential growth of magnetism; T1 measures how rapidly a tissue gains magnetism (Table 2–1)

    T2 = time constant of exponential decay of signal following an excitation pulse; a tissue with long T2 (such as water) maintains its signal (is bright on a T2-weighted image)(see Table 2–1)

    T2* = similar to T2 but includes the effects of magnetic field homogeneity

    TR = time to repetition; the time between successive excitation pulses; short TR is less than 80, long TR is greater than 80

    TE = time to echo; the time that an echo is formed by a refocusing pulse; short TE is less than 1000, long TE is greater than 1000

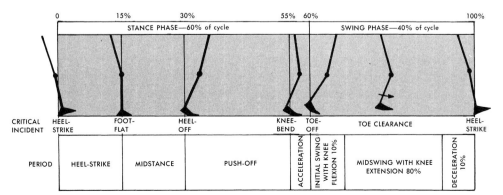

Figure 2–6 ■ The gait cycle. (From Tachdjian MO: Pediatric Orthopedics, 2nd ed. Philadelphia, WB Saunders, 1990, p 8.)

Table 2–1
MAGNETIC RESONANCE IMAGING SIGNAL INTENSITIES

Tissue	Appearance on T1-Weighted Image	Appearance on T2-Weighted Image
Cortical bone	Dark	Dark
Ligaments	Dark	Dark
Fibrocartilage	Dark	Dark
Hyaline cartilage	Gray	Gray
Meniscus	Dark	Dark
Meniscal tear	Bright	Gray
Yellow bone marrow (fatty-appendicular)	Bright	Gray
Red bone marrow (hematopoietic-axial)	Gray	Gray
Marrow edema	Dark	Bright
Fat	Bright	Gray
Normal fluid	Dark	Bright
Abnormal fluid (pus)	Gray	Bright
Acute blood collection	Gray	Dark
Chronic blood collection	Bright	Bright
Muscle	Gray	Gray
Tendon	Dark	Dark
Intervertebral disc (central)	Gray	Bright
Intervertebral disc (peripheral)	Dark	Gray

NEX = number of excitations; higher NEX results in decreased noise with better images

FOV = field of view

Spin echo = a commonly used pulse sequence in MRI

FSE = fast spin echo (a type of pulse sequence)

GRE = gradient-recalled echo (a type of pulse sequence)

Arthrography—instillation of radiopaque dye followed by plain radiography, CT, or MRI is used to outline intra-articular structures; although previously used more frequently, it is still useful for rotator cuff injuries and in conjunction with MRI

Nuclear medicine studies—help delineate areas of increased bony production (e.g., tumors, stress fractures, infection), but they are nonspecific tests

Technetium—labels osteoblastic activity and increased blood flow

Gallium—labels lymphocytes (chronic inflammation and infection)

Indium—labels leukocytes (acute infection)

Fluoroscopy—a useful tool for real-time static or dynamic visualization such as for intraoperative fracture management or evaluation of ligamentous injuries

Ultrasonography—can help in the identification of cysts, rotator cuff tears, and other pathology

Myelography—injection of radiopaque contrast into the epidural space to outline the spinal cord and roots; largely being replaced by MRI, but helpful in the identification of cord or root impingement, disc disease, spinal stenosis, and tumors

Discography—injection of radiopaque contrast into the nucleus pulposus of a disc results in pain and an abnormal disc contour in the patient with disc disease; injection with local anesthetic at the time of the study may give temporary relief, which may also be diagnostic of disc disease

Arteriography/venography—radiographs taken after parenteral administration of contrast; useful for the diagnosis of vascular injuries, thromboembolic disease, tumors, and others

Aspiration

Aspiration of fluid from any joint requires sterile preparation and a thorough knowledge of the local anatomy

Synovial fluid analysis (see Chapter 3)

Blood-fat droplets rise to the surface in a standing container, suggesting the presence of an intra-articular fracture

Injection

Injection of lidocaine can help localize the specific source of pain

Nerve Studies

Allow evaluation of peripheral nerves and their motor responses

Electromyography (EMG)—uses intramuscular needle electrodes to evaluate muscle units; denervation of muscles is demonstrated by fibrillations, sharp waves, and abnormal patterns

Nerve conduction studies (NCS)—latencies of more than 3.5 milliseconds or conduction velocities of less than 50 meters per second suggest nerve abnormalities

CHAPTER 3

Musculoskeletal Conditions of Adults

ARTHRITIC CONDITIONS (Tables 3–1 and 3–2)

Noninflammatory Arthritic Conditions

Osteoarthritis (OA) (Fig. 3–1)
  Also known as degenerative joint disease (DJD)
  Most common form of arthritis
  Loss and damage to articular cartilage
  Etiologies of OA
    Primary (age-related)
    Post-traumatic (such as following an intra-articular fracture)
    Iatrogenic (such as following an operative meniscectomy)
  Knee is the most common joint affected
  Radiographic findings
    Joint space narrowing
    Osteophytes (bone spurs)
  Biochemical changes (articular cartilage)
    Increased water content
    Collagen abnormalities
    Alterations in proteoglycans
  Treatment options
    Activity modification
    Supportive devices (cane)
    Nonsteroidal anti-inflammatory drugs (NSAIDs)
    Intra-articular injections
    Débridement of joint (open or arthroscopic)
    Interpositional (graft) arthroplasty
    Joint realignment procedure (via an osteotomy)
    Total joint arthroplasty
Neuropathic arthropathy (Fig. 3–2)
  Also known as Charcot's joint
  Caused by a disturbance in sensory innervation of a joint
  Causes
    Diabetes (foot)

Tabes dorsalis (lower extremity)—from syphilis
Syringomyelia (upper extremity)—fluid-filled cavity within the spinal cord
Hansen's disease (upper extremity)—from *Mycobacterium leprae*
Myelomeningocele (foot and ankle)—spina bifida
  Radiographs show advanced joint destruction
  Treatment options
    Braces and other types of supports
    Avoid surgery
Acute rheumatic fever (see Chapter 5)
Ochronosis
  A form of arthritis resulting from **alkaptonuria** (defect in homogentisic acid–oxidase enzyme system)

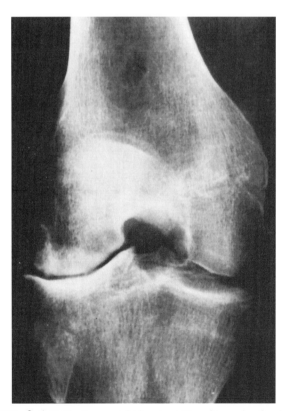

Figure 3–1 ■ Flexion weight-bearing PA radiograph of a knee demonstrating osteoarthritis (degenerative joint disease). Note osteophyte formation, sclerosis, and joint space narrowing of the medial and lateral compartments. (From Weissman BNW, Sledge CB: Orthopedic Radiology. Philadelphia, WB Saunders, 1986, p 542.)

Table 3–1
OVERVIEW OF ARTHRITIC CONDITIONS

Symmetric Findings	Asymmetric Findings
Inflammatory arthritides (except Reiter's syndrome, psoriatic arthritis, and the crystal deposition diseases)	Noninflammatory arthritides Infectious arthritides Hemorrhagic arthritides Reiter's syndrome Psoriatic arthritis Crystal deposition diseases

Table 3–2
JOINT FLUID ANALYSIS

Types of Arthritis	White Blood Cells	Polymorphonuclear Leukocytes (%)	Other Characteristics
Noninflammatory	200	25	Joint aspirate glucose and protein equal to serum values
Inflammatory	2000–75,000	50	↓ Joint aspirate glucose
Infectious	>80,000	>75	Thick cloudy fluid
			+ Gram stain
			+ Cultures
			↓ Joint aspirate glucose, ↑ joint aspirate protein

↓, decreased; ↑, increased, +, positive.

Excess homogentisic acid deposits into the large joints (and spine), polymerizes, and leads to early degenerative changes

Inflammatory Arthritic Conditions
(Table 3–3)

Rheumatoid arthritis (RA) (Fig. 3–3)
　Most common form of inflammatory arthritis
　Synovial and soft tissue inflammatory process, with later involvement of articular cartilage and bone
　Hand is the most common site affected
　Other common sites: wrist (collapse), elbows, and feet
　Clinical findings
　　Insidious onset
　　Morning stiffness

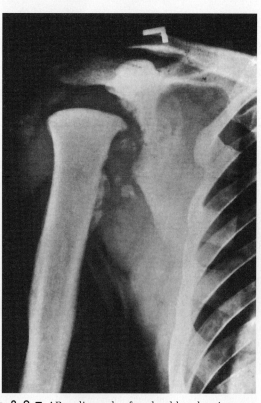

Figure 3–2 ■ AP radiograph of a shoulder showing severe destructive changes characteristic of neuropathic arthropathy. (From Weissman BNW, Sledge CB: Orthopedic Radiology. Philadelphia, WB Saunders, 1986, p 238.)

　　Multiple joint involvement
　　Subcutaneous nodules
　　Rheumatoid factor (RF) titer positive (80% of affected individuals) (see Table 3–3)
　Radiographic findings
　　Periarticular erosions
　　Osteopenia
　　Protrusio acetabuli (medial displacement of the femoral head within the acetabulum and into the pelvis)
　Systemic manifestations
　　Vasculitis
　　Pericarditis
　　Pulmonary disease
　Syndromes associated with RA
　　Felty's syndrome—RA with splenomegaly and leukopenia
　　Still's disease—acute-onset juvenile rheumatoid arthritis (JRA) with fever, rash, and splenomegaly
　　Sjögren's syndrome—an autoimmune exocrinopathy associated with RA; characterized by decreased salivary and lacrimal gland secretion
　Treatment options
　　Medications ("pyramidal approach")
　　Physical therapy
　　Surgery
　　Note: Must evaluate the cervical spine with flexion and extension radiographs to rule out instability and basilar invagination before surgery
Systemic lupus erythematosus
　Chronic inflammatory disease
　Immune-complex related
　Joint involvement very common
　Less destructive than RA
　Treatment is similar to that for RA
Polymyalgia rheumatica
　Aching stiffness (shoulder, pelvic girdle)
　Diagnosis of exclusion (of other disorders)
　Malaise, headaches, anorexia
　Increased erythrocyte sedimentation rate (ESR)
　Associated with temporal arteritis
Juvenile rheumatoid arthritis
　See Chapter 5
Relapsing polychondritis
　Progressive cartilage destruction with or without systemic vasculitis
　Rare disorder
　Self-limiting arthritis

Table 3-3
COMMONLY CONFUSED LABORATORY FINDINGS IN INFLAMMATORY ARTHRITIC CONDITIONS

Finding	May Be Positive For	Usually Negative For
Rheumatoid factor	Rheumatoid arthritis Sjögren's syndrome Sarcoid Systemic lupus erythematosus	Ankylosing spondylitis Gout Psoriatic arthritis Reiter's syndrome
HLA-B27	Ankylosing spondylitis Reiter's syndrome Psoriatic arthritis Enteropathic arthritis	
Antinuclear antibody	Systemic lupus erythematosus Sjögren's syndrome Scleroderma	

Diffuse involvement
Typically involves ears (thickened auricles)
Treatment is supportive
The spondyloarthropathies
  Ankylosing spondylitis (Fig. 3–4)
    Men
    Third to fourth decade of life
    Insidious onset of back and hip pain
    Morning stiffness
    HLA-B27 positive
    Progressive **spinal flexion deformities** (may progress to a **chin-on-chest deformity**)
    Spine becomes rigid (ankylosed)
    Bilateral sacroiliitis
    Hip involvement and young age at onset of disease are prognostic indicators of poor outcomes
    Radiographic findings
      Obliteration of the sacroiliac joints (100% of affected individuals have sacroiliitis)
      Vertical syndesmophytes (vertebrae)
      Squaring of vertebrae
      Protusio acetabuli
    Systemic manifestations
      Pulmonary fibrosis (restricted chest excursion)
      Iritis
      Aortitis
      Colitis
      Arachnoiditis
      Amyloidosis
      Sarcoidosis
    Treatment options
      Physical therapy
      NSAIDs
      Hip—total hip arthroplasty
      Spine—corrective osteotomies for flexion deformities
      Cervical spine fractures—high mortality rate
  Reiter's syndrome

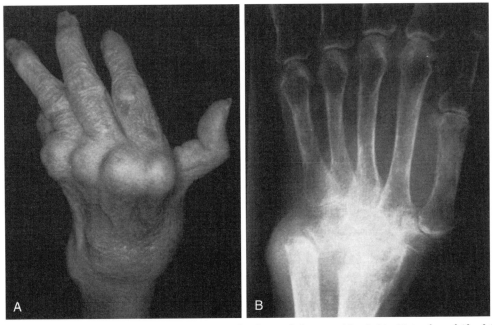

Figure 3–3 ■ *A*, Clinical photograph of the hand of a patient with advanced rheumatoid arthritis. Note ulnar drift of the metacarpophalangeal (MCP) joints caused by the ulnar shift of the extensor tendons, dislocations of the MCP joints, and thumb deformities. *B*, AP radiograph of the hand and wrist of a patient with rheumatoid arthritis. Note severe erosive destruction of the distal radioulnar joint and diffuse osteopenia. (From Bogumill GP: The hand. *In* Wiesel SW, Delahay JN, Connell MC [eds]: Essentials of Orthopaedic Surgery. Philadelphia, WB Saunders, 1993, p 228.)

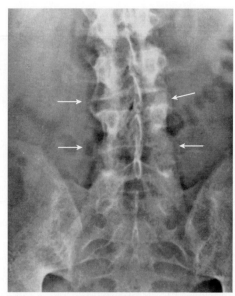

Figure 3–4 ■ AP radiograph of the lumbar spine and sacroiliac joints demonstrating marginal syndesmophytes (*arrows*) typical in ankylosing spondylitis. Note bilateral involvement of the sacroiliac joints. (From Bullough PG, Vigorita VJ: Atlas of Orthopaedic Pathology. Philadelphia, Gower Medical Publishing, 1984, p 8.11.)

Young men
Abrupt onset of arthritis
Asymmetric swelling
Classic triad
    Urethritis
    Conjunctivitis
    Oligoarticular arthritis
Other findings
    Oral ulcers (painless)
    Penile lesions
    Ulcers on the palms and soles of the feet (keratoderma blennorrhagicum)
    Plantar heel pain
Eighty percent of affected individuals are HLA-B27 positive
Sixty percent of affected individuals have sacroiliitis
Treatment—similar to ankylosing spondylitis
Psoriatic arthritis (Fig. 3–5)
    Affects 5% to 10% of patients with psoriasis
    Typically asymmetric involvement
    Small joints affected (hands, feet)
    Nail pitting
    Sausage digits
    "Pencil-in-cup" deformity (of phalanges)
    Treatment—similar to that for RA
Enteropathic arthritis
    Affects 10% to 20% of patients with Crohn's disease and ulcerative colitis
    Nondeforming arthritis
    Large, weight-bearing joints affected
    Fifty percent of affected individuals are HLA-B27 positive
    Arthritis may precede bowel symptoms
The crystal deposition diseases
    Gout
        Disorder of nucleic acid metabolism

Hyperuricemia leads to monosodium urate crystal (MSU) deposition in the joints (hyperuricemia may be from increased production or decreased excretion)
Inflammatory mediators are activated by crystals, which leads to joint destruction
Recurrent attacks of arthritis
Most common in men 40 to 60 years of age
Most common site is the great toe (podagra)
Radiographic findings (Fig. 3–6)
    Punched-out periarticular erosions
    Sclerotic overhangings bordering the joint
Diagnosis
    Elevated serum uric acid **is not** diagnostic of gout
    Must demonstrate MSU crystals in synovial fluid
    Crystals are thin and tapered, intracellular, and strongly negatively birefringent (Fig. 3–7)
Systemic manifestations
    Tophi—deposition of MSU crystals in the soft tissues (such as ear helix, olecranon)
    Kidney involvement
Treatment options
    Indomethacin—acute attacks (75 mg by mouth three times per day)
    Allopurinol—chronic gout (lowers serum uric acid levels); xanthine oxidase inhibitor (xanthine oxidase is responsible for converting xanthine oxidase to xanthine and xanthine to uric acid)

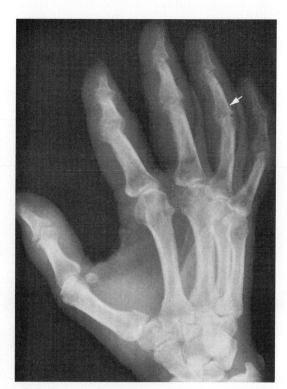

Figure 3–5 ■ AP radiograph of the hand of a patient with psoriatic arthritis. Note diffuse soft tissue swelling, periosteal reaction (*arrow*), and early "pencil-in-cup" deformity of the distal interphalangeal joint of the middle finger. (From Weissman BNW, Sledge CB: Orthopedic Radiology. Philadelphia, WB Saunders, 1986, p 81.)

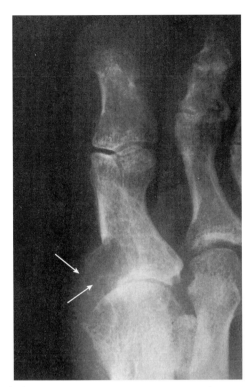

Figure 3–6 ▪ AP radiograph of the great toe of a patient with gout. Note soft tissue swelling and "punched out" periarticular erosions (*arrow*) and sclerotic overhangings bordering the joint. (From Bullough PG, Vigorita VJ: Atlas of Orthopaedic Pathology. Philadelphia, Gower Medical Publishing, 1984, p 5.4.)

Colchicine—prophylaxis after recurrent attacks
Chondrocalcinosis
  Etiologies
    Calcium pyrophosphate deposition disease (CPPD)
    Ochronosis

Hyperparathyroidism
Hypothyroidism
Hemochromatosis
CPPD is also known as **pseudogout**
  Calcium pyrophosphate crystals are deposited in joints
  Meniscus of the knee is the most common site for CPPD
  Calcium pyrophosphate crystals are short, blunt, rhomboid shaped, and weakly positively birefringent (see Fig. 3–7)
  Radiographs in cases of CPPD show fine linear calcifications in hyaline cartilage and diffuse calcification of fibrocartilage (such as meniscus) (Fig. 3–8)
Calcium hydroxyapatite crystal deposition disease
  Associated with chondrocalcinosis, a destructive degenerative joint disease, and Milwaukee shoulder (rotator cuff disease with shoulder arthritis and synovial fluid containing basic calcium phosphate crystals)

Infectious Arthritic Conditions

Pyogenic arthritis
  A purulent (pus-producing) infection (bacterial) within a joint
  Etiologies
    Open-joint traumatic injury
    Hematogenous spread (common in children)
    Extension of infection of bone (osteomyelitis) into a joint
  Risk factors
    Traumatic injuries
    Intravenous (IV) drug abuse
    Sexual activity (gonococcal infection)
    Diabetes
    RA

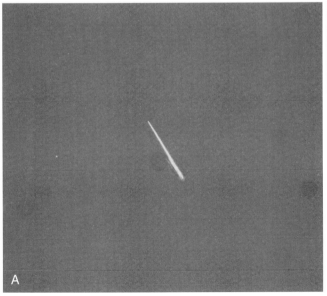
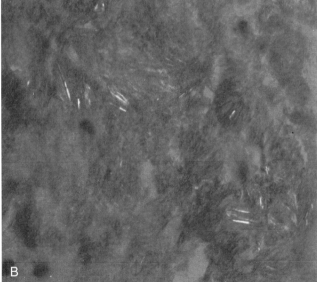

Figure 3–7 ▪ Photomicrographs demonstrating typical crystals of (*A*) gout and (*B*) pseudogout. Note the needle shape of the gout crystals and the rhomboid shape of the pseudogout crystals. (From Bullough PG, Vigorita VJ: Atlas of Orthopaedic Pathology. Philadelphia, Gower Medical Publishing, 1984, p 5.3.)

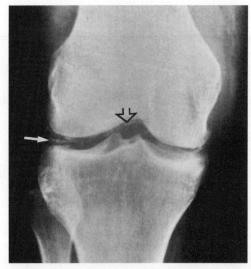

Figure 3–8 ■ AP radiograph demonstrating calcium pyrophosphate deposition disease (pseudogout) in the meniscus of the knee. Note the diffuse calcification within the (fibrocartilage) meniscus (*closed arrow*) and articular involvement with fine linear calcification of hyaline cartilage (*open arrow*). (From Weissman BNW, Sledge CB: Orthopedic Radiology. Philadelphia, WB Saunders, 1986, p 549.)

Clinical findings
  Fever
  Malaise
  Exquisite pain on even gentle attempted range of motion of the affected joint
  Increased ESR
  Increased white blood cell count
  Bone scans are usually positive
Treatment
  Joint aspiration before starting antibiotics to identify the organism and analyze the synovial fluid (see Table 3–2)
  Arthrotomy (surgical exposure and opening of the joint capsule)
  Arthroscopy
  Irrigation and débridement
  Antibiotics
Fungal arthritis
  Those at risk
    Neonates
    Patients with acquired immunodeficiency syndrome (AIDS)
    IV drug abusers
  Potassium hydroxide (KOH) preparation of synovial fluid shows fungi
  Amphotericin is the most common therapeutic agent used
Tuberculous arthritis
  Chronic granulomatous infection
  Caused by *Mycobacterium tuberculosis*
  Tuberculosis gets to joint via hematogenous spread
  Most often is a **monoarticular** arthritis
  Diagnosis
    Positive purified protein deriviative (PPD) test
    Acid-fast bacilli in joint fluid
  Treatment
    Irrigation and débridement

Long-term antibiotics
Lyme disease
  Characterized by acute self-limiting joint effusions
  Recurrent episodes
  Caused by the spirochete *Borrelia*
  Transmitted by tick *(Ixodes)* bites
    Transmission occurs in 10% of bites by infected ticks
  Immune complexes accumulate in the synovial fluid of affected individuals
  Diagnosis
    Enzyme-linked immunosorbent assay (ELISA) testing
  Systemic manifestations
    "Bull's-eye" rash (erythema chronicum migrans)
    Bell's palsy
    Cardiac abnormalities
  Treatment options
    Tetracycline/doxycycline
    Amoxicillin
    Cefuroxime

Hemorrhagic Arthritic Conditions

Hemophilic arthropathy
  X-linked recessive disorder
  Factor VIII (or IX) deficiency
  Etiology of arthritis (sequence of events)
    Repeated bleeds into joints caused by minor trauma
    Synovitis
    Enzymatic destruction of cartilage
    Joint deformities
  Knee is the most common site
  Nonoperative treatment options
    Correction of factor levels
    Splints, braces, compressive dressings
    Analgesics
  Operative treatment options (for cases refractive to nonoperative treatment)
    Synovectomy
    Arthroplasty (always total joint replacement, never hemiarthroplasty)
    Arthrodesis
Sickle cell arthropathy
  Hemoglobin SS
  Leads to osteonecrosis (ON), most commonly of the femoral head, which leads to joint destruction
  Treatment of ON of the femoral head is total joint arthroplasty
Pigmented villonodular synovitis (PVNS)
  Disease of synovium
  Exuberant proliferation of synovial villi (Fig. 3–9)
  Knee is the most common site
  Treatment is surgical excision of the affected synovium
  Recurrence rate is high

CONDITIONS AFFECTING BONE MINERALIZATION

Hypercalcemic Disorders

Clinical findings of hypercalcemia
  Polyuria

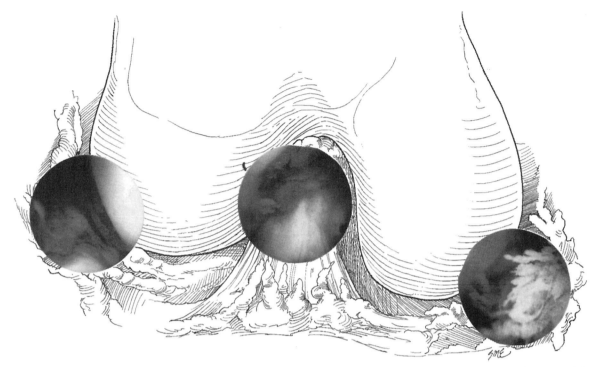

Figure 3–9 ■ Arthroscopic view of the left knee of a patient with pigmented villonodular synovitis. Note exuberant proliferation of synovial villi. (From Miller MD, Osborne JR, Warner JJP, et al: MRI-Arthroscopy Correlative Atlas. Philadelphia, WB Saunders, 1997, p 85.)

Kidney stones **(stones)**
Weakness
Lethargy **(groans)**
Disorientation
Areflexia
Central nervous system effects
Constipation
Gastrointestinal (GI) effects **(abdominal moans)**
Examples of hypercalcemic disorders
   Primary hyperparathyroidism
      Caused by overproduction of parathyroid hormone (PTH) (usually from a parathyroid adenoma)
      Excessive PTH causes a net increase in plasma calcium and a decrease in plasma phosphate (enhanced urinary excretion of phosphate) (Table 3–4)
      Bony changes

      Increased osteoclastic resorption of bone
      Osteopenia (radiolucencies seen on radiography)
      Osteitis fibrosa cystica—fibrous tissue replaces marrow
      Brown tumors (lytic lesion of bone [giant cells]) seen in patients with hyperparathyroidism
      Pathologic fractures
      Surgical parathyroidectomy is curative
   Other hypercalcemic disorders
      Multiple endocrine neoplasias
      Malignancy
      Hyperthyroidism
      Addison's disease
      Steroid administration
      Peptic ulcer disease
      Kidney disease
      Sarcoidosis

Table 3–4
LABORATORY FINDINGS IN ADULT CONDITIONS OF BONE MINERALIZATION

Condition	Serum Calcium	Serum Phosphate	PTH	Alkaline Phosphate	Other Findings
Primary hyperparathyroidism	↑	Nl or ↓	↑	Nl or ↑	↑ Urinary calcium
Primary hypoparathyroidism	↓	↑	↓	↑	
Pseudohypoparathyroidism	↓	↑	Nl or ↑		
Renal osteodystrophy	Nl or ↓	↑	↑	↑	↓ GFR, ↑ BUN, ↑ creatinine
Osteomalacia	Nl or ↓	↓	Nl or ↓ (↓ when serum calcium ↓)	↑	

↓, decreased; ↑, increased; Nl, normal; PTH, parathyroid hormone; GFR, glomerular filtration rate; BUN, blood urea nitrogen.

Hypocalcemic Disorders

Low serum calcium from
   Low PTH
   Low vitamin D_3
Clinical findings of hypocalcemia
   Hyperreflexia
   Tetany
   Seizures
   Cataracts
   Electrocardiographic changes
   Fungal infections of the nails
   Hair loss
   Pigment loss (vitiligo)
Examples of hypocalcemic disorders
   Primary hypoparathyroidism (see Table 3–4)
      Caused by decreased PTH (PTH underproduction)
      May be idiopathic
      Iatrogenic hypoparathyroidism may follow thyroidectomy
   Pseudohypoparathyroidism (see Table 3–4)
      Rare genetic disorder
      PTH has no effect on the target cells or organs (intestine, kidney, bone) because of a receptor abnormality (to PTH)
      PTH **level is normal**; PTH **action is blocked** because of a receptor abnormality
   Renal osteodystrophy (see Table 3–4)
      Chronic renal failure leads to inability to excrete phosphate
      High plasma phosphate leads to decreased plasma calcium
      High plasma phosphate also leads to hyperplasia of the parathyroid glands (in an effort to increase PTH production [which enhances urinary excretion of phosphate]), which may result in secondary hyperparathyroidism
      Treatment is directed at the renal pathology
   Osteomalacia (see Table 3–4)
      Failure of bone mineralization
      Leads to unmineralized osteoid
      Bone **qualitative** (not quantitative) defect
      Etiologies
         Nutritional deficiency
         GI absorption defects
         Defects in the renal tubules
         Renal osteodystrophy
         Medications (anticonvulsants, high-dose diphosphonates, sodium fluoride)
         Soft tissue tumors
         Heavy metal intoxication
         Hypophosphatasia
      Femoral neck fractures are common
      Diagnosis—transiliac bone biopsy shows **widened osteoid seams**
      Treatment—high-dose vitamin D
   Rickets (see Chapter 5)
      Childhood osteomalacia

CONDITIONS AFFECTING BONE MINERAL DENSITY

Bone mass is regulated by the relative rates of deposition and withdrawal

Conditions of Decreased Bone Mineral Density (Osteopenia)

Osteoporosis
   Age-related decrease in bone mass
   Usually associated with loss of estrogen in postmenopausal women
   Accounts for 1 million fractures per year in the United States
   Quantitative bone defect
   Quality of bone is fine; there is just not enough of it
   Risk factors
      Advanced age
      Women (especially those who breastfed their children)
      Sedentary lifestyle
      Thinness
      Caucasians
      Northern European descent
      Smokers
      Drinkers
      Phenytoin (impairs vitamin D metabolism)
      Low calcium/vitamin D diets
      Endocrine abnormalities
      Vitamin D deficiency/pathway abnormalities
      Renal tubular acidosis
      Hypophosphatemia/hypophosphatasia
   Cancellous bone is most markedly affected
   Clinical findings
      Vertebral compression fractures
      Kyphosis
      Hip fractures
      Distal radius fractures
   Radiographic findings (Fig. 3–10)
      Bone loss does not become visible until very advanced (40% bone loss)

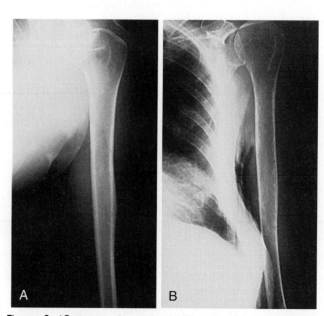

Figure 3–10 ■ AP radiograph of (*A*) a normal humerus demonstrating thick robust cortices and (*B*) a humerus of an elderly woman with postmenopausal osteoporosis demonstrating diffuse osteopenia (radiographic evidence of decreased bone density without implication of causality). (Courtesy of Fondren Orthopedic Group LLP, Texas Orthopedic Hospital, Houston, Texas.)

Diagnosis
  Dual energy x-ray absorptiometry (DEXA) is the best method of quantifying bone mineral density
  Laboratory findings are usually unremarkable **(normal)**
  Two types of osteoporosis
    Postmenopausal (type I)
      Affects cancellous bone primarily
    Age-related (type II)
      Seen in patients older than 75 years
      Affects both cancellous and cortical bone
      Related to poor calcium absorption
  Treatment options
    Methods that **increase bone mass**
      Fluoride with calcium, vitamin D, estrogen, or calcitonin (mass increases, but bone is brittle)
      Vigorous exercise (excellent treatment option)
    Methods that **halt bone loss**
      Calcium
      Vitamin D
      Estrogen
      Calcitonin
      Mild exercise
    Methods that **decrease (but do not halt) bone loss**
      Diphosphonate
      Phosphate
      Alendronate (Fosamax)
Osteomalacia (see section on Conditions of Bone Mineralization)
Scurvy
  Vitamin C (ascorbic acid) deficiency leads to defective collagen growth and repair
  Clinical findings
    Fatigue
    Gum bleeding
    Joint effusions
    Ecchymosis
    Iron deficiency
  Radiographic findings
    Thinning of cortices
    Metaphyseal clefts
  Laboratory values are normal
Osteogenesis imperfecta (see Chapter 5)
Marrow-packing disorders causing osteopenia
  Myeloma
  Leukemia

Conditions of Increased Bone Mineral Density

Osteopetrosis (Fig. 3–11)
  Marble bone disease
  Decreased osteoclastic function leads to decreased bone resorption
  Obliteration of the medullary canal (from decreased bone resorption) leads to anemia
  Although the bone has a marble-like appearance, it is brittle and therefore **pathologic fractures** are common
Osteopoikilosis
  Spotted bone disease

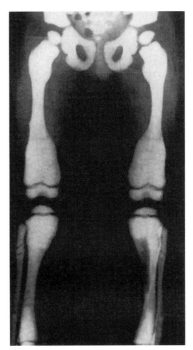

Figure 3–11 ■ Typical "marble bone" appearance in osteopetrosis. (From Tachdjian MO: Pediatric Orthopaedics, 2nd ed. Philadelphia, WB Saunders, 1990, p 795.)

Conditions That Display Both Increased and Decreased Bone Mineral Density

Paget's disease (Fig. 3–12)
  Three stages of Paget's disease
    Osteoclastic
    Osteoblastic
    Sclerotic
  Affects 3% of the older adult population
  Characterized by increased bone turnover with increased osteoclastic activity (bone resorption)
  Irregular bone formation leads to osteopenia
  Clinical findings
    Bowing of the extremities
    Skull widening (increased hat size)
    Kyphosis
    Cranial nerve abnormalities (from foraminal impingement caused by bony changes in the skull)
    High-output cardiac failure
  Radiographic findings
    Coarse prominent trabeculae
    Bone enlargement
  Laboratory findings
    Increased serum alkaline phosphatase
    Urinary hydroxyproline
  Treatment options
    Calcitonin
    Diphosphonates
    Cytotoxic agents
  Malignant degeneration of Paget's disease to osteosarcoma or chondrosarcoma occurs in 5% to 10% of patients and has a poor prognosis

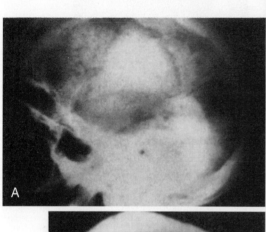

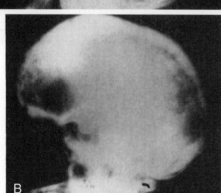

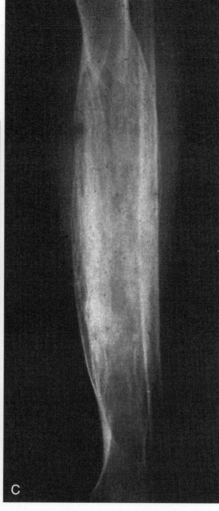

Figure 3–12 ■ Radiographic appearance of Paget's disease. *A*, Lateral radiograph of the skull demonstrating osteopenia characteristic of early stage (osteoclastic) disease. *B*, Late stage (sclerotic) Paget's disease. (From Merkow RL, Lane JM: Paget's disease of bone. Orthop Clin North Am 21:175, 1990.) *C*, AP radiograph of the tibia and fibula of a man with Paget's disease showing lytic destruction of the mid-shaft of the tibia. (From Bogumill GP, Schwamm HA: Orthopaedic Pathology: A Synopsis with Clinical and Radiographic Correlation. Philadelphia, WB Saunders, 1984, p 181.)

CONDITIONS AFFECTING BONE VIABILITY

Osteonecrosis

Also commonly referred to as **avascular necrosis** (AVN)

Represents death of bony tissue

Most common site involved is the **hip** (femoral head) (Table 3–5)

Death of subchondral bone leads to collapse of overlying cartilage and flattening of the femoral head **(crescent sign)** (Fig. 3–13)

Treatment options for ON of the hip include

Activity modification
NSAIDs
Cane
Core decompression (controversial)
Vascularized fibula graft (controversial)
Total hip arthroplasty for advanced cases that have failed conservative treatment

Bilateral hip involvement is very common (50% to 80%), so one needs to rule this out and follow over time in patients with **what appears to be** unilateral hip ON

Etiologies of hip ON

Idiopathic (Chandler's disease)

Table 3–5
CLASSIFICATION OF OSTEONECROSIS OF THE FEMORAL HEAD*

Stage	Pain	X-ray Findings	MRI Findings
0	None	Normal	Normal
I	Minimal	Normal	Early changes
II	Moderate	Sclerotic changes	Positive
III	Severe	Flattening of femoral head (crescent sign)	Positive
IV	Severe	Changes to femoral head and acetabulum	Positive

*Described by Ficat.

Table 3–6
SOFT TISSUE AND RELATED INFECTIONS

Type of Infection (Definition)	Common Organism(s)	Clinical Features/Aspects	Treatment
Cellulitis (infection of subcutaneous tissues)	Staphylococcus Streptococcus	Erythema Tenderness ↑ Warmth Lymphangitis Lymphadenopathy	Mild cases—oral antibiotics such as cephalexin (Keflex) Severe cases (high fever, toxicity) —IV antibiotics such as cefazolin (Ancef)
Erysipelas (a superficial, erythematous, sharply demarcated lesion)	Group A streptococci	Severe symptoms common Commonly occurs in Infants Diabetics Elderly Areas of preexisting skin ulcers	IV antibiotics
Necrotizing fasciitis (severe fascial infection)	Streptococcus Anerobes Polymicrobial	Aggressive Rapidly progressing Life threatening	Wide surgical débridement IV antibiotics
Gas gangrene	Clostridium species Others	Foul-smelling discharge X-rays show gas in tissues (Fig. 3–14) (organism produces gas)	Surgical I & D High-dose IV penicillin G
Tetanus (neuroparalytic disease caused by exotoxin)	Clostridium tetani	Tetanus-prone wound >6-hr old >1-cm deep Devitalized tissue present Gross contamination Frostbite wounds Crush injuries	Prophylaxis—proper wound care and tetanus toxoid if indicated (immunoglobin for severe wounds in patients without prior immunization) Late management—supportive
Toxic shock syndrome (toxemia, not septicemia)	Staphylococcus	Typically develops postoperatively Fever Hypotension Rash Serous exudate from wound	Emergent I & D IV antibiotics Fluid replacement
Surgical wound infection	Staphylococcus aureus Staphylococcus epidermitis	Fever Local signs and symptoms	I & D Antibiotics
Puncture wound to foot (through sole of sneaker)	Pseudomonas Staphylococcus aureus	Local signs and symptoms	I & D Antibiotics
Diabetic foot	Polymicrobial	Recurrent May be life-threatening Local signs and symptoms	Antibiotics I & D necrotic tissue
Paronychia (infection/ inflammation of the paronychial fold on the side of the nail)	Staphylococcus aureus Anaerobes Fungi Herpes simplex	Common in nail biters and dentists	Antibiotics, débridement, warm soaks Acyclovir for herpes simplex
Bite injuries Human	Anaerobic organisms Staphylococcus aureus Streptococcus viridans Eikenella	These injuries can be very serious and in general are worse than bites from other species	Amoxicillin trihydrate/clavulanate potassium (Augmentin)
Dog	Pasteurella Others	Local findings, cellulitis	Ampicillin Consider antirabies treatment
Cat	Pasteurella	Local findings, cellulitis	Amoxicillin trihydrate/clavulanate potassium (Augmentin)
Rat	Streptobacillus	Local findings, cellulitis	Ampicillin
Snake	Staphylococcus Anerobes Gram negatives	Can cause extensive soft tissue destruction and may even lead to a compartment syndrome Nausea, vomiting, neurologic dysfunction, local swelling, ecchymosis	First aid (tourniquet, suction of venom) Antivenom therapy Tetanus prophylaxis Ceftriaxone (Rocephin) Fasciotomy for compartment syndrome
Marine injuries	Anerobes (virulent organisms) Organisms difficult to culture		As per specific organism
Fungal infections (fungi are multicellular organisms that induce a hypersensitivity reaction in tissues)	Several	Chronic granulomas, abscess formation, tissue necrosis	Amphotericin B Others

Table continued on following page

Table 3–6
SOFT TISSUE AND RELATED INFECTIONS *Continued*

Type of Infection (Definition)	Common Organism(s)	Clinical Features/Aspects	Treatment
AIDS/HIV	HIV (virus) affects lymphocyte and macrophage cell lines ($\downarrow$ T helper cells [T_4 lymphocytes])	High incidence in homosexual males and hemophiliacs Increasing incidence in heterosexual population Advanced stages of HIV → AIDS HIV positivity is not a contraindication to performing required musculoskeletal operative procedures, but these patients may be at an increased risk for developing wound and nonwound-related complications	
Hepatitis	Hepatitis A	From poor sanitation Not from surgical transmission	
	Hepatitis B	200,000 cases per year in U.S. Surgical transmission risk	Vaccine for prophylaxis Immunoglobin for exposure
	Hepatitis C (non-A, non-B)	Most common transfusion-associated form of hepatitis	

IV, intravenous; I & D, irrigation and débridement; AIDS, acquired immunodeficiency syndrome; HIV, human immunodeficiency virus.

Post-traumatic
Steroid-induced
Alcohol-induced
Dysbarism (Caisson's disease)
Storage diseases (such as Gaucher's disease)
Other sites of ON
  Scaphoid (post-traumatic)
  Proximal humerus
  Talus (post-traumatic)
  Lunate (Kienböck's disease)
Evaluation
  Careful history for risk factors (to assess etiology)
  Physical examination
    Decreased joint range of motion

MUSCULOSKELETAL AND RELATED INFECTIONS

Soft Tissue and Related Infections
(Table 3–6)

Bone and Joint Infections (Table 3–7)

Overview of Antimicrobial Agents
(Table 3–8)

Antibiotics, Indications, and Side Effects
(Table 3–9)

MUSCULOSKELETAL TUMORS

Bone Tumors

Primary tumors of bone (Tables 3–10 and 3–11)
  Less common than metastatic tumors to bone
  Types of primary bone tumors
    Malignant bone tumors (sarcomas)
      Exhibit rapid growth

Destroy overlying cortex and spread into the surrounding soft tissues
May metastasize (via the blood stream or lymphatics) to other tissues (lung is the most common)
Benign bone tumors
  Generally have limited growth potential, but some types do have destructive potential
Bone tumor simulators
  Osteomyelitis
  Bone islands
  Others
Metastatic tumors to bone
  More common than primary bone tumors
  Most common sources of metastases to bone are from (mnemonic—"BLT with ketchup and pickle")
  Breast
  Lung
  Thyroid
  Kidney
  Prostate
  Metastases tend to go to the proximal portions of the skeleton (spine, pelvis, humerus, femur) and not the distal portions of the skeleton (forearm, tibia, hands, feet)
Evaluation of bone tumors
  History
    Pain (onset, quality, inciters versus relievers)
    Fevers/chills
    Weight loss
  Physical examination
    Inspection
      Size
      Skin changes
    Palpation
      Tenderness
      Mobility

Table 3–7
BONE AND JOINT INFECTIONS

Type of Infection (Definition)	Common Organism(s)	Clinical Features/Aspects	Treatment
Acute osteomyelitis (bone and bone marrow infection caused by direct inoculation of an open traumatic wound or by blood-borne organisms)	*Staphylococcus aureus* Anaerobes Others	Acute hematogenous osteomyelitis is most common in children (see Chapter 5)	As per specific organism
Chronic osteomyelitis (bone and bone marrow infection) (Fig. 3–15)	*Staphylococcus aureus* Others	May arise as a result of inappropriately treated acute osteomyelitis, trauma, or from soft tissue infection extension to bone (such as in diabetics, the elderly, immunocompromised individuals, and IV drug abusers) Skin and soft tissue involvement overlying infected bone is common Fistulous tracts (draining pus) can develop into epidermoid carcinoma Acute osteomyelitis is episodic with periods of quiescence followed by acute exacerbations (fever, toxicity, purulent drainage)	I & D IV antibiotics as per specific organism **This is a very difficult problem; cure is often not possible** Amputation is not uncommonly required
Septic arthritis	Bacterial Fungal Tuberculous Lyme (spirochete)	For adult septic arthritis see Infectious Arthritic Conditions (this chapter) For pediatric septic arthritis see Chapter 5	I & D Antimicrobials
Infected total joint arthroplasty	*Staphylococcus aureus* *Staphylococcus epidermidis* *Escherichia coli* *Pseudomonas* Others	A devastating complication of TJA Clinical findings similar to those of septic arthritis Incidence of infection increased with obesity, sickle cell disease, diabetes, alcoholism, osteonecrosis, rheumatoid arthritis, immunosupressed individuals, those on chronic steroids, ↑ operative time, revision procedures	Complex decision algorithm based on a variety of factors Treatment possibilities include a combination of the following: IV antibiotics I & D Exchange arthroplasty (remove implants and implant new ones) on either an immediate (same procedure) or a delayed (weeks to months) basis Resection arthroplasty (permanent removal of implants) Prophylaxis to prevent hematogenous seeding of a TJA in patients undergoing dental procedures is a complex matter, and the decision of whether to give antibiotics should be left to the treating orthopaedic surgeon
Septic bursitis	*Staphylococcus aureus* Others	Local pain Swelling Tenderness Fever	Penicillinase-resistant synthetic penicillins

I & D, irrigation and débridement; IV, intravenous; TJA, total joint arthroplasty.

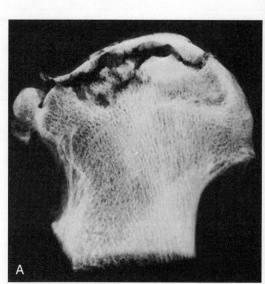 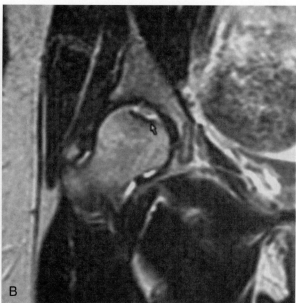

Figure 3–13 ■ *A,* Fine-grain radiograph demonstrating space between the articular surface and subchondral bone ("crescent sign") associated with avascular necrosis. (From Steinberg ME: The Hip and Its Disorders. Philadelphia, WB Saunders, 1991, p 630.) *B,* Coronal FSE T2 image demonstrating advanced osteonecrosis of the femoral head. *Arrow* points to the "crescent sign," suggestive of collapse and attempted repair of subchondral bone. (From Miller MD, Osborne JR, Warner JJP, et al: MRI-Arthroscopy Correlative Atlas. Philadelphia, WB Saunders, 1997, p 96.)

Radiographic evaluation (Figs. 3–16 and 3–17)
  Plain x-rays of the involved region
    Evaluate the effect of the tumor on the bone
    Evaluate the response of the bone to the tumor
  Technetium bone scan
    Search for occult malignancies
    Good screen for all anatomic sites of tumor
  Chest x-ray/CT scan
    In cases where bone malignancy (with possible metastases to the lung) is suspected
  CT scan of the lesion
    Evaluation of cortical involvement
  MRI of the lesion
    Evaluation of medullary involvement
    Screen for occult malignancies
    Search for skip lesions (tumor in the same extremity distant from a known tumor site)

    Useful for staging a tumor (based on grade [low versus high], delineating the tumor site, and metastases)
  Treatment of bone tumors
    Should be carried out by an orthopaedic surgeon with expertise in musculoskeletal oncology
    Biopsies
      Needle
      Incisional—removes a piece of the tumor (for microscopic study)
      Excisional—attempts to remove the entire tumor
    Definitive surgical procedures
      Intralesional resection
      Marginal resection—goes through the reactive zone (inflammatory cells) of the tumor
      Wide resection—takes a cuff of surrounding normal tissue with the tumor
      Radical resection—entire tumor and anatomic compartment(s) that the tumor lies within are removed
    Adjuvant therapies
      Chemotherapy
      Radiation therapy

Soft Tissue Tumors (Table 3–12)

OTHER ADULT MUSCULOSKELETAL CONDITIONS

Traumatic Disorders

Stress fracture (see Chapter 4 and Chapters 8 to 22 for stress fractures by specific anatomic region)

Figure 3–14 ■ Radiographic evidence of gas within the tissues (*arrow*) of an elderly diabetic patient with gas gangrene. (Courtesy of Fondren Orthopedic Group LLP, Texas Orthopedic Hospital, Houston, Texas.)

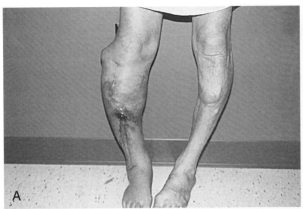
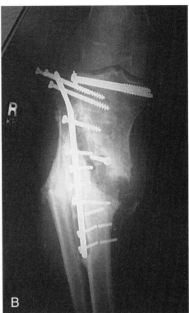

Figure 3–15 ■ Clinical photograph and AP radiograph of the tibia in a patient with an infected (chronic osteomyelitis) tibial nonunion. Clinical photograph (*A*) shows a sinus tract draining purulent material. Radiograph (*B*) demonstrates destructive changes of osteomyelitis with an obvious wide radiolucent line without evidence of fracture healing. Also note hardware failure (broken screws in the distal fragment) and loosening of screws in the proximal fragment caused by repetitive loading on the ununited fracture. (Courtesy of Fondren Orthopedic Group LLP, Texas Orthopedic Hospital, Houston, Texas.)

Sprain—soft tissue injury (tear) of a ligament
  Graded by severity
    First degree—an incomplete ligament tear involving a minimum number of fibers; does not result in joint instability
    Second degree—an incomplete ligament tear involving a greater number of fibers; results in minor joint instability
    Third degree—a complete tear of the ligament; results in major joint instability
Strain—a stretching or tearing of muscle or tendon
  Graded in a fashion similar to sprains (see above)
Tendon rupture—complete intrasubstance tearing of a tendon (resulting from trauma), often associated with a "mop-end" appearance of the two ends
Tendon laceration—injury to tendon caused by penetrating trauma
Ligament tear—represents a third-degree sprain
Bone bruise—represents a trabecular (bone) microfracture as the result of an axial load
Reflex sympathetic dystrophy (RSD)
  Neurologic vasomotor dysfunction with sustained efferent activity by sympathetic fibers
  Characterized by **intense burning pain** that is out of proportion with the traumatic or surgical insult
  Also characterized by delayed recovery and trophic changes to the extremity (cool hand, shiny skin)
  Common locations
    Shoulder
    Hand
    Knee
    Foot
  Treatment options
    Physical therapy
    Sympathetic block
    Sympathectomy
  This is a difficult entity to treat, and the prognosis is guarded

Causalgia
  RSD with a known nerve trunk injury
Nerve injuries (see Chapter 1)
  Regeneration of nerves occurs at 1 mm per day
  Tendon transfers are useful in cases where nerve function has failed to return to normal after injury
Thermal injuries
  Freezing injuries
    Most common cause of bilateral upper- and lower-extremity amputations
    Treatment regimen
      Restore core body temperature
      Rapid rewarming of the extremity
      Débridement
      Physical therapy
    Additional treatment options
      Anticoagulation
      Sympathectomy
  Burn injuries
    Treatment is based on the depth of the burn (Table 3–13)
  Electrical injuries
    Alternating current (AC) is more dangerous than direct current (DC)
    Treatment includes irrigation and débridement of all necrotic tissue (serial débridements every 48 hours) followed by plastic reconstructive procedures
    Acute amputation is sometimes required
Chemical burns
  Severity of injury depends on
    Specific chemical causing insult
    Concentration of chemical
    Duration of chemical contact
  Treatment
    Copious irrigation
    Other specific regimens based on specific chemicals (telephone Poison Control Center at 1-800-764-7661)

Table 3–8
OVERVIEW OF ANTIMICROBIAL AGENTS

Penicillins
  Natural
    Penicillin G
    Penicillin-VK
  Penicillinase Resistant (PRSP)
    Methicillin (Staphcillin, Celbenin)
    Nafcillin (Unipen, Nafcil)
    Oxacillin (Prostaphlin, Bactocill)
    Cloxacillin (Tegopen, Cloxapen)
    Dicloxacillin (Dynapen, Pathocil)
    Flucloxacillin (Floxapen, Ladropen, Staphcil)
  Aminopenicillins
    Ampicillin (Omnipen, Polycillin)
    Amoxacillin (Amoxil)
    Bacampicillin (Spectrobid)
    Amoxicillin/clavulanate (Augmentin)
    Ampicillin/sulbactam (Unasyn)
  Antipseudomonal Agents
    Indanyl carbenicillin (Geocillin)
    Ticarcillin (Ticar)
    Ticarcillin/clavulanate (Timentin)
    Mezlocillin (Mezlin)
    Piperacillin (Pipracil)
    Piperacillin/tazobactam (Zosyn)
Cephalosporins
  First Generation
    Cephalothin (Keflin, Seffin)
    Cefazolin (Ancef, Kefzol)
    Cephapirin (Cefadyl)
    Cephradine (Velosef)
    Cephalexin (Keflex, Keftab)
    Cefadroxil (Duricef, Ultracef)
  Second Generation
    Cefaclor (Ceclor)
    Cefamandole (Mandol)
    Cefoxitin (Mefoxin)
    Cefuroxime (Zinacef, Kefurox)
    Cefuroxime axetil (Ceftin)
    Cefmetazole (Zefazone)
    Cefotetan (Cefotan)
    Cefprozil (Cefzil)
    Cefonicid (Monocid)
    Loracarbef (Lorabid)
    Ceftibuten (Cedax)
  Third Generation
    Cefetamet pivoxil (R. 15-8075)
    Cefoperazone (Cefobid)
    Cefotaxime (Claforan)
    Ceftizoxime (Cefizox)
    Ceftriaxone (Rocephin, Nitrocephin)
    Ceftazidime (Fortaz, Tazicef, Tazidime)
    Cefixime (Suprax)
    Cefpodoxime proxetil (Vantin)
  Fourth Generation
    Cefpirome (HR 810)
    Cefepime (Maxipime)
Carbapenems
    Imipenem + cilastatin (Primaxin)
    Meropenem (Merrem)
Monobactams
    Aztreonam (Azactam)
Aminoglycosides
    Amikacin (Amikin)
    Gentamicin (Garamycin)
    Kanamycin (Kantrex)

Netilmicin (Netromycin)
Tobramycin (Nebcin)
Fluoroquinolones
  Norfloxacin (Noroxin)
  Ciprofloxacin (Cipro)
  Ofloxacin (Floxin)
  Enoxacin (Penetrex)
  Lomefloxacin (Maxaquin)
  Pefloxacin
  Grepafloxacin (Raxar)
  Levofloxacin (Levaquin)
  Sparfloxacin (Zagam)
  Trovafloxacin (Trovan)
Macrolides
  Azithromycin (Zithromax)
  Clarithromycin (Biaxin)
  Erythromycin
Other Antibacterial Agents
  Chloramphenicol (Chloromycetin)
  Clindamycin (Cleocin)
  Vancomycin (Vancocin, Vancoled)
  Teicoplanin (Targocid)
  Doxycycline (Vibramycin)
  Minocycline (Minocin)
  Tetracycline (Terramycin)
  Polymyxin B (Aerosporin)
  Fusidic acid (Fucidin)
  Fosfomycin (Monurol)
  Sulfisoxazole (Gantrisin)
→ Trimethoprim/sulfamethoxazole (Bactrim, Septra)
  Metronidazole (Flagyl)
Antifungal Agents
  Amphotericin B (Fungizone)
  Fluconazole (Diflucan)
  Flucytosine (Ancobon)
  Ketoconazole (Nizoral)
  Itraconazole (Sporanox)
Antimycobacterial Agents
  Isoniazid [INH (Nydrazid)]
  Rifampin (Rifadin)
  Ethambutol (Myambutol)
  Streptomycin
  Pyrazinamide
  Ethionamide
  Cycloserine (Seromycin)
  Amikacin (Amikin)
  Capreomycin (Capastat)
  Thioacetazone
  Rifabutin (Mycobutin)
Antiparasitic Agents
  Albendazole (Zentel)
  Atovaquone (Mepron)
  Dapsone
  Mefloquine (Lariam)
  Pentamidine (Pentam 300)
  Pyrimethamine (Daraprim)
  Praziquantel (Biltricide)
Antiviral Agents
  Acyclovir (Zovirax)
  Amantadine (Symmetrel)
  Didanosine (Videx)
  Foscarnet (Foscavir)
  Ganciclovir (Cytovene)
  Zalcitabine (Hivid)
  Zidovudine [AZT (Retrovir)]

Adapted from Gilbert DN, Moellering RC, Sande MA: The Sanford Guide to Antimicrobial Therapy, 28th ed. Virginia, Antimicrobial Therapy, Inc., 1998, pp 55–71. Reprinted by permission.

Table 3–9
ANTIBIOTICS, INDICATIONS, AND SIDE EFFECTS

Antibiotic	Indications	Side Effects
Cell Wall Synthesis Inhibitors		
Penicillin	*Streptococcus*, G+	Hypersensitivity/resistance, hemolytic
Methicillin/oxacillin/nafcillin	Penicillinase-resistant organisms	Same as penicillin; nephritis (methicillin); subcutaneous skin slough (nafcillin)
Carbenicillin/ticarcillin/piperacillin	Better against G−	Bleeding diathesis (carbenicillin)
Cephalosporins		
First generation	Prophylaxis (surgical)	
Second generation	Some G+/G−	
Third generation	G−, fewer G+	Hemolytic anemia (bleeding diathesis [moxalactam])
Inhibitors of Cell Membrane Function		
Polymyxin/nystatin	GU	Nephrotoxic
Amphotericin	Fungi	Nephrotoxic
Inhibitors of Protein Synthesis		
Aminoglycosides	G−, PM	Nephrotoxicity, ototoxicity (dose-related)
Clindamycin	G+, anaerobes	Pseudomembranous enterocolitis
Chloramphenicol	*Haemophilus influenzae*, anaerobes	Bone marrow aplasia
Erythromycin	G+ (patients with PCN allergy)	Ototoxic
Tetracycline	G+ (patients with PCN allergy)	Stains teeth/bone (up to age 8)
Fluoroquinolones		
Ciprofloxacin	G−, methicillin-resistant *Staphylococcus aureus*	Cartilage erosion (children); oral therapy increases theophylline levels; antacids reduce absorption
Inhibitors of Nucleic Acid Synthesis		
Vancomycin	Methicillin-resistant *Staphylococcus aureus*, *Clostridium difficile*	Ototoxic, erythema with rapid IV delivery
Sulfonamides	GU	Hemolytic anemia
Carbapenems		
Imipenem	G+, some G−	Resistance, seizures
Azactam	G−, no anaerobes	

G+, gram positive; G−, gram negative; GU, genitourinary; PM, polymicrobial; PCN, penicillin; IV, intravenous.
From Miller MD: Review of Orthopedics, 2nd ed. Philadelphia, WB Saunders, 1996.

Compartment syndrome

Increased pressure within a soft tissue (fascial) compartment of the extremities leads to compression of tissue capillaries (and venules), leading to tissue necrosis

Typically follows a traumatic injury to an extremity (crush injury, fracture, etc.)

Occurs most commonly in the leg (tibia) and forearm, but may occur in any other area where fascial compartments are present (buttock, thigh, foot, arm, etc.)

Clinical findings ("The 5 Ps")
Pain—the earliest and most reliable indicator
Pallor
Paralysis
Paresthesia
Pulselessness

Diagnosis
Pain on passive motion that puts the compartment muscles being tested on stretch
Example: to test for a compartment syndrome of the anterior compartment of the leg (tibia), one should passively plantarflex the ankle; this will put the muscles of the anterior compartment on stretch and will cause severe pain if a compartment syndrome exists

Compartment pressure measurement
Measure compartment pressures using a commercially available instrument or a homemade device constructed from sterile tubing and a sphygmomanometer (Fig. 3–18)

Continuous measurements should be performed using an indwelling compartment catheter in those patients at high risk for developing a compartment syndrome (significant trauma) who are unable to adequately be evaluated (such as head-injured or unconscious individuals)

All compartments in the anatomic region in question should be evaluated

Abnormal compartment pressures are **greater than 30 mm Hg** or within 30 mm Hg of the diastolic blood pressure

Treatment of a compartment syndrome
A surgical emergency
Fasciotomy (surgical release of fascial compartments) within 4 hours of onset of compartment syndrome typically prevents muscle necrosis

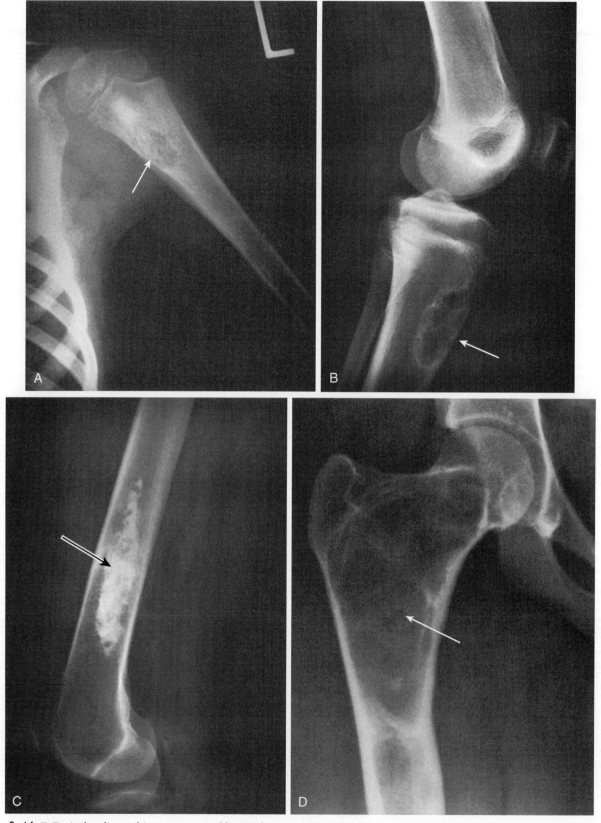

Figure 3–16 ■ Typical radiographic appearance of benign bone tumors. *A,* Well-circumscribed lytic lesion (*arrow*) (osteoblastoma) in the proximal humerus without significant bony destruction. *B,* Lateral radiograph of the knee showing a "scalloped," well-circumscribed nondestructive lesion (*arrow*) (nonossifying fibroma) of the proximal tibia. *C,* Lateral radiograph of the distal femur showing a densely mineralized medullary lesion (*arrow*) (enchondroma) that is not eroding the bony cortices. (*A–C* from Frassica FJ, McCarthy EF: Orthopaedic pathology. *In* Miller MD [ed]: Review of Orthopaedics, 2nd ed. Philadelphia, WB Saunders, 1996, p 307.) *D,* AP radiograph of the proximal femur showing a well-circumscribed lytic lesion (*arrow*) (fibrous dysplasia) without destruction of the cortex. (From Wold LE, McLeod RA, Sim FH, et al: Atlas of Orthopaedic Pathology. Philadelphia, WB Saunders, 1990.)

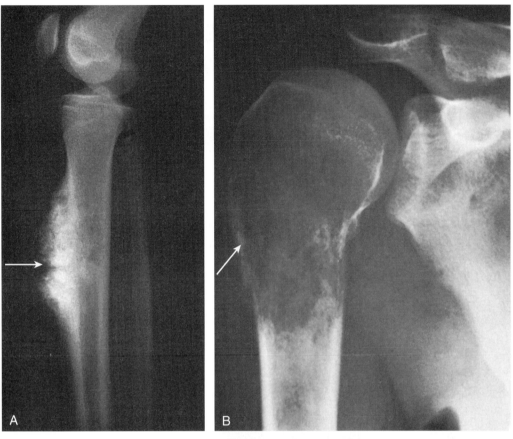

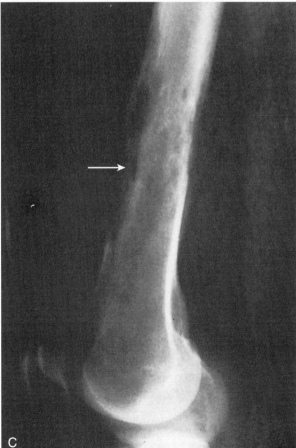

Figure 3–17 ■ Typical radiographic appearance of malignant bone tumors. *A,* Lateral radiograph of the tibia showing a densely mineralized, rapidly expanding lesion (*arrow*) (periosteal osteosarcoma) demonstrating cortical destruction. (From Frassica FJ, McCarthy EF: Orthopaedic pathology. *In* Miller MD [ed]: Review of Orthopaedics, 2nd ed. Philadelphia, WB Saunders, 1996, p 306.) *B,* AP radiograph of the proximal humerus showing an aggressive lesion (*arrow*) (fibrosarcoma of bone) with marked cortical disruption. *C,* Lateral radiograph of the distal femur demonstrating marked osteopenia and cortical destruction (*arrow*) (metastatic thyroid cancer). (*B* and *C* from Wold LE, McLeod RA, Sim FH, et al: Atlas of Orthopaedic Pathology. Philadelphia, WB Saunders, 1990.)

Table 3–10
TUMORS OF BONE

	Benign Tumors (see Fig. 3–16)	Malignant Tumors (see Fig. 3–17)
Effect of the Tumor on the Bone	Spread slowly but can invade soft tissues	Spread rapidly through medullary cavity Early cortical destruction Spread of tumor to soft tissues
Response of the Bone to the Tumor	Host bone forms periosteal rim of new bone or cortex thickens in an effort to contain tumor	Host bone unable to mount a response to contain rapidly expanding tumor Rapid bone destruction

Table 3–11
ADULT BONE TUMORS

Age (yr)	Benign	Malignant
20–40	Osteoma Enchondroma Giant cell tumor Periosteal chondroma Aneurysmal bone cyst Chondromyxoid fibroma Fibrous dysplasia Hemangioma Neurilemmoma Lipoma	Osteosarcoma (parosteal) Chondrosarcoma Malignant fibrous histiocytoma Lymphoma Leukemia Adamantinoma Fibrosarcoma Angiosarcoma Hemangiopericytoma Metastases to bone
>40	Paget's disease Hemangioma Neurilemmoma Lipoma Hyperparathyroidism (brown tumors)	Metastases to bone Multiple myeloma Lymphoma Chondrosarcoma Malignant fibrous histiocytoma Fibrosarcoma Angiosarcoma Hemangiopericytoma Chordoma Paget's sarcoma Postradiation sarcoma

Table 3–12
ADULT SOFT TISSUE TUMORS

Benign	Malignant
Superficial fibromatoses	Malignant fibrous histiocytoma
Nodular fasciitis	Fibrosarcoma
Lipoma	Liposarcoma
Neurilemmoma (peripheral nerve)	Neurofibrosarcoma
Neurofibroma	Leiomyosarcoma
Leiomyoma	Rhabdomyosarcoma (extremities)
Hemangioma	Angiosarcoma (extremities)
Glomus tumor	Kaposi's sarcoma
Ganglia	Synovial sarcoma
Pigmented villonodular synovitis	Lymphangiosarcoma
Synovial chondromatosis	Epithelioid sarcoma
Giant cell tumor of tendon sheath	Clear cell sarcoma
Lymphangioma	Alveolar cell sarcoma (skeletal muscle)

Table 3–13
BURN INJURIES

Degree	Depth	Findings	Treatment
First	Epidermis	Edema, erythema	Symptomatic
Second	Dermis	Blisters, blanching	Topical antibiotics, splint, range-of-motion exercises
Third	Subcutaneous	Waxy, dry	Excision, split-thickness skin graft
Fourth	Deep	Exposed tissues	Amputation vs. reconstruction

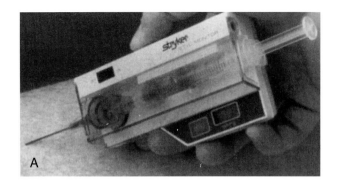

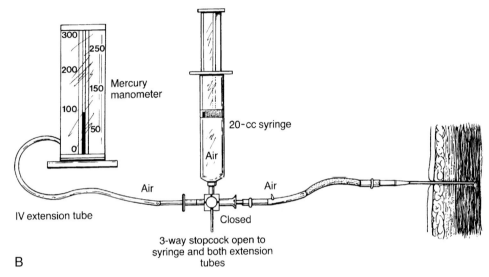

Figure 3–18 ■ *A,* Commercially available instrument for measuring compartment pressures. (From Rorabeck CH: Compartment syndromes in skeletal trauma. *In* Browner BD, Jupiter JB, Levine AM, et al [eds]: Skeletal Trauma. Philadelphia, WB Saunders, 1992, p 297.) *B,* Homemade device for measuring compartment pressures using sterile tubing and a sphygmomanometer. (From Rorabeck CH: Compartment syndromes in skeletal trauma. *In* Browner BD, Jupiter JB, Levine AM, et al [eds]: Skeletal Trauma. Philadelphia, WB Saunders, 1992, p 292.)

(Fig. 3–19) (see compartment anatomy for each anatomic region in Chapters 8 to 22)

Débridement of necrotic tissues as needed; signs of necrotic tissues include abnormal color, consistency, contraction, and capacity to bleed

Atraumatic Disorders

Exertional compartment syndrome
  Induced by exercise
  This is a chronic condition of increased compartment pressures related to exercise
  Typically involves the anterior or deep posterior compartment of the leg (tibia)
  Diagnosis is made based on clinical findings and compartment pressure measurements (pressures increase significantly during exercise but fail to return to normal for more than 30 minutes with rest)
  Treatment—not a surgical emergency but may require an elective fasciotomy if physical therapy (stretching, rest, strengthening) fails to resolve symptoms
Postexercise muscle pain
  Caused by eccentric (muscle lengthens) muscle contraction
  Results in acute injury to fast twitch muscle fibers
Drug abuse

  Can lead to increased risk of sudden death
  Common drug problems in athletes include
    Stimulants
    Narcotics
    β-blockers
    Diuretics
    Anabolic steroids (see Chapter 1)
Tendinitis
  Inflammation and degeneration within a tendon sheath
  Typically a chronic condition
  May lead to tendon rupture
  Treatment depends on the anatomic location; treatment options include
    Rest
    Ice
    Elevation
    Splinting, casting
    Tendon sheath injection **(on a limited basis only)**
    Surgical débridement
Tenosynovitis
  Tendon sheath inflammation
Peritendinitis
  Inflammation around a tendon that has no tendon sheath
Menstrual cycle irregularities
  Common in female athletes (particularly runners)
    Female athlete triad
      Menstrual cycle irregularities

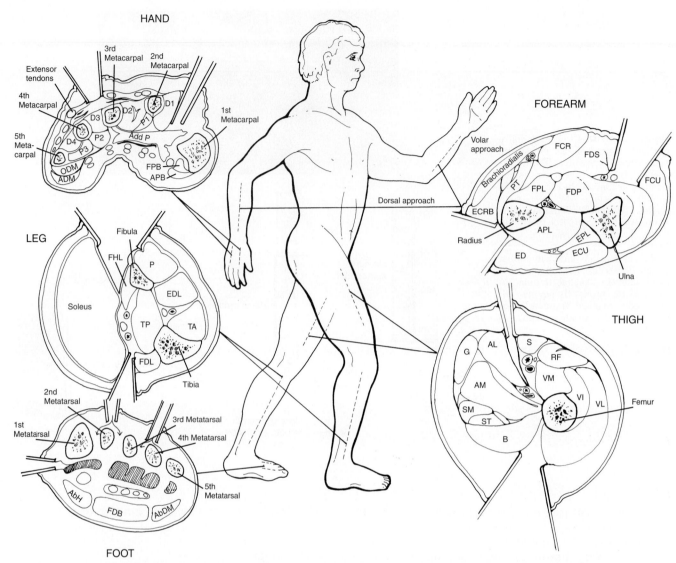

Figure 3–19 ■ Cross-sectional anatomy and techniques for fasciotomy of some of the more common compartment syndromes: hand, leg, foot, forearm, thigh. *Hand:* D1, D2, D3, D4 = dorsal interossei; P1, P2, P3 = palmar interossei; Add P = adductor pollicis; ODM = opponens digiti minimi; ADM = abductor digiti minimi; FPB = flexor pollicis brevis; APB = abductor pollicis brevis. *Leg:* P = peroneus longus and brevis; EDL = extensor digitorum longus; TA = tibialis anterior; TP = tibialis posterior; FHL = flexor hallucis longus; FDL = flexor digitorum longus. *Foot:* AbH = abductor hallucis; FDB = flexor digitorum brevis; AbDM = abductor digiti minimi. *Forearm:* ECRB = extensor carpi radialis brevis; PT = pronator teres; FCR = flexor carpi radialis; FPL = flexor pollicis longus; FDS = flexor digitorum superficialis; FDP = flexor digitorum profundus; FCU = flexor carpi ulnaris; APL = abductor pollicis longus; EPL = extensor pollicis longus; ED = extensor digitorum; ECU = extensor carpi ulnaris. *Thigh:* G = gracilis; AL = adductor longus; S = sartorius; RF = rectus femoris; AM = adductor magnus; VM = vastus medialis; VI = vastus intermedius; VL = vastus lateralis; SM = semimembranosus; ST = semitendinosus; B = biceps femoris.

Eating disorders
Osteoporosis
Related to changes in body fat composition and sex hormone production
Associated with decreased bone mineral density and stress fractures
Eating disorders
Anorexia nervosa

Fear of becoming obese
Excessive exercise
Inadequate caloric intake
Twenty percent mortality rate
Bulemia
Weight fluctuations
Binge eating
Sleep abnormalities

CHAPTER 4

General Principles of Fractures and Dislocations

Contrary to popular ideas, the operative treatment of fractures is much simpler than is the non-operative. At operation the fracture lies open for all to see, and the mechanical procedures which may be needed are obvious in the extreme.

Sir John Charnley, Manchester, 1950

INTRODUCTION

The general principles of fractures and dislocations are reviewed in this chapter
Specific injuries are covered by anatomic region in Chapters 8 through 22
Injuries in children are reviewed by anatomic region in Chapter 5

FRACTURE DESCRIPTION

In order for health care providers to accurately communicate with one another, clarity and precision in fracture description are essential
A fracture (or dislocation) is described based on the findings of the examination of the injured body part and a review of pertinent radiographs
Fractures should be described in a number of ways, as outlined below

Anatomic Location of Fracture

Name of bone(s) fractured

Regional Location of Fracture (Fig. 4–1)

Diaphysis—located between the metaphyses of a long bone; shaft of a tubular bone
  Proximal third
  Middle third
  Distal third
Metaphysis—located between the epiphysis and diaphysis; widened end of a tubular bone
Epiphysis—located between the joint and the epiphyseal plate (physis) in children or the epiphyseal scar in adults
  Extra-articular—fracture does not extend into the joint
  Intra-articular—fracture does extend into the joint

Physis—growth plate; the growth plate is found only in children and is responsible for longitudinal growth of the long bones (see Chapter 5)
Note: A fracture may span several regional locations to include two or more adjacent regions

Direction of Fracture Line(s) (Fig. 4–2)

Transverse
Oblique
Spiral

Condition of Bone (Fig. 4–3)

Comminuted fracture—a fracture with three or more fragments

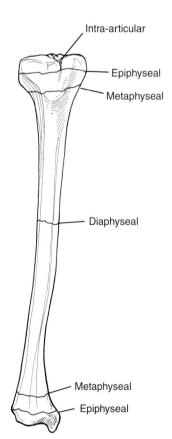

Figure 4–1 ■ Regional locations for adult long bone fractures.

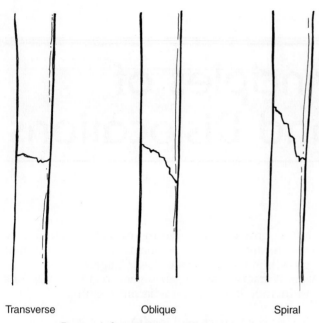

Transverse   Oblique   Spiral

Figure 4–2 ■ Direction of fracture lines.

Pathologic fracture—a fracture through an area of pre-existing disease with weakened bone (primary bone tumors, metastases to bone, bone infections, osteoporosis, metabolic bone disease, others)

Incomplete fracture—one in which the bone is not broken into separate fragments
  The fracture does not span the entire cross-section of the bone
Segmental fracture—one in which there is a middle fragment of bone surrounded by a proximal and a distal segment
  The middle fragment usually has an impaired blood supply
  These injuries are typically high-energy injuries with soft tissue stripping (muscle and periosteum) from bone and are therefore prone to poor healing (delayed union or nonunion)
Fracture with bone loss—may be caused by an open fracture where bone is left at the scene of the injury (a high-energy open injury) or a closed fracture where a segment is comminuted so severely that from a practical standpoint there is bone missing
Fracture with a butterfly fragment—similar to a segmental fracture except that the butterfly segment does not span the entire cross-section of the bone
Stress fracture—a fracture caused by repeated loading such as in military recruits (who march all day) or ballet dancers
  Common sites of stress fractures include the metatarsals, calcaneus, and tibia (other sites are possible)
Avulsion fracture—caused by the pull of a tendon or ligament at its site of bony insertion

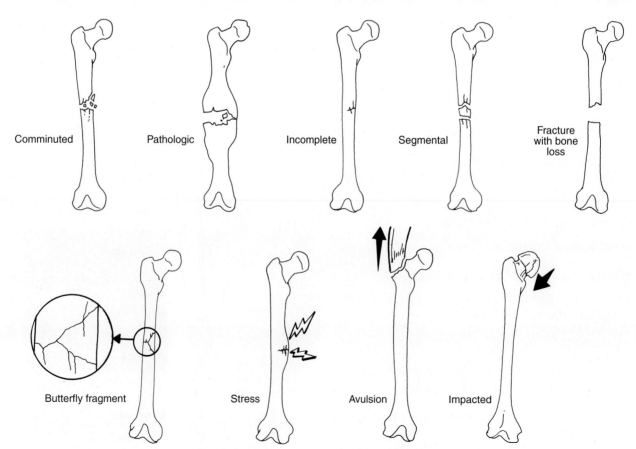

Comminuted   Pathologic   Incomplete   Segmental   Fracture with bone loss

Butterfly fragment   Stress   Avulsion   Impacted

Figure 4–3 ■ Condition of bone in fractures: comminuted fracture, pathologic fracture, incomplete fracture, segmental fracture, fracture with bone loss, fracture with a butterfly fragment (*inset*), stress fracture, avulsion fracture, and impacted fracture.

Acute fractures display irregular borders on radiography

These should not be confused with sesamoid bones (hands, foot, others) or an unfused center of ossification (bipartite patella, accessory navicular, os trigonum)

Impacted fracture—the fracture fragments are compressed together (generally the result of an axial load)

Condition of Soft Tissues

Closed fracture—fracture is not exposed to the external environment

Open fracture—fracture is exposed to the external environment as a result of damage to the overlying skin and soft tissues (the term *compound fracture* is of historical interest only and should not be used) (Fig. 4–4)

Open fractures have been classified (based on the size of the wound, amount of soft tissue injury, and a variety of other factors) by Gustilo into types I, II, IIIA, IIIB, and IIIC

Type I—open wound less than 1 cm

Type II—open wound 1 to 10 cm

Type IIIA—open wound greater than 10 cm

Other factors that make an open fracture a type III irrespective of the size of the open wound

High-velocity (> 2000 ft/sec) gunshot wounds (IIIA)

Segmental fractures (IIIA)

Fractures with significant periosteal stripping (IIIA)

Open fracture more than 8 hours old without treatment (IIIA or B)

Barnyard injuries with gross contamination (IIIB)

Fractures with a vascular injury requiring repair (IIIC)

Open joint injury

A surgical emergency that mandates irrigation and débridement regardless of the size of the wound

To determine whether an open wound communicates with an adjacent joint (in cases that are not obvious), a dilute methylene blue solution can be injected into the joint; leakage of blue solution from the open wound is diagnostic of communication between the joint injected and the open wound

Deformities of a Fracture (Fig. 4–5)

Displacement (translation) of a fracture—describes the position of the **distal fragment** in relation to the proximal fragment

Displacement (translation) in the anterior or posterior direction can be seen only on a lateral radiograph

Displacement (translation) in the medial or lateral direction can be seen only on the anteroposterior (AP) radiograph

Naturally, displacement (translation) of a fracture can occur in an oblique plane

Example: posterolateral displacement

Angulation of a fracture—describes the direction in which the apex of the angulated fracture points

Anterior or posterior angulation is seen on a lateral radiograph; medial or lateral angulation is seen on an AP radiograph

Varus describes angulation whereby the apex points away from the midline

Valgus describes angulation whereby the apex points toward the midline

Like displacement, angulation can occur in an oblique plane

Rotation of a fracture—rotation is a term used to describe the turning of fracture fragments along the long axis of a bone

Rotation is generally measured by physical examination (internal or external rotation)

For practical purpose we generally describe a fracture as rotated (and specify in which direction) or not rotated

Shortening of a fracture—describes a state in which the ends of the fracture fragments overlap

Shortening is measured in millimeters (or centimeters)

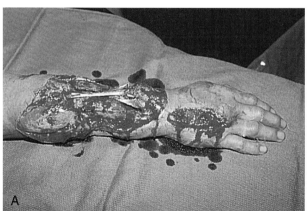
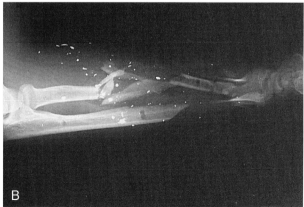

Figure 4–4 ■ Clinical photograph (*A*) and radiograph (*B*) of a comminuted, open (Gustilo type IIIA) forearm fracture sustained from a high-velocity gunshot wound. Note significant soft tissue and bone loss. (Courtesy of Fondren Orthopedic Group LLP, Texas Orthopedic Hospital, Houston, Texas.)

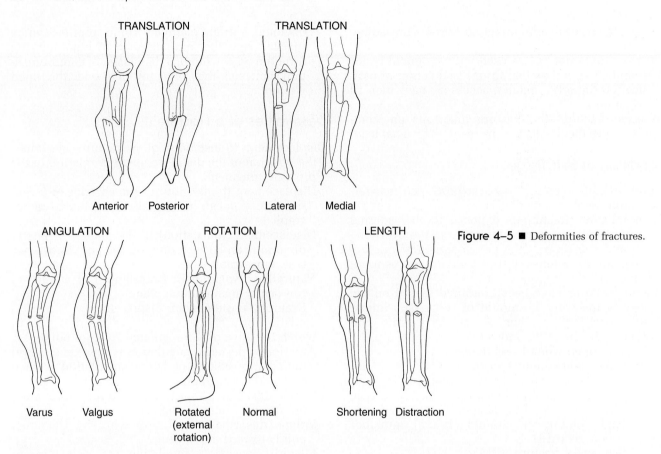

TRANSLATION   TRANSLATION

Anterior   Posterior   Lateral   Medial

ANGULATION   ROTATION   LENGTH

Varus   Valgus   Rotated   Normal   Shortening Distraction
                   (external
                   rotation)

Figure 4–5 ■ Deformities of fractures.

Distraction of a fracture—describes a state where the ends of the fracture fragments are separated, leaving a gap

   Distraction is generally caused by excessive traction and is measured in millimeters (or centimeters)

   Distraction can lead to a fracture nonunion

OVERVIEW OF THE MANAGEMENT OF FRACTURES

Goals of Fracture Management

Achieve anatomic reduction
Restore stability
Promote joint range of motion
Create an environment conducive to fracture healing
Return the patient to preinjury function
Achieve acceptable cosmesis

Principles of Fracture Management

To create an **environment conducive to fracture healing**, the treating physician must consider both the **biologic** and **mechanical** aspects of the injury (the *S's* of fracture healing)

  Biologic aspects

    Soft tissue envelope—the soft tissue attachments to bone are an important source of the blood supply (periosteal) to bone that is so important for fracture healing; in general, open fractures are more prone to soft tissue stripping, which increases the likelihood of problems with fracture healing

    Sterile—sterility at the fracture site is crucial; an infection at the fracture site may arise as a result of an open fracture or from an operative (invasive) procedure; an infection at a fracture site increases the likelihood of problems with fracture healing

    Sickless—fractures heal better in healthy patients than in patients with chronic illness (diabetics, immunosuppressed individuals, others)

    Smokeless—smoking increases the likelihood of problems with fracture healing

    Stimulated—a fracture site needs biologic stimulation to heal; this generally occurs with growth factors that are present in the fracture hematoma

    Spatially oriented—bony contact with interdigitation of fragments at the fracture site (without a significant gap) promotes fracture union; **osteoblasts do not jump**

  Mechanical aspects

    Soft tissue envelope—the soft tissue attachments to bone are responsible for the position of bone fragments; displacement, angulation, rotation, and shortening of fracture fragments can be thought of as the sum of the vector forces (pulls) of those soft tissues still attached to the bone fragments and the absence of pulls of the soft tissues no longer attached

    Stability—stability at the fracture site is important

for healing and can be achieved via a variety of nonoperative and operative methods; instability at a fracture site increases the likelihood of problems with fracture healing

Straight—alignment of fracture fragments aids in transmission of mechanical forces across the fracture and promotes bony union

Specific Methods of Fracture Management

Provisional modes of treatment

Splinting/bracing

A fracture may be immobilized using a conventional splint/brace or an improvised one constructed from any available rigid body (sticks, rolled-up newspaper, etc.) when conventional splinting material is unavailable

Splinting/bracing should be performed by trained emergency medical service technicians at the scene of an accident when possible or by a physician upon arrival to the emergency room

Benefits of splinting/bracing

Facilitates patient transport and evaluation

Reduces pain

Decreases the likelihood of further soft tissue injury (such as converting a closed fracture to an open one)

Provides rigid immobilization of a fracture yet allows for the soft tissue swelling that commonly occurs after an acute fracture (casts are completely circumferential, do not allow for swelling, and increase the risk of a compartment syndrome in an acute fracture)

Useful for initial stabilization of an acute fracture **(do not use a cast for an acute fracture for the initial 3 to 5 days)**

Types of splints/braces (see Chapter 7)

Traction

Skin traction—such as Buck's traction for the presurgical treatment of a femoral neck fracture (Fig. 4–6)

Skeletal traction—a metallic pin (Steinmann pin)

Table 4–1
COMPARISON OF PLASTER OF PARIS AND FIBERGLASS CASTING MATERIALS

	Plaster of Paris	Fiberglass
Composition	Calcium sulfate	Polyurethane resin in fiberglass
Advantages	Easier to mold cast for 3-point fixation	Lightweight Durable Easier for beginners to apply
Disadvantages	Heavy May cause soft tissue problems	More difficult to mold cast for 3-point fixation Finished cast may have sharp edges May cause soft tissue problems

is placed through a bone to apply traction to a fracture (which is proximal to the pin) by a weight/pulley system

Example: skeletal traction for a femoral shaft fracture is used to keep the femur from shortening (out to proper length)—a proximal tibial pin is used to suspend weight to apply traction to the femur) (Fig. 4–7)

Definitive modes of treatment

Closed reduction

Manual manipulation of the extremity to align the fracture fragments; this should be performed as early as possible (preferably within 6 hours of the injury)

Technique

Evaluate radiographs to understand the fracture deformity

Apply manual traction

Reverse the mechanism of injury

Align the distal fragment on the proximal fragment

Casting

Application of circumferential plaster or fiberglass for the purpose of stabilizing a fracture site while bony union occurs (Table 4–1)

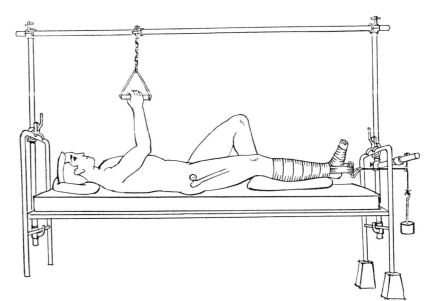

Figure 4–6 ■ Buck's traction. (From Schmeisser G Jr: A Clinical Manual of Orthopedic Traction Techniques. Philadelphia, WB Saunders, 1963.)

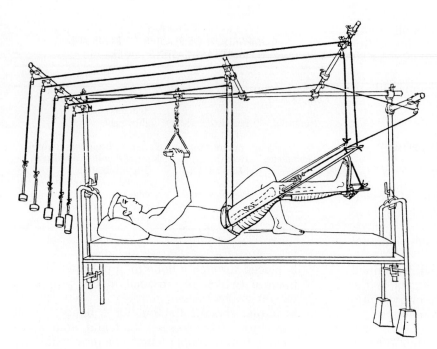

Figure 4–7 ■ Skeletal traction with balanced suspension. Traction is applied through a proximal tibial pin to maintain the length and alignment of the fractured femur. (From Schmeisser G Jr: A Clinical Manual of Orthopedic Traction Techniques. Philadelphia, WB Saunders, 1963.)

Casting should not be performed on an acute fracture because of the risk of continued swelling within the initial 3 to 5 days, leading to a compartment syndrome (use a splint initially and convert to a cast at 3 to 5 days after injury)

Casting principles
  A **curved** cast is needed to make a straight limb (Fig. 4–8)
  A cast should be molded to allow for **3-point fixation**, which holds the fracture fragments reduced

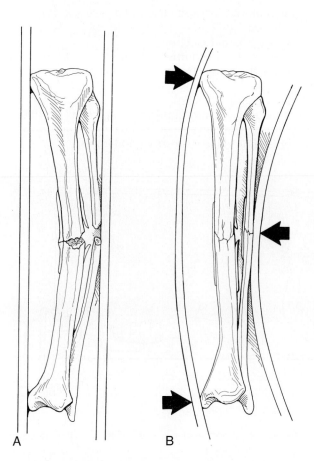

Figure 4–8 ■ *A*, Without proper molding, an adequate reduction cannot be maintained. *B*, Using the technique of cast molding with 3-point fixation, a curved cast achieves a straight limb by applying tension to the soft tissue hinge that is generally intact on the concave (compression) side of the fracture.

A   B

A fracture that displaces in a well-applied cast is probably unsuitable for casting and is better treated with another method (such as open reduction with internal fixation [ORIF])

Technique of cast application (Fig. 4–9)—casting is a demanding technique that is mastered over time and best learned from one experienced in the art (apprenticeship); **those inexperienced in cast application should not attempt to apply a cast without expert supervision**

Examine the limb and practice the manual maneuvers required to reduce the fracture fragments

Apply cast padding from distal to proximal, overlapping a 50% width of the cast padding with each turn; cast padding should be applied smoothly (without wrinkles) to avoid soft tissue pressure that could lead to skin breakdown; a stockinette can be placed between the skin and cast padding, but this is optional

Apply casting material; turns of cast material should overlap 50%; proper "tensioning" of turns of cast material is learned with experience; "tucking" to accommodate the tapering of a limb is another technique mastered over time

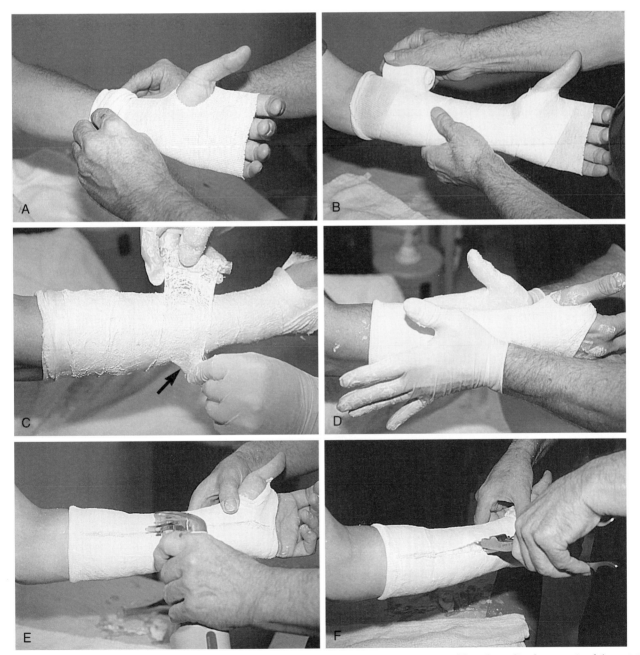

Figure 4–9 ■ Technique of cast application. *A*, Apply stockinette (optional). *B*, Apply cast padding from distal to proximal (note 50% overlap with each turn). *C*, Apply cast material and tuck (*arrow*) excess material as the limb tapers distally. *D*, Cast molding for 3-point fixation. The cast is then trimmed with a cast saw and/or bandage scissors, and the edges are smoothed. *E*, Removal of the cast using a cast saw. *F*, Cast spreader technique.

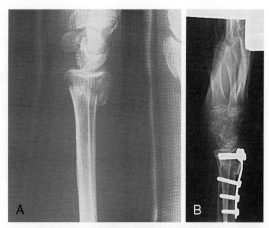

Figure 4–10 ■ *A*, Injury film shows a distal radius fracture. *B*, Postoperative films after open reduction and internal fixation using a plate and screws. (Courtesy of James B. Bennett, MD, Fondren Orthopedic Group LLP, Texas Orthopedic Hospital, Houston, Texas.)

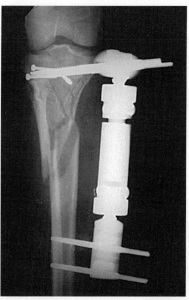

Figure 4–12 ■ Postoperative film (AP view) after closed reduction and placement of a unilateral external fixator in a patient with a high-energy (comminuted) fracture of the proximal tibia involving the tibial plateau, metaphysis, and diaphysis. (Note the patient also had placement of cannulated screws to stabilize the tibial plateau fracture.)

While the cast is setting, perform fracture reduction maneuvers, mold the cast for 3-point fixation, and hold until the cast hardens

Cast trimming (proximally and distally) as needed is done with a cast saw

Splinting/bracing

A fracture may be treated to healing via closed reduction and splinting/bracing

Example: distal radius fracture

Note: For specific types of casts, splints, and braces, see Chapter 7

Skeletal traction

Under certain circumstances, traction may be used to treat a fracture to healing

Example: certain acetabular fractures

Pins in plaster

Pins are placed percutaneously through bone; pins are then manipulated to allow for fracture reduction; once reduction is obtained, pins are incorporated in a plaster cast to maintain reduction

Used more frequently in the past and is no longer a preferred method of treatment

ORIF (Fig. 4–10)

Is a preferred treatment of certain fractures that are not amenable to nonoperative stabilization

Example: adult both-bone forearm fractures

Surgical dissection down to bone; fracture fragments are reduced to an anatomic position and held using bone reduction forceps (open reduction); internal fixation is performed using orthopaedic hardware (such as interfragmentary screws, plates and screws, pins, K wires [Kirschner wires], tension band wiring)

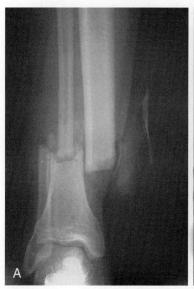
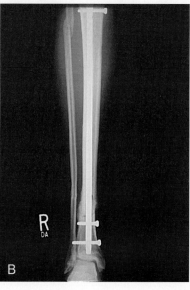

Figure 4–11 ■ *A*, Injury film (AP radiograph) shows a displaced (lateral translation) distal third tibia fracture. *B*, Radiograph several months after closed reduction with internal fixation using an intramedullary nail (rod) shows fracture union. Note that interlocking screws that traverse the cortical bone and holes through the nail are placed proximal and distal to the fracture and therefore control (do not allow) rotation. (Courtesy of Fondren Orthopedic Group LLP, Texas Orthopedic Hospital, Houston, Texas.)

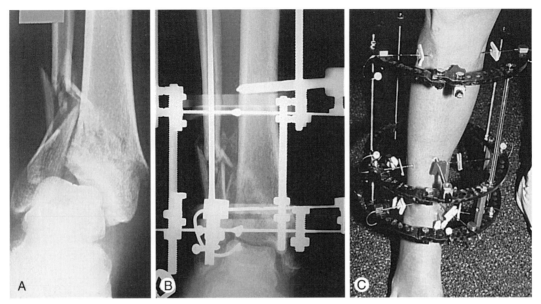

Figure 4-13 ■ *A*, Injury film (AP radiograph) shows a high-energy distal tibia fracture (pilon fracture) with severe angulation (valgus). *B*, Postoperative films after closed reduction and placement of a circular external fixator show anatomic reduction of the distal tibia. The patient also had closed reduction with internal fixation of the fibula fracture using an intramedullary rod. *C*, Clinical photo of the patient with the circular external fixator in place. (Courtesy of Fondren Orthopedic Group LLP, Texas Orthopedic Hospital, Houston, Texas.)

Soft tissue stripping (of muscle and periosteum from the bone surface) during the surgical dissection should be minimized to preserve the blood supply to bone, which is important for fracture healing

Closed reduction with internal fixation (Fig. 4–11)

The fracture is reduced via manual manipulation; internal fixation is then performed using an intramedullary nail (rod), K wires, cannulated screws, and others

External fixation (Figs. 4–12 and 4–13)

Pins or wires are placed percutaneously through bone; pins or wires are attached to an external frame that stabilizes the extremity

Useful treatment for open fractures because it facilitates treatment of the soft tissue injuries

May also be useful for treatment of intra-articular and periarticular (near joint) fractures

Challenges in Fracture Management

Open fractures

Require thorough irrigation and débridement that is repeated every 48 to 72 hours until the wound is clean and is safe to close or cover with a soft tissue graft

Prophylactic antibiotic regimen

Gustilo types I and II—cefazolin (Ancef)

Gustilo type IIIA—cefazolin (Ancef) and gentamicin

Gustilo types IIIB and IIIC—cefazolin (Ancef), gentamicin, and penicillin

Tetanus prophylaxis

Intra-articular fractures

Require anatomic reduction and early range of motion to promote return to preinjury function (Fig. 4–14)

Figure 4-14 ■ *A*, Injury film shows an olecranon fracture extending into the elbow joint. *B*, Open reduction and internal fixation using tension band wire technique allows for restoration of the articular surface and early range of motion exercises. (Courtesy of Fondren Orthopedic Group LLP, Texas Orthopedic Hospital, Houston, Texas.)

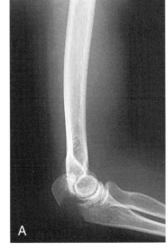
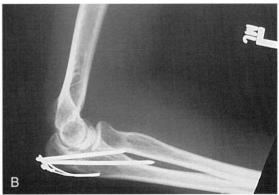

Anteroposterior View   Lateral View

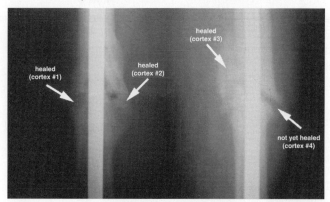

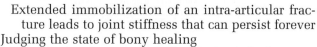

Figure 4–15 ■ AP and lateral radiographs of a femoral shaft fracture (4 months following treatment with an intramedullary nail) showing bridging callus in three of four cortices at the fracture site. (Courtesy of Fondren Orthopedic Group LLP, Texas Orthopedic Hospital, Houston, Texas.)

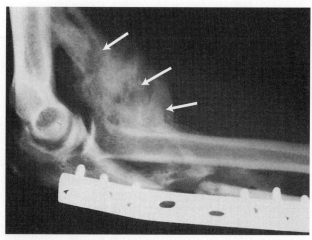

Figure 4–17 ■ Extensive ectopic bone (*arrows*) after open reduction and internal fixation of a proximal ulna fracture. (From Frassica FJ, Coventry MB, Morrey BF: Ectopic ossification about the elbow. In Morrey BF [ed]: The Elbow and Its Disorders, 2nd ed. Philadelphia, WB Saunders, 1993, p 507.)

Extended immobilization of an intra-articular fracture leads to joint stiffness that can persist forever

Judging the state of bony healing

In general, a fracture is said to be healed when

There is no pain to palpation at the fracture site

There is no pain upon mechanical stressing (using manual techniques) of the fracture site

There is bridging callus seen on at least three of the four cortices (seen on the AP and lateral radiographs) (Fig. 4–15)

Complications of Fractures and Their Treatments

Delayed union—a fracture that cannot yet be classified as a nonunion but is showing slow (if any) callus formation

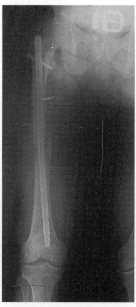

Figure 4–16 ■ AP radiograph of the femur of a patient involved in a motor vehicle accident who underwent immediate closed reduction and intramedullary nailing. At 3 years after injury, he continues to have severe midthigh pain, and his radiograph is consistent with a femoral shaft nonunion. Note rounding of the ends of the bone at the fracture site, the persistent radiolucency at the fracture site, and the absence of callus bridging the fracture site.

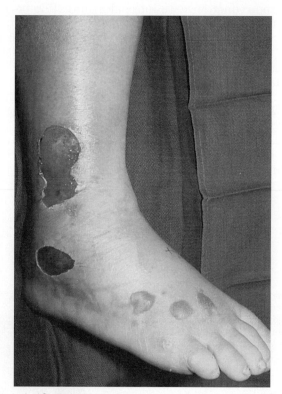

Figure 4–18 ■ Fracture blisters on the dorsum of the right foot of a patient with a high-energy distal tibia fracture. Note the two large fracture blisters on the lateral aspect of the right foot and ankle that have been unroofed and show the injured soft tissues. (Courtesy of Fondren Orthopedic Group LLP, Texas Orthopedic Hospital, Houston, Texas.)

Table 4–2
TABLE OF ACCEPTABLE REDUCTIONS FOR VARIOUS LONG BONE FRACTURES (MAXIMUM ALLOWABLE DEFORMITY)

Bone	Shortening	Varus/Valgus Angulation	Anterior/Posterior Angulation	Displacement	Rotation
Humeral shaft	30 mm	30 degrees	20 degrees		15 degrees
Radial shaft	Anatomic reduction is required				
Ulnar shaft			10 degrees	50% (overlap)	
2nd and 3rd metacarpal shafts	5 mm		20 degrees		
4th and 5th metacarpal shafts	5 mm		50 degrees		
Femoral shaft	10 mm	8 degrees	15 degrees		15 degrees
Tibial shaft	5 mm	5 degrees	10 degrees		0 degrees
2nd, 3rd, and 4th metatarsal shafts		45 degrees	10 degrees		
1st and 5th metatarsal shafts		10 degrees	10 degrees		

Nonunion—a fracture that no longer shows clinical or radiographic signs of progression to bony union (Fig. 4–16)

Infection—occurs most commonly in open fractures or after open treatment of a closed fracture

Neurovascular injury—can arise as a result of the injury or the treatment (injury caused by closed manipulation with the bony fragments contacting neurovascular structures or from a surgical dissection)

Heterotopic ossifications—ectopic bone forms in the soft tissues in response to an injury (especially in head-injured patients) or a surgical dissection (such as following ORIF of an elbow fracture) (Fig. 4–17); **myositis ossificans** is a form of heterotopic ossification that occurs specifically when the ossification is in muscle

Limited range of motion—caused by prolonged immobilization of a joint that is near a fracture (occurs commonly in fractures of the distal humerus)

Reflex sympathetic dystrophy—may arise after a fracture; a vasomotor dysfunction of the sympathetic nervous system characterized by pain, swelling, stiffness, and shiny atrophic skin

Fracture blisters—represent superficial edema between the layers of the epidermis that presents as fluid-filled blisters; they are generally a sign of a severe soft tissue crush injury, but the blisters themselves are generally not a problem (Fig. 4–18)

Cast sores—arise from poorly applied or improperly padded casts (Fig. 4–19)

Fracture and Dislocation Management Algorithm (Fig. 4–20)

Acceptable Reductions for Various Long Bone Fractures (Table 4–2)

Fracture Patterns of Various Loading Modes (Table 4–3)

Types of Fracture Healing (Table 4–4)

DISLOCATIONS (Fig. 4–21)

Dislocation of a joint usually results from high-energy trauma, but in certain instances it may result from

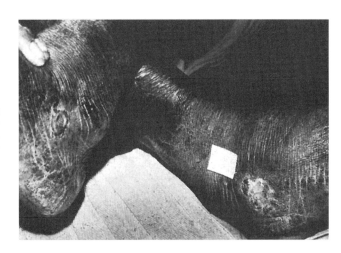

Figure 4–19 ■ Ulcers seen on the medial malleolus of both legs from cast pressure. (From Selvapandian AJ, Sundararaj GD: Infections of the foot and ankle, including leprosy, mycetoma, and yaws. *In* Jahss MH [ed]: Disorders of the Foot and Ankle, 2nd ed. Philadelphia, WB Saunders, 1991, p 1965.)

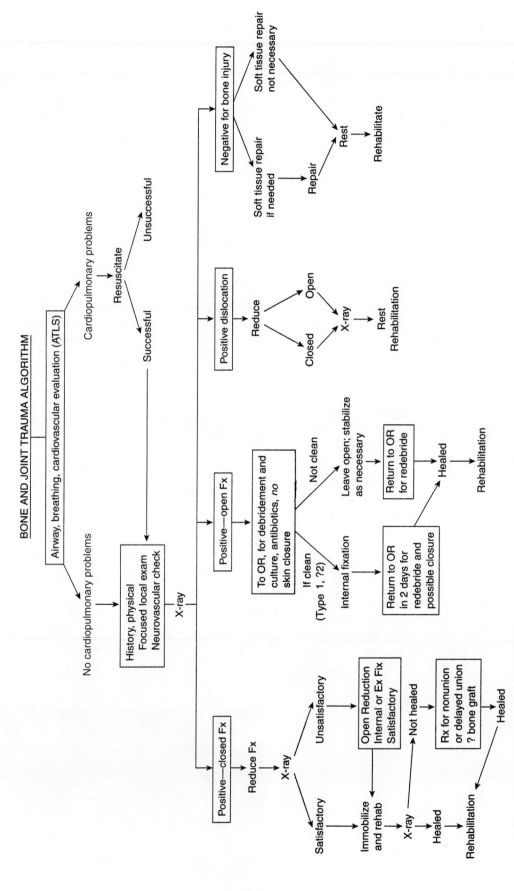

Figure 4–20 ■ Fracture and dislocation management algorithm. ATLS, advanced trauma life support; Ex Fix, external fixation; Fx, fracture; Rx, treatment; OR, operating room. (Modified from Wiesel SW, Delahay JN: Essentials of Orthopaedic Surgery, 2nd ed. Philadelphia, WB Saunders, 1997, p 57.)

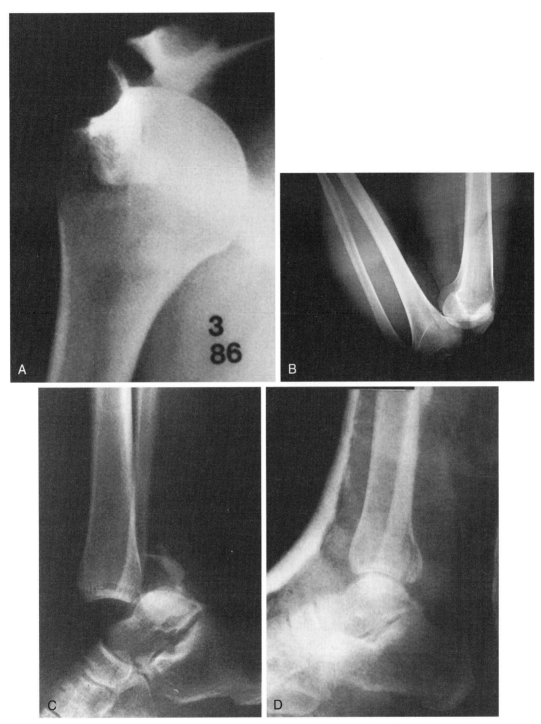

Figure 4–21 ■ *A,* AP radiograph of a subcoracoid anterior dislocation of the shoulder. (From Pagnani MJ, Galinat BJ, Warren RF: Glenohumeral instability. *In* DeLee JC, Drez D Jr [eds]: Orthopaedic Sports Medicine: Principles and Practice. Philadelphia, WB Saunders, 1994, p 592.) *B,* Knee dislocation. (Courtesy of Robert H. Fain, Jr., MD, Fondren Orthopedic Group LLP, Texas Orthopedic Hospital, Houston, Texas.) Prereduction *(C)* and postreduction *(D)* lateral radiographs of a posterior ankle dislocation. Note that the posterior malleolar fragment reduces with closed reduction. (From Pankovich AM: Trauma to the ankle. *In* Jahss MH [ed]: Disorders of the Foot and Ankle, 2nd ed. Philadelphia, WB Saunders, 1991, p 2370.)

Table 4–3
CHARACTERISTIC FRACTURE PATTERNS OF VARIOUS LOADING MODES

Loading Mode	Fracture Pattern	Figure
Tension	Transverse	See Fig. 4–2
Compression	Oblique	See Fig. 4–2
Torsion	Spiral	See Fig. 4–2
Bending	Butterfly	See Fig. 4–3
High energy	Comminuted	See Fig. 4–3

Table 4–4
TYPES OF FRACTURE HEALING

Method of Treatment	Type of Fracture Healing
Closed (casting)	Enchondral healing Periosteal bridging callus Visible callus
Rigidly fixed fracture (compression plating)	Direct osteonal primary bone healing No visible callus

lower-energy forces (such as in recurrent shoulder dislocations)

A joint is said to be **dislocated** when there is sufficient disruption that the articular surfaces of the apposing bones (such as the distal femur and proximal tibia of the knee) are no longer in contact

A joint is said to be **subluxated** when a portion of the articular surfaces of the joint remains in contact

Dislocations and subluxations can occur in conjunction with a fracture

The most common clinical signs and symptoms of a dislocation include pain, deformity, and loss of joint motion

CHAPTER 5

Pediatric Orthopaedics

Children are not just small adults.
Mercer Rang, MD

COMMON CHILDHOOD MUSCULOSKELETAL CONDITIONS

General Principles of Fractures and Dislocations in Children

Children's bones bend more before fracture than do adults' bones (children's bones are more ductile)

The periosteum in children is thicker and more highly developed and often remains intact on the concave side of a fracture

Children's fractures heal more rapidly and, therefore, require shorter immobilization time than do adults' fractures

Stiffness across joints after immobilization is less of a problem in children than in adults

Children's bones remodel to a greater extent than adults' do and, therefore, a greater amount of angulation and displacement is acceptable in children than in adults (except intra-articular fractures; angulation or displacement of intra-articular fractures is not acceptable in adults or children)

Specific pediatric fractures are discussed by anatomic region within this chapter

Physeal (growth plate) fractures

Classically occur through the zone of hypertrophy of the growth plate but can involve other zones

Usually caused by a torsion (not tension) at the growth plate

Complications of physeal fractures include

Limb length discrepancies

Malunions

Physeal bars (leading to angular or longitudinal deformities)

Most common sites for physeal fractures are the distal radius and distal tibia

Classification of physeal fractures (Salter-Harris classification [SH]) (Fig. 5–1)

General treatment guidelines for physeal fractures

SH I fractures—initial attempt at gentle closed reduction (may require general anesthesia)

SH II fractures—initial attempt at gentle closed reduction (may require general anesthesia)

SH III fractures—intra-articular; often require open reduction to properly align the growth plate

SH IV fractures—intra-articular; often require open reduction to properly align the growth plate

SH V fractures—generally identified late and have a high complication rate

Growth plate arrest (Fig. 5–2)

Physeal bars (bridges) arise as a result of a growth plate injury that leads to an arrest of growth of a portion of the physis; an uninjured portion of the physis may continue to grow

Centrally located bars within the physis lead to arrest of longitudinal growth with resultant shortening of the extremity

Peripheral bars lead to angular deformities

Treatment options include operative resection of the bar or ipsilateral completion of a growth arrest in conjunction with an epiphysiodesis to the contralateral extremity (to equalize the growth disturbance in both extremities)

Greenstick fracture—fractures in children commonly are incomplete and leave a hinge of intact bone and soft tissues similar to the manner in which a green stick from a tree branch breaks (Fig. 5–3)

Torus (buckle) fracture—occurs in children at the metaphyseal diaphyseal junction of a long bone (most commonly distal radius) as a result of an axial load (see Fig. 5–3)

Child abuse (battered child syndrome)

A high index of suspicion is needed to make the diagnosis

Most common in children younger than 3 years of age

Unusual histories are a tip-off

Physical exam may show multiple healing skin bruises, burns, etc.

The most common locations for fractures in child abuse are the humerus, tibia, and femur

Skull fractures are also common

Skeletal survey (x-rays of the skull, thoracolumbar spine, chest and ribs, pelvis, femur, knees, tibias, fibulas, ankles, wrists, and hands) to search for other fractures in suspected cases (fractures may be healed)

A technetium bone scan may also be helpful to search for other skeletal injuries

Bone Dysplasias

Definition—deformities caused by an intrinsic disturbance of bone

Leads to dwarfism

Dwarfing can be **disproportionate** or **proportionate**

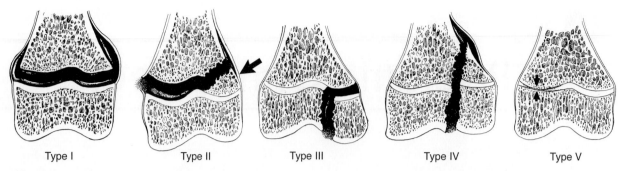

Type I   Type II   Type III   Type IV   Type V

Figure 5–1 ■ Salter-Harris classification of physeal fractures. *Type I:* transverse fracture through the physis. *Type II:* fracture through the physis with a metaphyseal (Thurston-Holland) fragment (*arrow*). *Type III:* fracture through the physis and into the epiphysis (intra-articular). *Type IV:* fracture through the epiphysis, physis, and metaphysis. *Type V:* crush injury of the physis. (Redrawn after Salter RB, Harris WR: Injuries involving the epiphyseal plate. J Bone Joint Surg 45A:587, 1963. From Tachdjian MO: Pediatric Orthopedics, 2nd ed. Philadelphia, WB Saunders, 1990, vol 4, p 3023.)

Disproportionate dwarfing conditions
  Asymmetric dwarfing between trunk and limbs
  Short-trunk varieties
    Kneist syndrome (autosomal dominant)
    Spondyloepiphyseal dysplasia (three forms)
      Congenita form (autosomal dominant)
      Tarda form (X-linked recessive)
      Pseudoachondroplastic dysplasia (autosomal dominant or recessive)
    Others
  Short-limb varieties (subdivided by region of limb that is short: rhizomelic = proximal; mesomelic = middle; acromelic = distal)
    Achondroplasia (autosomal dominant or spontaneous mutation) (Fig. 5–4)
    Diastrophic dysplasia (autosomal recessive)
    Chondroectodermal dysplasia (Ellis-van Creveld syndrome) (autosomal recessive)
    Others
Proportionate dwarfing conditions
  Symmetric dwarfing of trunk and limbs
  Examples

Cleidocranial dysostosis (autosomal recessive)
Mucopolysaccharidoses (four syndromes)
  I. Hurler's syndrome (autosomal recessive)
  II. Hunter's syndrome (X-linked recessive)
  III. Sanfilippo's syndrome (autosomal recessive)
  IV. Morquio's syndrome (autosomal recessive)
Others

Chromosomal Disorders

Down syndrome
  Trisomy 21
  The most common chromosomal abnormality
  Associated with older age (40 years or more) of mother
  Clinical findings
    Ligament laxity
    Mental impairment
    Heart disease
    Endocrine disorders
    Premature aging
  Orthopaedic problems
    Spinal abnormalities

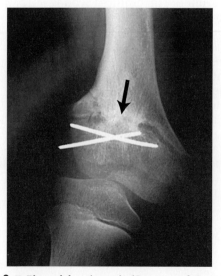

Figure 5–2 ■ Physeal bar (*arrow*). (Courtesy of Gary T. Brock, MD, Fondren Orthopedic Group LLP, Texas Orthopedic Hospital, Houston, Texas.)

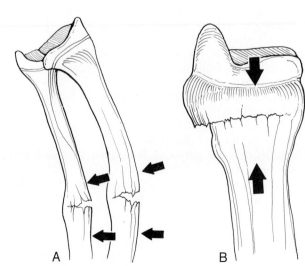

A   B

Figure 5–3 ■ *A,* Greenstick fracture of a child's forearm. *B,* Torus fracture of a child's distal radius. *Arrows* indicate the direction of forces that produce the injury.

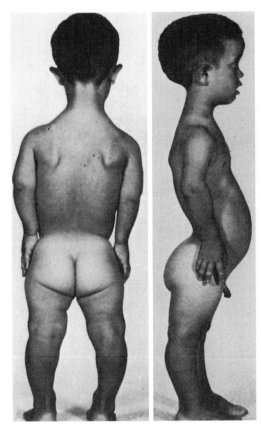

Figure 5–4 ■ Short-limbed (achondroplastic) dwarf. (From Bogumill GP, Schwamm HA: Orthopaedic Pathology: A Synopsis with Clinical and Radiographic Correlation. Philadelphia, WB Saunders, 1984, p 48.)

Cervical spine instability (atlantoaxial instability: evaluate with flexion-extension radiographs of the cervical spine)
Hip instability
Slipped capital femoral epiphysis (SCFE)
Turner's syndrome
45,XO female
Short stature
Sexual infantilism
Web neck
Noonan's syndrome
Short stature
Web neck
Prader-Willi syndrome
Chromosome 15 abnormality
Floppy hypotonic infant
Intellectual impairment
Adults generally obese with insatiable appetite
Menkes' syndrome
X-linked recessive disorder of copper transport
Affects bone growth
Patients have characteristic kinky hair
Rett syndrome
Progressive impairment with abnormal hand movements

Teratologic Disorders

Fetal alcohol syndrome
Growth disturbances
Central nervous system (CNS) problems
Abnormal facies
Spine abnormalities
Maternal diabetes
Other teratogens
Thalidomide
Phenytoin
Others

Hematopoietic Disorders

Gaucher's disease
Autosomal recessive
Lysosomal storage disease
Accumulation of cerebroside in cells of the reticulo-endothelial system
Common findings
Osteonecrosis of the femoral head
Erlenmeyer-flask deformity of the distal femur
Niemann-Pick disease
Accumulation of phospholipid in reticuloendothelial cells
Bone involvement includes marrow expansion, cortical thinning, and coxa valga
Sickle cell anemia
Affects 1% of African Americans
Characterized by
Pain crises
Skeletal immaturity
Osteonecrosis of the femoral head
Osteomyelitis (most commonly diaphyseal); *Salmonella* is a characteristic infecting organism
Septic arthritis
Thalassemia
Hemophilia
X-linked recessive disorder
Factor VIII (or IX) deficiency
Hemarthrosis leads to painful swelling and limited range of motion (ROM)
Clotting factor levels should be kept above 25% during bleeding episodes
A large percentage of hemophiliacs are human immunodeficiency virus (HIV) positive
Leukemia
The most common pediatric malignancy
Acquired immunodeficiency syndrome (AIDS)
Caused by HIV
(For more information on AIDS, see Chapter 3)

Pediatric Conditions Affecting Bone Mineralization, Bone Mineral Density, and Bone Viability

Rickets
Failure of **mineralization** leads to changes in the physis (increased width and disorganization of the physis)
Also leads to changes in bone (Fig. 5–5)
Cortical thinning
Bowing of the long bones
Brittle bones
Physeal cupping

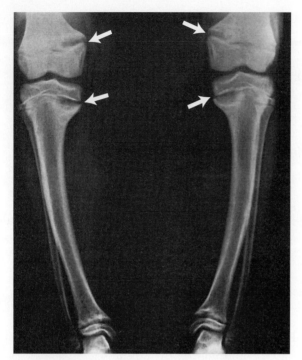

Figure 5–5 ■ Radiographs of the lower extremity of a patient with rickets. Note typical bowing and physeal widening (*arrows*). (From Gartland JJ: Fundamentals of Orthopaedics, 4th ed. Philadelphia, WB Saunders, 1986, p 106.)

Physeal widening
Coxa vara
Rickets is known as osteomalacia in the adult (see Chapter 3)
Vitamin D–deficiency rickets
Almost eliminated in the United States after addition of vitamin D to milk
Still seen in immigrants from Asia
Laboratory studies
Low/normal calcium
Low phosphate
Increased parathyroid hormone (PTH)
Low levels of vitamin D
Treatment—vitamin D and calcium (most deformities will resolve)
Hereditary vitamin D–dependent rickets
Rare autosomal recessive disorder
Defect in 1-hydroxylation of vitamin D_3 in the kidney, which leads to abnormality of the active form of vitamin D_3
Clinical features are similar to those of vitamin D–deficiency rickets but may be more severe
Treatment—high doses of vitamin D
Familial hypophosphatemic rickets (vitamin D–resistant rickets [phosphate diabetes])
X-linked dominant disorder
Caused by impaired renal tubular reabsorption of phosphate
Treatment—phosphate replacement and vitamin D_3
Hypophosphatasia
Autosomal recessive disorder
Caused by low levels of alkaline phosphatase

Clinical features are similar to those of rickets
Increased urinary phosphoethanolamine is diagnostic
Treatment—phosphate therapy
Osteogenesis imperfecta (OI) (Fig. 5–6)
Defect in type I collagen
Leads to brittle bones and **multiple fractures that often lead to angular deformities of the limbs**
Disease represents a spectrum of inheritance patterns and severity
Clinical findings—depending on type—include
Blue sclerae
Dentinogenesis imperfecta (teeth abnormalities)
Hearing abnormalities
Fractures occur less frequently with increasing age
Spinal deformities are common
Sillence classification of OI
Type I (autosomal dominant)
Milder form
Blue sclerae
Type II (autosomal recessive)
Nearly always lethal in the neonatal period
Blue sclerae
Type III (autosomal recessive)
Severe type
Normal sclerae
Birth fractures
Short stature

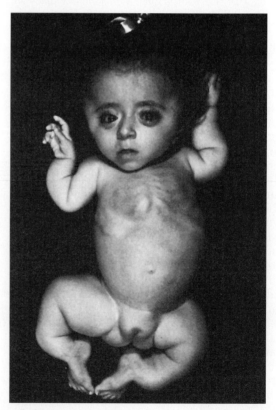

Figure 5–6 ■ Clinical photograph of a child with severe osteogenesis imperfecta (type III). Note angular limb deformities from multiple malunited long-bone fractures. (From Gertner JM, Root L: Osteogenesis imperfecta. Orthop Clin North Am 21:153, 1990.)

Type IV (autosomal dominant)
  Milder form
  Normal sclerae
Treatment goal is fracture management and long-term rehabilitation
Idiopathic juvenile osteoporosis
  Rare
  Self-limiting disorder
  Differential diagnosis
    OI
    Malignancy
    Cushing's disease
Osteopetrosis (see Chapter 3)
  Mild form is autosomal dominant (Albers-Schönberg disease)
  Malignant form is autosomal recessive
  Bone-within-bone appearance on radiographs
  Hepatosplenomegaly
  Aplastic anemia
  Bone marrow transplantation can be lifesaving during childhood
Infantile cortical hyperostosis (Caffey's disease)
  Characterized by soft tissue swelling and bony cortical thickening
  Follows febrile illness in infants
  Radiographs show characteristic periosteal reaction
  Differential diagnosis
    Hypervitaminosis A
    Infection
    Scurvy
    Progressive diaphyseal dysplasia
Scurvy
  (See Chapter 3)
Osteochondroses (Table 5–1)
  Pathologic condition is similar to osteonecrosis but occurs at traction apophyses in children

Arthritic Conditions of Children

Juvenile rheumatoid arthritis (JRA)
  Also known as juvenile chronic arthritis
  A persistent noninfectious arthritis that lasts more than 6 weeks after other possible etiologies have been excluded

Table 5–1
OSTEOCHONDROSES

Anatomic Site	Disease
Elbow (capitellum)	Panner's disease
Phalanges of hand	Thiemann's disease
Spine	Scheuermann's disease
Ischiopubic synchondrosis	Van Neck's disease
Femoral head	Legg-Calvé-Perthes disease
Inferior patella	Sinding-Larsen-Johansson disease
Proximal tibial epiphysis	Blount disease
Tibial tuberosity	Osgood-Schlatter disease
Calcaneus	Sever's disease
Tarsal navicular	Köhler's bone disease
Metatarsal head	Freiberg's disease

Diagnosis (affected individuals will have one or more of the following)
  Rash
  Positive rheumatoid factor
  Iridocyclitis
  Cervical spine involvement
  Pericarditis
  Tenosynovitis
  Episodic fevers
  Morning stiffness
Girls are more commonly affected with JRA than are boys
Areas involved
  Knee (most common)
  Wrist/fingers
  Ankle
  Cervical spine (kyphosis, facet ankylosis, and atlantoaxial subluxation)
Lower extremity problems
  Flexion contractures of the hip, knee, and ankle
  Deformities—protrusio acetabuli, valgus knees, equinovarus feet
  Joint subluxations
Synovial proliferation leads to destruction of the joint (chondrolysis) and soft tissue destruction
Clinical picture
  50%—symptoms resolve without sequelae
  25%—slightly disabled
  25%—have crippling arthritis and/or blindness
Five types of JRA have been described
  Systemic JRA (25% of cases)
    Involves many joints
    Characterized by fever, rash, and organomegaly
  Seronegative polyarticular JRA (15% of cases)
    Rheumatoid factor–negative
    Five or more joints are involved
    More frequently seen in girls
  Seropositive polyarticular JRA (15% of cases)
    Rheumatoid factor–positive
    Involves five or more joints
    More frequently seen in girls
    Exhibits destructive degenerative joint disease
    Frequently develops into adult RA
  Early-onset pauciarticular JRA (30% of cases)
    Involves four or fewer joints
    More frequently seen in girls
    Is associated with **iridocyclitis**
  Late-onset pauciarticular JRA (15% of cases)
    Involves four or fewer joints
    Is seen more commonly in boys
Treatment of JRA
  Night splinting
  Salicylates
  Synovectomy (for chronic painful swelling refractory to conservative treatment)
  Arthrodesis or total joint arthroplasty may be required in severe cases of JRA
  Slit lamp examination of the eye is required every 6 months (progressive iridocyclitis can lead to rapid loss of vision if left untreated)
Ankylosing spondylitis (see Chapter 3)

Affects adolescent boys, who typically present with hip and back pain
Asymmetric lower-extremity large joint involvement
HLA-B27 positive in 95% of involved patients
Treatment
   Nonsteroidal anti-inflammatory medications
   Physical therapy
Acute rheumatic fever
   One form of childhood arthritis
   Follows untreated streptococcal infection
   Diagnosis via Jones criteria (preceding streptococcal infection plus two major criteria or one major criterion and two minor criteria)
   Arthritis is **migratory**
   Affects multiple **large joints** (polyarthritis) (major criterion)
   Arthralgia (minor criterion)
   Other findings
      Carditis (heart murmur) (major criterion)
      Skin rash (erythema marginatum) (major criterion)
      Chorea (major criterion)
      Electrocardiogram (ECG) changes (minor criterion)
      Elevated sedimentation rate (minor criterion)
      Elevated antistreptolysin O (ASO) titer
      Subcutaneous nodules (major criterion)
      Fever (minor criterion)
      Previous history of rheumatic fever (minor criterion)

Disorders of the Connective Tissues

Marfan syndrome
   Autosomal dominant
   Abnormal collagen synthesis
   Clinical findings
      Arachnodactyly
      Scoliosis
      Pectus deformities
      Cardiac abnormalities
      Ocular abnormalities (lens dislocation)
      Joint laxity
      Protrusio acetabuli
Ehlers-Danlos syndrome
   Autosomal dominant
   Hyperextensibility of skin
   Joint hypermobility
   Joint dislocations/subluxations
   Bone fragility
   Soft tissue fragility
   Soft tissue calcification
   Several subtypes have been described
Homocystinuria
   Autosomal recessive
   Inborn error of methionine metabolism
   Accumulation of the intermediate metabolite homocysteine can lead to osteoporosis, marfanoid habitus, lens dislocation (lens typically dislocates inferiorly in homocystinuria and superiorly in Marfan syndrome)

Clinical findings
   CNS effects
   Mental retardation
Diagnosis made by demonstrating increased homocysteine in the urine

Cerebral Palsy (CP) (Fig. 5–7)

Nonprogressive neuromuscular disorder
Typical onset before 2 years of age
Results from some type of brain injury
Patients have static encephalopathy
Etiology
   Prematurity (most common)
   Perinatal infections
   Traumatic head injuries
   Anoxic brain injuries
   Meningitis
Children present with a wide spectrum of musculoskeletal problems (the most common is joint contractures)
Classifications (two types)
   Physiologic classification
      Spasticity—increased muscle tone, hyperreflexia (the most common form of CP)
      Athetosis—slow, writhing, involuntary movements
      Ataxia—poor coordination of muscles for voluntary motion
      Mixed—most commonly a combination of spasticity and athetosis

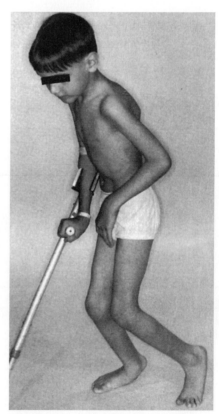

Figure 5–7 ■ Clinical photograph of a young patient with spastic cerebral palsy. (From Gartland JJ: Fundamentals of Orthopaedics, 4th ed. Philadelphia, WB Saunders, 1986, p 172.)

Topographic classification

Hemiplegia—involves both the upper extremity and lower extremity on the same side

Diplegia—lower extremities more involved than upper extremities

Totally involved—extensive involvement, typically nonambulators

Evaluation of the CP child

Birth and developmental history on physical examination

Primitive reflexes (normally disappear by 4 to 5 months of age)

Persistence of primitive reflexes is suggestive that the child will be a nonambulator

Moro (startle) reflex

Parachute reflex

Specific CP disorders

Gait disorders

The most common musculoskeletal problem in the CP child

Diplegia—crouched gait, toe walking, knee flexion deformity

Hemiplegia—usually toe walkers

Spinal disorders

Scoliosis is the most common spine disorder seen in the child with CP

Kyphosis is also common

Hip disorders

Hip subluxation and dislocation is very common in the child with CP

Windswept hips—abduction of one hip and adduction of the contralateral hip

Knee disorders

Typically involve flexion contractures with decreased range of motion

Foot and ankle disorders

Common in CP

Equinovalgus foot

Caused by spasticity of the peroneal muscles

More common in spastic diplegics

Equinovarus foot

Caused by overpull of the posterior and/or anterior tibialis tendons

More common in spastic hemiplegics

Note: The treatment of specific disorders in CP is beyond the scope of this textbook

Neuromuscular Disorders

Myelodysplasia—represents a disorder of spinal cord development, neural tube closure, or a rupture of a developing cord, most commonly caused by hydrocephalus (Fig. 5–8)

Spina bifida occulta—defect in the vertebral arch (spinal cord and meninges are not exposed)

Meningocele—defect with bulging sac but without protrusion of neural elements through the defect

Myelomeningocele (spina bifida)—defect with protrusion of the neural elements

Rachischisis—neural elements exposed without any coverings

Myelodysplasia may be diagnosed in utero by increased α-fetoprotein

Sudden changes in functional capacity, a rapid increase in a scoliotic curve, worsening spasticity, or new or worsening neurologic defects suggest the development of hydrocephalus (most common), hydromyelia (increased fluid in the central canal of the spinal cord), or a tethered cord (scarring of the neural elements within the spinal canal that causes stretching [tethering] of the spinal cord)

Function in the patient with myelodysplasia is primarily related to the level of the defect and other associated congenital abnormalities

Myelodysplasia level is based on the lowest functioning level

L4 is a key level because the quadriceps can function and allow community ambulation

Level is based on physical examination of **motor function**

Cervical—upper extremity motor function is abnormal

Thoracic—no motor activity in the muscles crossing the hip joint

Upper lumbar—active adduction or flexion of the hips is present; active extension of the knees is present; active abduction of the hips is absent; active flexion of the knees and dorsiflexion of the ankles are absent

Lower lumbar—active abduction of the hips is present; active flexion of the knees and dorsiflexion of the ankles are present; active extension of the hips and active plantar flexion of the ankles and toes are absent

Sacral—active extension of the hips is present; active plantar flexion of the ankles and toes is also present

Functional levels of walking

Community ambulators—walk indoors or outdoors (with or without crutches or braces), but may use a wheelchair for long trips

Household ambulators—walk indoors only with crutches or braces, and use a wheelchair for some indoor and all outdoor activities

Nonfunctional ambulators—walk only during therapy sessions and use a wheelchair for transportation

Nonambulators—are wheelchair-bound but may be able to transfer from chair to bed

Fractures in myelodysplasia

Occur as a result of insensate portions of the lower extremities

Traumatic episode leading to fracture may go unnoticed because of insensate lower extremities

Patient may present with redness, warmth, and swelling of the lower extremity

X-rays to confirm fracture

Treatment approach in the patient with myelodysplasia

Requires a team approach—orthopaedic surgeon, pediatrician, neurologist, neurosurgeon, urolo-

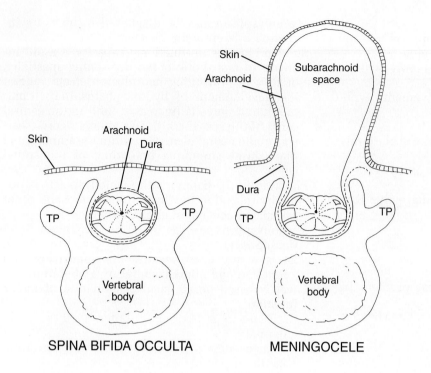

SPINA BIFIDA OCCULTA

MENINGOCELE

Figure 5–8 ■ Characteristics of the various types of myelodysplasia. See text for a detailed description of each type of myelodysplasia. TP, transverse process.

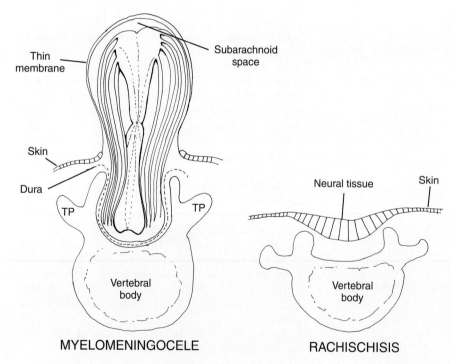

MYELOMENINGOCELE

RACHISCHISIS

gist, physical therapist, social services, orthotist, prosthetist, and others

Specific disorders of myelomeningocele

  Hip disorders

    Hip dislocation occurs frequently in myelodysplasia because of unopposed hip flexors and adductors (hip abductors and extensors are paralyzed)

    Hip dislocation is most common in patients with myelodysplasia with an L3 or L4 level

Knee disorders

  Quadriceps weakness

  Flexion deformities

  Recurvatum

Foot and ankle disorders

  Valgus foot deformities

  Valgus ankle deformities

  Rotational deformities of the distal tibia

  Subtalar angular deformities

Spinal disorders

Scoliosis
  May result from the spine defect itself
  May be paralytic
  Rapid curve progression may be associated with hydrocephalus, hydromyelia, or a tethered cord
  Kyphosis is not uncommon and is difficult to treat
  Pelvic obliquity may occur in myelodysplasia as a result of prolonged unilateral hip contractures or scoliosis
Note: The treatment of specific disorders in myelodysplasia is beyond the scope of this textbook
Arthrogryposis multiplex congenita
  Nonprogressive disorder
  Characterized by multiple congenitally rigid joints
  May be myopathic, neuropathic, or mixed
  Upper-extremity involvement
    Humerus—adducted and internally rotated
    Elbow—extension
    Wrist—flexion, ulnar deviation
  Lower-extremity involvement
    Foot—rigid clubfoot
    Hip—dislocation
    Knee—contractures
  Fractures are common
Larsen's syndrome
  Clinical picture similar to that in arthrogryposis but joints are less rigid
Multiple pterygium syndrome

Autosomal recessive
Cutaneous flexor surface webs
Congenital vertical talus
Scoliosis
Muscular dystrophies—noninflammatory inherited disorders characterized by progressive muscle weakness
  Several types of muscular dystrophy have been classified based on their inheritance pattern
  Duchenne's
    X-linked recessive
    Young men
    Decreased motor skills, clumsy walking, lumbar lordosis, calf pseudohypertrophy
    Physical exam reveals positive **Gowers' sign** (patient arises from the sitting position by walking the hands up the legs to compensate for gluteus maximus and quadriceps weakness) (Fig. 5–9)
    Patients have a markedly elevated creatine phosphokinase (CPK)
    Children usually die of cardiorespiratory complications
  Becker's
    X-linked recessive
    Clinical picture similar to that in Duchenne's but less severe
    Affected individuals are typically red-green color-blind males
  Facioscapulohumeral

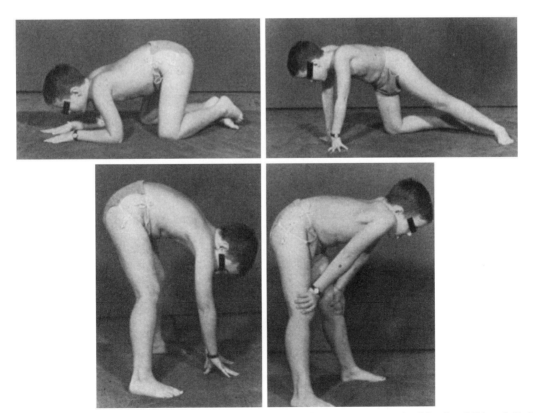

Figure 5–9 ■ Gowers' sign. In a child with muscular dystrophy, a series of maneuvers is required for the child to "climb up his legs" in order to stand up from a sitting position because of pelvic and trunk weakness. (From Drennan JC: Neuromuscular disorders. *In* Lovell WW, Winter RB [eds]: Pediatric Orthopaedics, 2nd ed. Philadelphia, JB Lippincott, 1985, p 265.)

Autosomal dominant
Facial muscle abnormalities
Normal CPK
Winging of the scapulae
Limb-girdle
Autosomal recessive
Others
Ocular
Oculopharyngeal
Myotonic myopathies
Autosomal dominant
Characterized by inability of muscles to relax after contracture
Three basic types
Myotonia congenita (Thomsen's)
Dystrophic myotonia (Steinert's)
Paramyotonia congenita (Eulenburg's)
Congenital myopathies
Autosomal dominant
Nonprogressive disorder; affected infant presents as a "floppy baby"
Polymyositis, dermatomyositis
Characterized by a febrile illness
Hereditary neuropathies
Friedreich's ataxia
Degenerative disease of the cerebellum
Typical onset before age 10 years
Affected child presents with staggering, wide-based gait
Involves both motor and sensory defects

Charcot-Marie-Tooth disease (peroneal muscle atrophy)
Autosomal dominant
Involves motor defects only
Myasthenia gravis
Chronic disease
Develops insidiously
Muscle fatigue caused by competitive inhibition of acetylcholine receptors at the motor end plate
Disorders of the anterior horn cells
Poliomyelitis
Viral destruction of anterior horn cells in the spinal cord and brain stem
Has nearly disappeared in the United States after vaccine development
Spinal muscle atrophy (Werdnig-Hoffmann disease)
Autosomal recessive
Loss of anterior horn cells from the spinal cord
Associated with progressive scoliosis
Four types of spinal muscle atrophy (types I–IV) have been described
Guillain-Barré syndrome
Acute idiopathic postinfectious polyneuropathy
Symmetric ascending motor paresis
Caused by demyelination after viral infection
Usually self-limiting
Overgrowth syndromes
Proteus syndrome
Klippel-Trénaunay-Weber syndrome
Hemihypertrophy

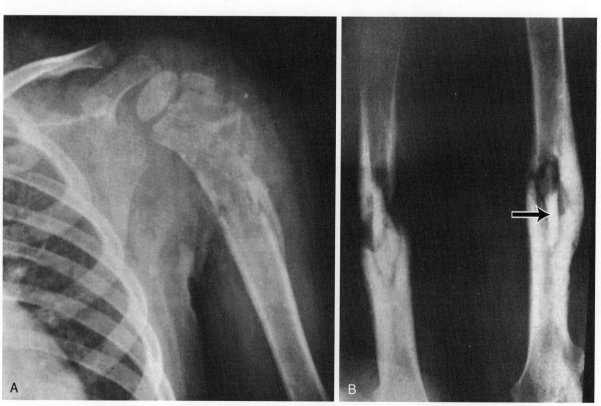

Figure 5–10 ■ *A,* Acute hematogenous osteomyelitis of the proximal humerus of a young child. *B,* Sequelae of acute hematogenous osteomyelitis of the femur with destructive changes and sequestrum (dead bone) (*arrow*). (From Gartland JJ: Fundamentals of Orthopaedics, 4th ed. Philadelphia, WB Saunders, 1986, pp 152–153.)

Infections in Children

Acute hematogenous osteomyelitis (and sequelae) (Fig. 5–10)

Infection of bone and bone marrow

Most common cause in children is **blood-borne organisms**

Boys more commonly affected than girls

Staphylococcus aureus is the most common infecting organism in patients >4 years of age

The most characteristic pathogen in the **newborn** is group B streptococci

The most characteristic pathogens in those who are not newborns but are ≤4 years of age are *S. aureus* and *Haemophilus influenzae*

The most common site for infection in acute hematogenous osteomyelitis is the **metaphysis** or the **epiphysis**

Epiphyseal osteomyelitis is caused almost exclusively by *S. aureus*

Infection typically does not cross (traverse) the physis

Sequestrum = dead bone with surrounding granulation tissue

Involucrum = periosteal new bone formation

Clinical findings of acute hematogenous osteomyelitis include

Pain

Loss of function

Soft tissue erythema, warmth, and sometimes abscess

Laboratory findings include

Elevated white blood cell (WBC) count

Elevated erythrocyte sedimentation rate (ESR)

Positive blood cultures

Radiographs and imaging

Technetium bone scan with or without gallium or indium scan is helpful

Magnetic resonance imaging (MRI) shows bone changes earlier than x-rays (which may be normal for up to 2 weeks)

Treatment of acute hematogenous osteomyelitis

Identification of organism

Selection of appropriate antibiotics

Delivery of antibiotics to the site of infection

Halting of tissue destruction

Subacute osteomyelitis

May arise as a result of a partially treated osteomyelitis or in a fracture hematoma

WBC count and ESR may be normal

Radiographs typically show a localized radiolucency (Brodie's abscess)

Unlike acute osteomyelitis, subacute osteomyelitis can cross (traverse) the physis

Treatment—surgical drainage (if pus present) and 6 weeks of intravenous (IV) antibiotics

Septic arthritis

Often follows hematogenous spread or extension of metaphyseal osteomyelitis in children

The metaphyses of the proximal femur, proximal humerus, radial neck, and distal fibula are within their respective joint capsules; metaphyseal osteomyelitis can rupture into the joint in these areas

The most common site in which septic arthritis follows an episode of acute osteomyelitis is the proximal femur/hip

Treatment—surgical drainage and IV antibiotics

Discitis

Disc space infection

Child refuses to walk or sit

Physical examination shows decreased ROM of the spine

ESR is elevated

MRI is diagnostic early

Late (2–3 weeks after onset) disc space narrowing seen on x-rays

Treatment—bed rest without traction, immobilization, antibiotics

Pediatric Bone Tumors

Table 5–2 lists pediatric bone tumors by age group.

PEDIATRIC CONDITIONS BY ANATOMIC REGION

UPPER EXTREMITY

The Pediatric Shoulder

Brachial plexus birth injuries (Fig. 5–11)

In approximately 1 in 500 births, the infant sustains a brachial plexus stretch or contusion injury

Injuries more common with larger children, shoulder dystocia, forceps delivery, breech position, and prolonged labor

Table 5–2
PEDIATRIC BONE TUMORS

Age (yr)	Benign	Malignant
0–5	Eosinophilic granuloma Osteofibrous dysplasia Osteomyelitis	Leukemia Metastatic neuroblastoma Wilms' tumor (metastases to bone) Fibrosarcoma Metastatic rhabdomyosarcoma
5–10	Osteoid osteoma Simple bone cyst Fibrous cortical defect Fibrous dysplasia Eosinophilic granuloma Osteomyelitis	Osteosarcoma (types: central, periosteal, high-grade surface) Ewing's sarcoma Leukemia
10–20	Osteoid osteoma Osteoblastoma Osteoma Osteochondroma Chondroblastoma Aneurysmal bone cyst Fibroma Ossifying fibroma Eosinophilic granuloma Osteomyelitis Fibrous dysplasia Fibrous cortical defect* Enchondroma	Osteosarcoma (types: central, periosteal, high-grade surface) Ewing's sarcoma Leukemia

*Also known as a nonossifying fibroma (NOF).

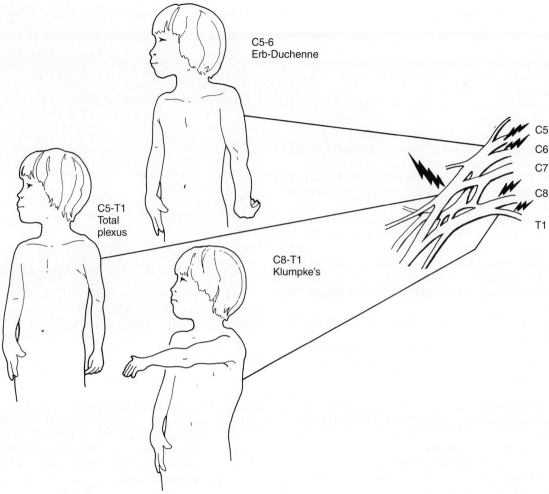

C5-6
Erb-Duchenne

C5-T1
Total
plexus

C8-T1
Klumpke's

C5
C6
C7
C8
T1

Figure 5–11 ■ Composite figure demonstrating the anatomic location of various brachial plexus birth injuries (Erb-Duchenne, Klumpke's, and total plexus) and associated clinical deformities.

Three types of brachial plexus palsies
  Erb-Duchenne
    C5 and C6 roots (upper trunk distribution) involved
    "Waiter's tip" deformity
    Best prognosis
  Klumpke's
    C8 and T1 roots (ulnar nerve distribution) involved
    Wrist flexion is weak (flexor carpi ulnaris motor activity is absent), and motor activity of intrinsics of the hand is absent
    Intermediate prognosis
  Total plexus
    C5 to T1 roots involved
    Flaccid arm
    Worst prognosis
Treatment of brachial plexus birth injuries
  Physical therapy to maintain passive ROM while awaiting return of motor function (which can occur for up to 18 months)
  More than 90% of brachial plexus palsies resolve without intervention

  Lack of biceps function 3 months after birth injury carries a poor prognosis
Congenital pseudoarthrosis of the clavicle
  Represents failure of union of the medial and lateral ossification centers
  Clinical presentation—enlarging nontender mass over the involved clavicle
  X-rays show rounded sclerotic margins at the pseudoarthrosis site
  Should not be confused with a fracture of the clavicle (which will develop callus; pseudoarthrosis will not develop callus over time)
  Treatment—typically none needed unless the pseudoarthrosis becomes painful
Sprengel's deformity (Fig. 5–12)
  Undescended scapula
  Often associated with scapular winging
  The most common anomaly of the shoulder
  Associated with Klippel-Feil syndrome, kidney disease, scoliosis, and diastematomyelia
Deltoid fibrotic bands
  Fibrous bands replace the deltoid muscle
  Shoulder demonstrates abduction contracture

Traumatic injuries of the pediatric shoulder
 Pediatric proximal humerus injuries (Fig. 5–13)
  Growth plate injuries are classified based on the Salter-Harris (SH) scheme
  SH type I—most common in preschoolers
  SH type II—most common in grade schoolers
   Reduction with more than 50% opposition and less than 45 degrees of angulation acceptable; otherwise, reduce and percutaneously pin or perform open reduction with internal fixation (ORIF)
  Metaphyseal injuries are not uncommon and often heal without sequelae even in cases with significant displacement of the fragments
  Stress fractures (Little Leaguer's shoulder)—treat with activity modification
 Pediatric glenohumeral dislocations
  Treated as in adults
  Avoid reconstructive procedures until childhood laxity resolves or until skeletal maturity, if possible
 Pediatric clavicle injuries
  Unique because the childhood periosteal "sleeve" has abundant healing capacity, even for widely displaced fractures
  Clavicle fractures and acromioclavicular (AC) injuries—treat with a sling or a figure-of-8 splint
Tumors of the pediatric shoulder
 Chondroblastoma
 Osteosarcoma
 Simple bone cyst

The Pediatric Arm

Traumatic injuries of the pediatric arm
 Humeral shaft fractures

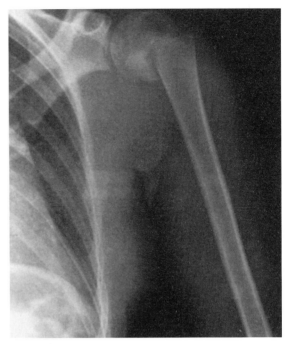

Figure 5–13 ■ Salter-Harris type II proximal humeral fracture. (From Curtis RJ Jr, Rockwood CA Jr: Fractures and dislocations of the shoulder in children. *In* Rockwood CA Jr, Matsen FA III [eds]: The Shoulder. Philadelphia, WB Saunders, 1990, p 996.)

Treatment based on patient age (Table 5–3)
Tumors of the pediatric arm (humerus)
 Osteochondroma

The Pediatric Elbow

Congenital dislocation of the radial head
 Abnormally formed radial head
 Abnormal contour to ulna
 Associated with connective tissue disorders
 Look for abnormal contour of the capitellum
Traumatic injuries of the pediatric elbow
 May be subtle; extremely painful elbow in children should be assumed to be a fracture until proved otherwise
 Radiographic lines have been described to help identify displaced fractures that are often difficult to appreciate in the pediatric elbow (Fig. 5–14)
 "Fat pad" sign (presence of soft tissue shadow(s), especially posteriorly) suggests the presence of an intra-articular effusion (and fracture) (Fig. 5–15)

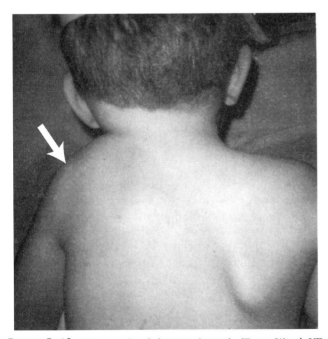

Figure 5–12 ■ Sprengel's deformity (*arrow*). (From Wood VE, Marchinski L: Congenital anomalies of the shoulder. *In* Rockwood CA Jr, Matsen FA III [eds]: The Shoulder. Philadelphia, WB Saunders, 1990, p 104.)

Table 5–3
TREATMENT OF HUMERAL SHAFT FRACTURES

Age	Treatment
Neonate	Bind arm to side (elastic wrap)
<3 years	Collar and cuff sling
3–12 years	Sling and swathe
>12 years	Sugar-tong splint

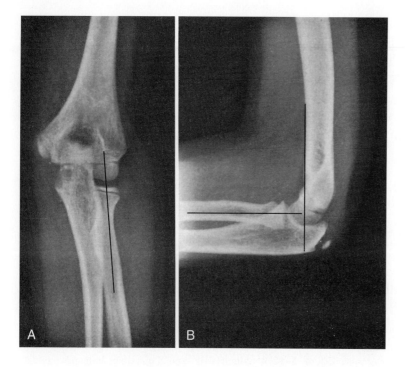

Figure 5–14 ■ Radiographic lines for evaluation of pediatric elbow injuries. A line drawn along the long axis of the proximal radius should bisect the capitellum on both the anteroposterior (*A*) and lateral (*B*) radiographic views. A line drawn along the anterior cortex of the distal humerus on the lateral radiographic view (*B*) (anterior humeral line) should bisect the capitellum. (Modified from Gartland JJ: Fundamentals of Orthopaedics, 4th ed. Philadelphia, WB Saunders, 1986, p 249.)

Overview of pediatric elbow injuries (Fig. 5–16)
  Supracondylar fractures
    Classification
      Type I—minimally displaced; slight loss of distal angulation of the condyle
      Type II—displaced; posterior cortex intact
      Type III—totally displaced; no contact between fragments
    Treatment
      Type I—reduction and immobilization in flexion

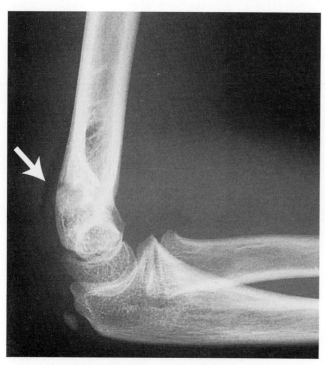

Figure 5–15 ■ Posterior fat-pad sign (*arrow*).

      Type II—closed reduction and percutaneous pinning
      Type III—closed reduction and percutaneous pinning (ORIF if not reducible using closed manipulation)
    Complications
      Inadequate reduction (deformity or loss of motion)
      Nerve injury (important to recognize these before treatment!)
      Vascular insult (excessive flexion to maintain reduction can cut off the radial pulse (if this goes unrecognized it can result in disastrous sequelae—Volkmann's ischemic contracture)
  Lateral condyle physeal fractures
    Location—SH type IV (Milch I) or SH type II (Milch II)
    Displacement—undisplaced, moderately displaced, displaced and rotated
    Treatment—based on the degree of displacement
      Undisplaced—cast
      Displaced—closed reduction and pinning or ORIF
    Complications
      Cubitus valgus (gunstock deformity)
      Ulnar nerve problems (can occur late—"tardy" ulnar nerve palsy)
      Physeal arrest
      Osteonecrosis
  Medial condyle physeal fractures
    Rare injury
    Location—SH type IV (Milch I) or SH type II (Milch II)
    Displacement—undisplaced, moderately displaced, displaced and rotated
    Treatment—similar to that for lateral condyle physeal fractures

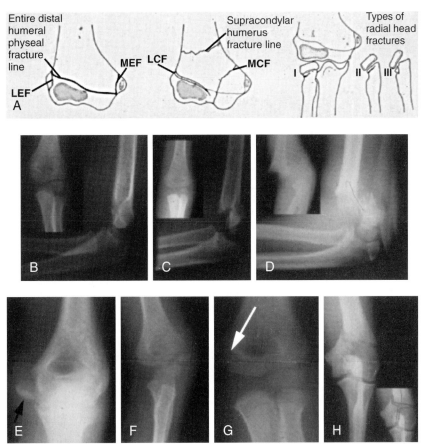

Figure 5-16 ■ Pediatric elbow fractures. *A,* Schematic representation of various pediatric elbow injuries. LEF, lateral epicondylar apophyseal fracture line; MEF, medial epicondylar apophyseal fracture line; LCF, lateral condylar physeal fracture line; MCF, medial condylar physeal fracture line. Pediatric supracondylar elbow fractures are quite common. Extension-type injuries (the distal fragment is posterior to the proximal fragment) account for greater than 95% of pediatric supracondylar fractures; flexion-type injuries (the distal fragment is anterior to the proximal fragment) are exceedingly rare. Pediatric supracondylar elbow fractures are easiest to classify on the lateral radiograph. *B,* AP and lateral radiographs of a type I (extension) pediatric supracondylar elbow fracture. *C,* AP and lateral radiographs of a type II (extension) pediatric supracondylar elbow fracture. *D,* AP and lateral radiographs of a type III (extension) pediatric supracondylar elbow fracture. *E,* AP radiograph showing a medial epicondylar apophyseal fracture (*arrow*). *F,* AP radiograph showing a lateral condylar physeal fracture. *G,* AP radiograph showing a medial condylar physeal fracture (*arrow*). *H,* AP radiograph showing a pediatric T-condylar fracture; note that the fracture lines have been outlined on the insert. (Radiographs courtesy of Joseph J. Gugenheim, MD, Gary T. Brock, MD, and Howard R. Epps, MD, Fondren Orthopedic Group LLP, Texas Orthopedic Hospital, Houston, Texas.)

Complications
  Missed diagnosis
  Osteonecrosis
  Valgus deformity
Entire distal humeral physeal fracture—treated like a supracondylar fracture; **these injuries are difficult to recognize and are often missed!**
Medial and lateral epicondylar apophyseal fractures—usually treated with early ROM; excision of the fragment is recommended only if it is in an intra-articular position
T-condylar fractures—require ORIF if significantly displaced
Radial head/neck fractures—treatment involves ORIF only if the fragments are angulated greater than 60 degrees
Olecranon fractures—rare injury; treatment similar to that for fractures in adults
Elbow dislocations
  Classification—based on the position of the forearm relative to the distal humerus (posteromedial, posterolateral, anterior, medial, and lateral); posterior dislocations are the most common
  Treatment—closed reduction
  Complications—median nerve entrapment, associated injuries, myositis ossificans
Tumors of the pediatric elbow
  Uncommon

The Pediatric Forearm

Congenital radial-ulnar synostosis
  Congenital union of the forearm bones
  Most commonly occurs proximally in the forearm
  Blocks pronation and supination of the forearm
  Associated with congenital abnormalities of the hip or foot, chromosomal abnormalities, and fetal alcohol syndrome
  This entity is difficult to treat

Traumatic injuries of the pediatric forearm
  Classification of fractures—based on the degree of injury (see Fig. 5–3)
    Greenstick (incomplete)
    Compression/torus (buckle)
    Complete
  Treatment—closed manipulation and casting (Fig. 5–17)
  Associated injuries must be addressed
    Monteggia's fracture = ulna shaft fracture with a radial head dislocation
    Galeazzi's fracture = radial shaft fracture with distal radioulnar subluxation/dislocation
Tumors of the pediatric forearm
  Uncommon

The Pediatric Wrist

Madelung's deformity
  Abnormal growth of the distal radial epiphysis with premature closure of the ulnar half of the distal radius
  May lead to progressive volar and ulnar angulation of the wrist
  May arise as a congenital deformity (autosomal dominant) or may be post-traumatic
  Occurs in girls more often than boys
Radial clubhand (radial aplasia) (Fig. 5–18)
  Disorder of radial development
  Results in radial deviation of the hand
  May be associated with absent scaphoid, abnormal thumb development, and stiff fingers
  May be associated with gastrointestinal and genitourinary abnormalities; aplastic anemia; thrombocytopenia; and heart anomalies

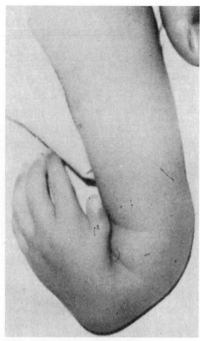

Figure 5–18 ■ Clinical photo of radial clubhand. (From Gartland JJ: Fundamentals of Orthopaedics, 4th ed. Philadelphia, WB Saunders, 1986, p 71.)

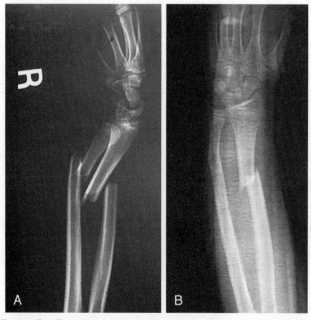

Figure 5–17 ■ Pediatric both-bone forearm fracture. *A*, Injury. *B*, Reduction with interosseous molding in a cast. (Courtesy of Joseph J. Gugenheim, MD, Fondren Orthopedic Group LLP, Texas Orthopedic Hospital, Houston, Texas.)

Ulnar clubhand
  Less common than radial clubhand
  Not associated with systemic disorders
Traumatic injuries of the pediatric wrist
  Usually involve the distal radius
  Classification
    SH types I to V
    Torus
    Greenstick
    Complete
  Treatment—closed reduction and casting in supination for displaced fractures
Tumors of the pediatric wrist
  Uncommon

The Pediatric Hand

Congenital hand disorders (Fig. 5–19)
  Syndactyly (joined digits)
    Description (based on what's involved [skin/bone] and the extent of involvement)
      Simple = only skin involvement
      Complex = bony involvement
      Complete = entire length of digit involved
      Incomplete = does not involve entire length of digit
    Syndactyly associated with a variety of anomalies: Poland's syndrome, Streeter's dysplasia, Apert's syndrome
    Surgical release works well
  Polydactyly (duplicated digits)
    May represent only a soft tissue nubbin or a completely developed, functional, duplicated digit
  Brachydactyly = short digits
  Macrodactyly = enlarged digits

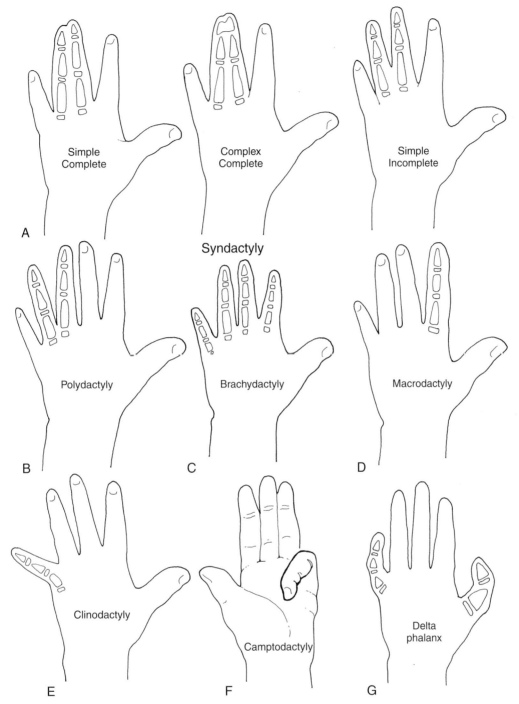

Figure 5–19 ■ Spectrum of congenital hand disorders. *A*, Syndactyly. *B*, Polydactyly. *C*, Brachydactyly. *D*, Macrodactyly. *E*, Clinodactyly. *F*, Camptodactyly. *G*, Delta phalanx.

May be isolated or associated with disorders such as neurofibromatosis

Clinodactyly = skeletal abnormality with digit deviated in the medial/lateral plane

Camptodactyly = soft tissue abnormality with digit deviated in the anterior/posterior plane

Symphalangism = congenital ankylosis of the proximal interphalangeal (PIP) joint

Delta phalanx = triangular phalanx and physis lead to angular deviation of the finger

Congenital thumb anomalies

Congenital hypoplastic thumb

Clasped thumb disorder

Floating thumb

Congenital trigger finger

Congenital stenosing tenosynovitis at the A1 pulley

Many cases resolve spontaneously

Streeter's dysplasia

Fibrous amniotic bands result in intrauterine constriction of digits

Associated with other congenital abnormalities

Congenital amputation
  May be caused by constriction bands or failure of development
Traumatic injuries of the pediatric hand
  Phalangeal and metacarpal fractures—closed treatment with splinting is usually successful
  Dislocations—treatment and classification similar to those in adults
Tumors of the pediatric hand
  Enchondroma

SPINE AND PELVIS

The Pediatric Cervical Spine

Torticollis (Fig. 5–20)
  Congenital deformity caused by contraction of the sternocleidomastoid muscle
  Associated with other "uterine packing" problems (hip dysplasia, metatarsus adductus, and others)
  Child presents with head rotated toward the uninvolved side and laterally flexed toward the involved side
  Must differentiate from atlantoaxial rotatory instability, other cervical spine anomalies, and eye disorders

Klippel-Feil syndrome—multiple fused cervical vertebrae (Fig. 5–21)
  Caused by failure of segmentation of cervical somites during development
  Associated with congenital scoliosis, renal abnormalities, Sprengel's deformity, congenital heart disease, brain stem abnormalities, congenital cervical stenosis, synkinesis
  Classic triad of Klippel-Feil syndrome = webbed neck, decreased cervical range of motion, low posterior hairline
  These children should not participate in sports activities
Os odontoideum—bony ossicle of the tip of the odontoid process (of C2) that is not attached to the base of the odontoid (Fig. 5–22)
  Previously thought to represent a failure of fusion; now believed to arise from a prior traumatic event
  May lead to significant anterior/posterior instability
  X-ray evaluation important (lateral flexion/extension view [active motion only] of the cervical spine to look for translation of C1 on C2)
Atlantoaxial instability
  Caused by C1-2 ligamentous laxity
  Anterior/posterior instability

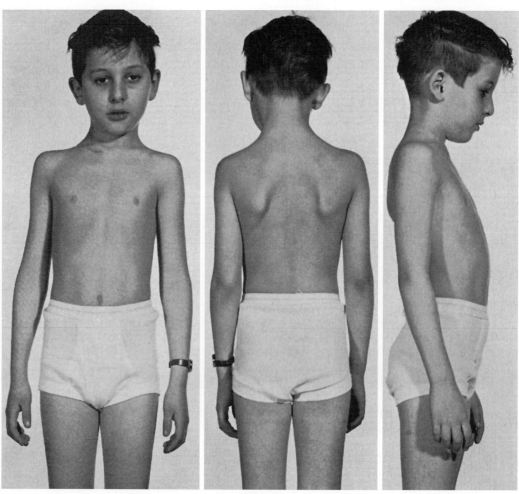

Figure 5–20 ■ Torticollis. In this child, the right sternocleidomastoid muscle is contracted. (From Tachdjian MD: Pediatric Orthopedics. Philadelphia, WB Saunders, 1972, p 76.)

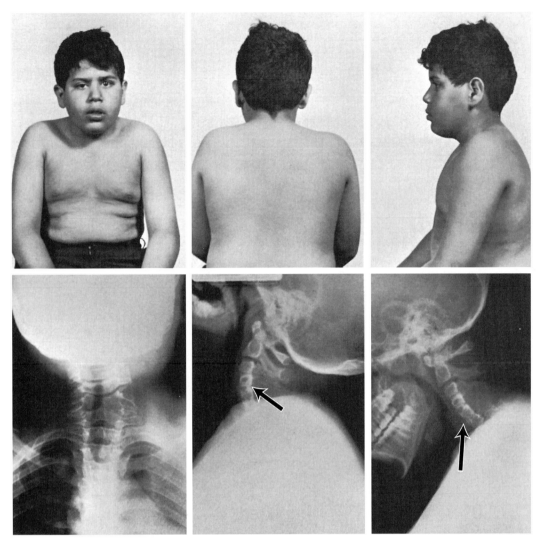

Figure 5–21 ■ Klippel-Feil syndrome. Clinical photos (*top*) and radiographs (*bottom*). Note the fusion of the lower cervical vertebrae into a single bony mass (*arrows*). (From Tachdjian MD: Pediatric Orthopedics. Philadelphia, WB Saunders, 1972, p 77.)

Associated with trisomy 21, JRA, os odontoideum, and other abnormalities

Evaluate with flexion/extension x-rays as in os odontoideum

Rotatory atlantoaxial subluxation

Abnormal rotation of C1 on C2

May present as torticollis

May arise as a result of a retropharyngeal inflammation (Grisel's syndrome)

May also be caused by ligamentous laxity

Evaluate with computed tomography (CT) scan with the neck actively rotated in different positions to evaluate rotational instability between C1 and C2

Pseudosubluxation of the cervical spine (Fig. 5–23)

Subluxation of C2 on C3 of up to 4 mm (or as much as 40%) can be normal in children less than 8 years of age

To differentiate pseudosubluxation from a true acute injury, evaluate soft tissue swelling both clinically and radiographically

Basilar impression

Bony deformities at the base of the skull cause upward migration of the odontoid into the foramen magnum

Contact of the odontoid on the brain stem can cause weakness, paresthesias, and hydrocephalus

Traumatic injuries of the pediatric cervical spine

Children most frequently sustain fractures of the upper cervical spine (C1 and C2), as opposed to adults, who more commonly sustain fractures of the lower cervical spine

Injuries in children can be fatal

Tumors of the pediatric cervical spine

Osteoblastoma

Aneurysmal bone cyst

Eosinophilic granuloma

The Pediatric Thoracolumbar Spine

Idiopathic scoliosis—lateral deviation of the spine without an identifiable cause; the spine is also rotated in idiopathic scoliosis (Fig. 5–24)

Curve description—a curve is described by its apex (position and direction [right or left] that it points to) (Fig. 5–25)

Right thoracic curves—apex at T7 or T8 (the most common type)

Double major curves—right thoracic curve with a left lumbar curve

Left lumbar curves

Right lumbar curves

Curve measurement (see Fig. 5–25)

Most commonly curves are measured using the method of Cobb

Measurements are made on standing posteroanterior (PA) radiographs

Measurements are made by constructing intersecting lines that are perpendicular to the end plates of the most tilted vertebrae

Determination of skeletal maturity (see Fig. 5–25)

Risser staging—based on the ossification of the iliac crest apophysis

Risser staging is graded 0 (least mature) to 5 (most mature)

Adolescent idiopathic scoliosis

Typically presents between ages 10 and 18 years

This is the most common form of idiopathic scoliosis

Curve progression is most likely with

Curve magnitudes of greater than 20 degrees

Age at diagnosis of less than 12 years

A Risser stage of 0 or 1

Approximately 75% of immature patients with curves of 20 to 30 degrees progress at least 5 degrees

Severe curves of 90 degrees or more are associated with significant cardiac and pulmonary impairment

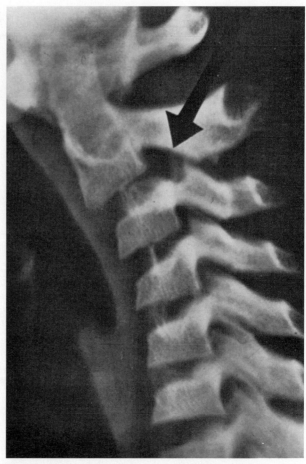

Figure 5–23 ■ Pseudosubluxation of the cervical spine (C2 displaced anteriorly on C3). (From Fielding JW: *In* Ahstrom JP Jr [ed]: Current Practice in Orthopaedic Surgery, Vol. 5. St. Louis, CV Mosby, 1973.)

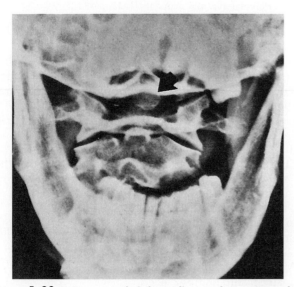

Figure 5–22 ■ Open-mouth (odontoid) view shows an os odontoideum. Arrow points to the bony ossicle of the tip of the odontoid process that is not attached to the base of the odontoid. The ossicle's edges have a rounded-off appearance, which differentiates it from an acute fracture. (From Fielding JW, Hawkins RJ, Ratzan SA: Spine fusion for atlantoaxial instability. J Bone Joint Surg 58A:405, 1976.)

Left thoracic curves are rare and necessitate evaluation of the spinal cord using MRI

Treatment options include observation, bracing, and surgery (spinal arthrodesis with instrumentation)

Treatment decisions are based on the likelihood of curve progression (based on natural history studies) from known factors such as curve magnitude, age at diagnosis, skeletal maturity (as assessed using the Risser staging method), the presence of menarche, and curve progression during the period of time that the patient has been followed

Physical findings of adolescent idiopathic scoliosis include shoulder or pelvic asymmetry and an asymmetric rib hump seen on forward bending (see Fig. 5–24)

Adolescent idiopathic scoliosis is typically not painful, and the child presenting with a painful curvature should be given a thorough work-up

Infantile idiopathic scoliosis

Typically presents within the first 3 years of life with a left-sided thoracic curvature

This condition is associated with other congenital defects

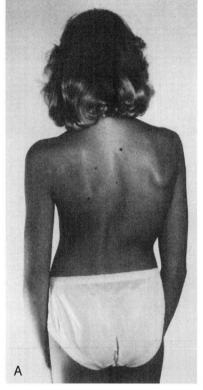 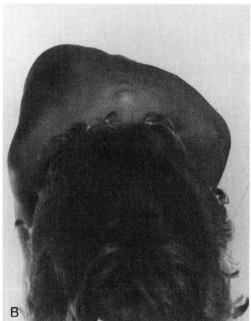

Figure 5–24 ■ Patient with right thoracic scoliosis. *A,* Observation from behind shows right scapular elevation and asymmetry of the triangles formed between the upper extremity and the trunk. The abnormal spinal curvature is also apparent. *B,* Forward bending, a useful technique of physical examination, accentuates this patient's deformity. In this right thoracic curvature, forward bending demonstrates a prominent right rib hump deformity. (From Sabiston DC Jr: Essentials of Surgery. Philadelphia, WB Saunders, 1987, p 774.)

Juvenile idiopathic scoliosis
    Typically presents between 3 and 10 years of age
    Presentation is similar to that in adolescent idiopathic scoliosis
Neuromuscular scoliosis
    Many children with neuromuscular disorders develop scoliosis

As compared with idiopathic curves, neuromuscular curves progress more rapidly, involve more vertebral segments (curves are longer), are more often associated with pelvic obliquity, and generally do not have a rotational component
Pulmonary complications in these patients are common
Treatment options include wheelchair modification, orthoses and braces, and operative arthrodesis procedures
Rapid progression of a curve in an individual with a neuromuscular disorder necessitates an investigation for spinal cord abnormalities or tethering of the spinal cord; MRI is a useful diagnostic test
Congenital scoliosis (Fig. 5–26)
    The most common congenital disorder of the spine
    Congenital scoliosis is caused by abnormally formed vertebral bodies (vertebral anomalies)
    A variety of anomalies have been described and include
        Unilateral unsegmented bar—the most common and most likely to progress
        Hemivertebra—"half a vertebra" (has only one pedicle)
        Wedge vertebra—incomplete vertebra (has at least a portion of both pedicles)
        Block vertebra—nonsegmentation of two or more adjacent vertebral bodies
Congenital kyphosis
    Humpback deformity resulting from abnormal vertebra (differs from congenital scoliosis in that a kyphotic deformity is in the sagittal plane)
May arise as a result of failure of formation, failure of segmentation, or a combination of the two

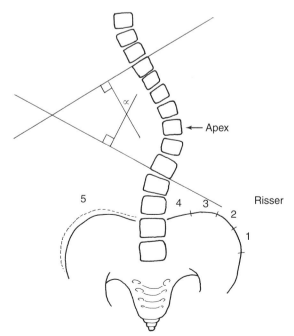

Figure 5–25 ■ Scoliosis curve measurement (Cobb method) and determination of skeletal maturity via Risser staging.

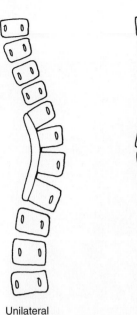

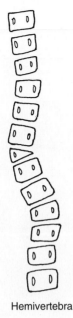

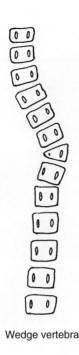

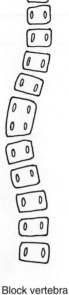

Unilateral unsegmented bar

Hemivertebra

Wedge vertebra

Block vertebra

Figure 5–26 ■ Vertebral anomalies of congenital scoliosis.

Neurofibromatosis
  Autosomal dominant disorder of neural crest cells
  Diagnostic criteria of neurofibromatosis
    Café au lait spots (six or more)
    Neurofibromas (two or more)
    Axillary or inguinal freckles
    Bony lesions
    Optic gliomas
    Lisch nodules (two or more)—lesions of the iris (detected by slit lamp examination)
    Family history
  The spine is the most common site of skeletal involvement in neurofibromatosis

Diastematomyelia (Fig. 5–27)
  A longitudinal cleft in the spinal cord secondary to a fibrous, cartilaginous, or bony bar
  Most commonly occurs in the lumbar spine
  May lead to tethering of the cord with associated neurologic abnormalities
Lower back pain in children
  Although lower back pain is a common complaint in adults, it is very uncommon in children and should be taken seriously
  Differential diagnosis includes spondylolysis, discitis, osteomyelitis, herniated nucleus pulposus, spinal cord tumor, and others

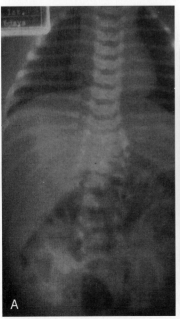

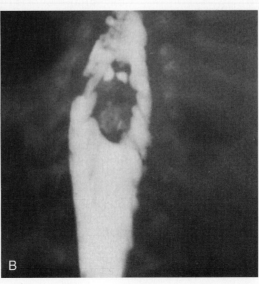

Figure 5–27 ■ Radiograph (A) and myelogram (B) of diastematomyelia in an infant. Note the longitudinal cleft in the spinal cord (the myelographic material is divided into two columns). (From Tachdjian MO: Pediatric Orthopedics. Philadelphia, WB Saunders, 1972, p 884.)

Scheuermann's disease
  Hyperkyphosis that does not reverse on attempts at hyperextension
  Most common in adolescent males
  Diagnosis made by x-ray measurement—thoracic kyphosis increased to more than 45 degrees, with 5 degrees or more of vertebral wedging at three sequential vertebrae
  Treatment options include bracing and surgery
Spondylolysis—a defect in the pars interarticularis
  The most common cause of lower back pain in children and adolescents
  The pars defect is the result of a fatigue fracture from repetitive hyperextension
  Most common in gymnasts and football linemen
Spondylolisthesis—forward slippage of one vertebra on another
  Usually occurs at the L5-S1 level in children
  Most common in children involved in hyperextension activities
Traumatic injuries of the pediatric thoracolumbar spine
  Findings similar to those in adults
  Radiographic abnormality may not be detectable on plain radiographs
  Spinal cord injury without radiographic abnormality (SCIWORA)—MRI indicated
Tumors of the pediatric thoracolumbar spine
  Osteoblastoma
  Aneurysmal bone cyst
  Eosinophilic granuloma

The Pediatric Pelvis, Sacrum, Coccyx

Sacral agenesis
  Partial or complete absence of the sacrum (and lower lumbar spine)
  Associated with maternal diabetes
Traumatic injuries of the pediatric pelvis, sacrum, coccyx
  Pelvic ring disruptions in children are similar to those of adults
  Avulsion fractures
    Anterior superior iliac spine (ASIS)—sartorius avulsion
    Anterior inferior iliac spine (AIIS)—rectus femoris avulsion
    Ischium—hamstring origin avulsion
    Treatment—symptomatic, crutches, nonoperative
Tumors of the pediatric pelvis, sacrum, coccyx
  Osteoblastoma
  Aneurysmal bone cyst
  Eosinophilic granuloma
  Ewing's sarcoma

LOWER EXTREMITY
Examination and Evaluation

The lower extremity should be examined as a unit in the child with lower-extremity abnormalities
The physical examination should include the hips, thigh, knee, leg, ankle, and foot
Rotational problems
  Rotational problems of the lower extremities include femoral anteversion, tibial torsion, and metatarsus adductus
  Rotational problems may arise as a result of "intrauterine packing" problems (positioning); affected children most commonly present with an in-toeing gait
  Physical examination techniques for rotational problems of the lower extremity (Table 5–4) include
    Foot progression angle—the angle the foot makes with a straight line on the floor during walking (Fig. 5–28)
    Internal rotation—ROM of the hip in the prone position
    External rotation—ROM of the hip in the prone position
    Thigh-foot angle—the angle the foot makes with the thigh with the patient in the prone position and the knee flexed to 90 degrees
    Lateral border of the foot
Leg length discrepancy
  Causes of leg length discrepancy include hemihypertrophy, proximal femoral focal deficiency, developmental dysplasia of the hip, abnormalities of the tibia and fibula, polio, infections involving the growth plate, tumors, and trauma

Table 5–4
ROTATIONAL PROBLEMS OF THE LOWER EXTREMITY (IN-TOEING)

Physical Exam	Femoral Anteversion	Tibial Torsion	Metatarsus Adductus
Hip rotation	Passive internal rotation of the hip is increased (abnormal), and passive external rotation is decreased	Normal	Normal
Thigh-foot axis	Normal	The angle the foot makes with the thigh is decreased (to less than 10 degrees) because of the internal rotation (torsion) of the tibia (and foot)	Normal
Lateral border of the foot	Normal	Normal	Apex lateral angulation (medial side of the foot may have a crease)

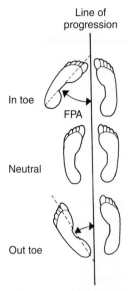

Line of
progression

In toe

FPA

Neutral

Out toe

Figure 5–28 ■ Foot progression angle (FPA) is a useful tool in evaluating rotational problems of the lower extremity.

Long-term problems associated with leg length discrepancy include lower back pain, postural spinal curvatures, equinus contractures of the ankle, and an abnormal gait pattern

The degree of discrepancy can be measured using physical exam techniques and/or radiographic measurements

Estimation of leg length discrepancy

Boys continue to grow until age 16; girls continue to grow until age 14

The proximal femur grows ⅛th of an inch per year until skeletal maturity

The distal femur grows ⅜th of an inch per year until skeletal maturity

The proximal tibia grows ⅝th of an inch per year until skeletal maturity

More precise estimates of growth to maturity can be calculated using the Mosley graphic method or the Green-Anderson method

General treatment guidelines for leg length discrepancies at maturity (or the discrepancy that is predicted at the time of maturity)

Discrepancy less than 2 cm—shoe lift

Discrepancy of 2 to 5 cm—epiphysiodesis of the contralateral unaffected side

Discrepancy greater than 5 cm—leg lengthening using the Ilizarov principles (metaphyseal corticotomy [cutting bone] with distraction osteogenesis at a rate of 1 mm per day), physeal distraction for lengthening can also be accomplished using the technique of **chondrodiastasis,** which allows for distraction across the growth plate with lengthening at this site without a corticotomy

The limping child (Table 5–5)

A thorough, timely evaluation is mandatory

A limp (or inability to walk) may arise as a result of a number of pediatric conditions

The diagnostic work-up of the limping child should include

History

Recent trauma

Fever

Recent infections

Developmental history

Onset of symptoms

Changes in family situations

Physical examination

Observation (walking, sitting)

Inspection (erythema, deformity, swelling, skin changes)

Palpation (masses, crepitus, tenderness, increased warmth, joint effusion)

ROM examination (limited and painful in infectious processes and toxic synovitis)

Laboratory work

Complete blood count (CBC) with differential (mandatory)

ESR (mandatory)

ASO titer (as indicated)

Rheumatoid factor (as indicated)

X-rays

Hip

Other regions of the lower extremity and spine as dictated by physical findings (pain, limitation to ROM, others)

Special studies

Ultrasonography—detects the presence of joint fluid (does not differentiate sterile from septic effusion)

Technetium bone scan—detects bony infection; may also be useful in detecting osteonecrosis of the femoral head (such as in Legg-Calvé-Perthes disease) or bone tumors

Aspiration of joint fluid or from metaphyseal bone—for the work-up of septic arthritis or metaphyseal osteomyelitis

MRI—aids in the diagnosis of discitis or tumors

Table 5–5
POSSIBLE ETIOLOGIES OF THE LIMPING CHILD

Fever Absent	Fever Present
Toxic synovitis	Septic arthritis (hip, knee, ankle)
Fracture	Acute osteomyelitis
Soft tissue injuries	Discitis
Leg length discrepancy	Toxic synovitis
Legg-Calvé-Perthes disease	Fracture
Developmental dysplasia of the hip	Systemic malignancies (such as leukemia)
Slipped capital femoral epiphysis	Acute rheumatic fever
Juvenile rheumatoid arthritis	
Subacute (partially treated) osteomyelitis	
Local tumors (benign or malignant)	
Systemic malignancies (such as leukemia)	
Psychologic disturbances	
Child abuse	
Sexual abuse	
Neuromuscular disorders	

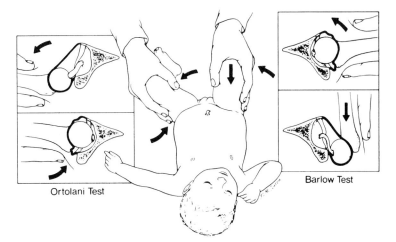

Figure 5–29 ■ Ortolani's and Barlow's tests for developmental dysplasia of the hip. In Ortolani's test, elevation and abduction of the femur relocates a dislocated hip. In Barlow's test, adduction and depression of the femur dislocates a dislocatable hip. (From Sabiston DC Jr: Essentials of Surgery. Philadelphia, WB Saunders, 1987, p 776.)

Ortolani Test

Barlow Test

The Pediatric Hip

Developmental dysplasia of the hip (DDH)
  Previously known as congenital dysplasia of the hip (CDH)
  Represents aberrant development of the hip resulting from capsular laxity
  Commonly associated with dislocation of the hip
  DDH is commonly associated with other "uterine packing" problems such as metatarsus adductus and torticollis
  DDH includes a spectrum of complete dislocation, hip subluxation, hip instability, and hip dysplasia
  DDH occurs more commonly in the left hip, in females, and in those with a positive family history
  Three phases of DDH are commonly recognized
    Dislocated hip
    Dislocatable hip
    Subluxatable hip
  Diagnosis of DDH (Fig. 5–29)
    Ortolani's test—elevation and abduction of the femur relocates a dislocated hip
    Barlow's test—adduction and depression of the femur dislocates a dislocatable hip
    Galeazzi's sign—asymmetry of the lower extremities demonstrated with the knees flexed and the feet together; the knee on the affected side will be lower (Fig. 5–30)
  Physical examination of the newborn hip is essential, and repeat examinations in the infant are important
  Radiographic examination is helpful in the symptomatic child older than 3 months (Fig. 5–31)
  Other useful tests include arthrography and ultrasonography
  Treatment of DDH (Table 5–6)
    Reconstructive osteotomies of the femur or pelvis may be necessary in the older child with DDH
    Pelvic osteotomies include Salter, Steel, Sutherland, Dial, Pemberton, and Chiari
Congenital coxa vara (Fig. 5–33)
  Represents a decreased neck shaft angle caused by a defect in the ossification of the femoral neck

The child may have a painless waddling gait or limp
Less severe cases correct spontaneously, but many cases require operative reconstruction
Legg-Calvé-Perthes disease (Fig. 5–34)
  Noninflammatory deformity of the weight-bearing surface of the femoral head
  Arises as a result of a vascular insult or abnormality
  The vascular insult leads to osteonecrosis of the proximal femoral epiphysis
  Most commonly presents in boys 4 to 8 years of age
  Symptoms include pain in the hip **or knee** and decreased ROM of the hip (particularly limited abduction and internal rotation)
  Can occur bilaterally
  Differential diagnosis includes septic arthritis, epiphyseal dysplasia, blood dyscrasias, and hypothyroidism
  The pathologic process includes necrosis of bone, followed by revascularization and resorption of bone via creeping substitution that allows for remodeling

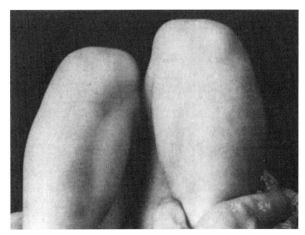

Figure 5–30 ■ Galeazzi's sign. Comparison of the relative heights of the femoral condyles by holding the hips in flexion. In this example, the right femur appears shorter because of a right hip dislocation. (From Sabiston DC Jr: Essentials of Surgery. Philadelphia, WB Saunders, 1987, p 777.)

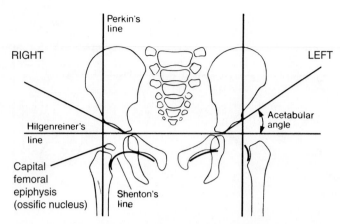

Figure 5–31 ■ Radiographic features of developmental dysplasia of the hip. In this example, the left hip is dislocated and the right hip is normal. There is a delay in ossification of the left capital femoral epiphysis. **Shenton's line,** a smooth continuation of an imaginary line drawn along the inferior aspect of the femoral neck and superior margin of the obturator foramen, is normal on the right side but is interrupted in the dysplastic left hip. **Hilgenreiner's line** is a horizontal line that connects the two triradiate cartilages. **Perkin's line** is a line drawn perpendicular to Hilgenreiner's line that passes through the superolateral edge of the acetabulum. In the normal right hip, the ossific nucleus lies in the inferomedial quadrant defined by the intersection of these lines. The ossific nucleus in a dysplastic hip can be absent (shown here on the left) or displaced from the inferomedial quadrant. The **acetabular angle** is measured at the intersection of Hilgenreiner's line and a line drawn from the triradiate cartilage to the lateral edge of the acetabulum. This angle defines the shape of the bony acetabulum and is normally less than 25 degrees. (Modified from Sabiston DC Jr: Essentials of Surgery. Philadelphia, WB Saunders, 1987, p 777.)

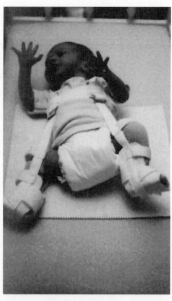

Figure 5–32 ■ The Pavlik harness is a dynamic splint that directs the femoral head toward the acetabulum and promotes concentric reduction of the hip over time. (From Tachdjian MO: Pediatric Orthopedics, 2nd ed. Philadelphia, WB Saunders, 1990, vol 1, p 331.)

Radiographic findings vary with the stage of disease; different staging systems have been defined by Caterall and by Salter-Thompson

Salter-Thompson stage A—no involvement of the lateral pillar of the femoral head; prognosis generally good

Salter-Thompson stage B—lateral pillar of the femoral head is involved; prognosis generally poor

The **crescent sign** represents a pathologic fracture with collapse of subchondral bone in the resorbing femoral head (see Chapter 3)

Treatment of Legg-Calvé-Perthes disease

The goal in treating Legg-Calvé-Perthes disease is to maintain the sphericity of the femoral head

Radiographic findings associated with a poor prognosis have been described by Caterall ("head at risk" signs) and include

Lateral calcification

Gage's sign (V-shaped lateral defect)

Lateral subluxation

Metaphyseal cysts

Horizontal growth plate

Treatment for Caterall stage I and stage II disease (Salter-Thompson stage A) is usually observation

Treatment for Caterall stage III and stage IV (Salter-Thompson stage B) is early ROM followed by containment of the femoral head

Table 5–6
TREATMENT OF DEVELOPMENTAL DYSPLASIA OF THE HIP

Hip Abnormality	Findings	Treatment
Newborn		
Dislocated	Positive Ortolani's test	Pavlik harness (Fig. 5–32)
Dislocatable	Positive Barlow's test	Pavlik harness (Fig. 5–32)
Subluxatable	Barlow's test rides up edge	Supportive/Pavlik harness (Fig. 5–32)
<6 Months Old		
Dislocatable/reducible	Positive Ortolani's test	Pavlik harness (Fig. 5–32)
Unreducible	Negative Ortolani's test	Pavlik harness (Fig. 5–32), traction, closed reduction
≥6 Months Old		
Unreducible	Negative Ortolani's test	Traction and closed reduction
Failed closed reduction	Medial dye pool >5 mm on arthrography	Operative tratement
>3 Years Old		
Dislocated	Trendelenburg gait, leg asymmetry (Galeazzi's sign)	Operative treatment

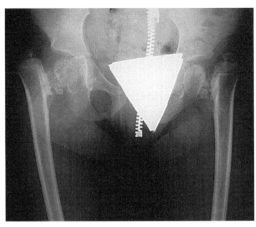

Figure 5–33 ■ Radiograph of patient with bilateral congenital coxa vara. (Courtesy of Joseph J. Gugenheim, MD, Fondren Orthopedic Group LLP, Texas Orthopedic Hospital, Houston, Texas.)

within the acetabulum using an abduction brace or surgery

Slipped capital femoral epiphysis (SCFE)

The femoral head remains in the acetabulum, and the neck displaces through the growth plate in the anterior direction

Caused by weakness of the perichondrial ring and a slip through the hypertrophic zone of the developing growth plate

SCFE is most commonly seen in obese, African American adolescent boys

It is more common in individuals with a positive family history

Bilateral involvement is not uncommon

SCFE is also associated with hypothyroidism and renal disease

Patients present with hip or knee pain and an externally rotated lower extremity with decreased ROM of the hip (internal rotation is particularly limited)

Radiographs show the slip, which is classified

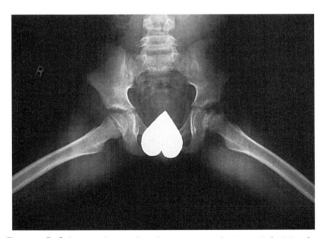

Figure 5–34 ■ Radiograph of patient with Legg-Calvé-Perthes disease of the left hip. (Courtesy of Joseph J. Gugenheim, MD, Fondren Orthopedic Group LLP, Texas Orthopedic Hospital, Houston, Texas.)

based on the degree of slippage and best seen on the frog-leg lateral view (Fig. 5–35)

Grade I—0% to 33% slip

Grade II—33% to 50% slip

Grade III—greater than 50% slip

Treatment is in situ pinning across the capital femoral epiphysis to prevent further slippage

Proximal femoral focal deficiency (PFFD)

A developmental defect of the proximal femur

The child is born with a short, bulky thigh

Deformities include flexion, abduction, and external rotation of the thigh

PFFD is commonly associated with coxa vara and fibula hemimelia

Proximal femoral deficiency has been classified into four classes by Aiken

Class A—femoral head present, acetabulum normal, short femur, at maturity the femoral shaft and femoral head are connected

Class B—femoral head present, acetabulum normal or nearly normal, short femur, at maturity the femoral shaft and femoral head are not connected

Class C—femoral head absent or nearly absent, acetabulum severely dysplastic, short femur

Class D—femoral head absent, acetabulum absent, short deformed femur

Treatment is based on the degree of leg length discrepancy, extent of hip bony abnormality, condition of the proximal thigh musculature, degree of femoral rotation, and amount of hip joint stability

Excessive femoral anteversion (Fig. 5–36)

Normally, the femoral neck and head sit 15 to 25 degrees anterior of the horizontal (where the horizontal would be neutral version) and therefore are said to be anteverted

Excessive femoral anteversion is a condition in which the femoral neck and head have abnormal version in the anterior direction (greater than 25 degrees)

Patients with excessive femoral anteversion have an internal rotation deformity of the femur that is seen most commonly in 3- to 6-year-olds (an easy way to remember or to understand this is the following logic: If the femoral neck and head have excessive femoral anteversion, the femur must internally rotate because the femoral head is located within the acetabulum)

Physical exam shows increased internal rotation and decreased external rotation of the lower extremity with an in-toeing gait and internally rotated patellas

Children with excessive femoral anteversion commonly sit in the "W" position

This condition most commonly spontaneously corrects by age 10 years

Femoral retroversion (see Fig. 5–36)

These individuals present with increased external rotation and decreased internal rotation of the lower extremity

Toxic (transient) synovitis of the hip

Joint pain from a nonbacterial infectious process

Etiology unknown

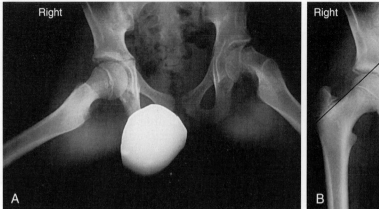

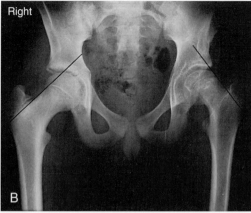

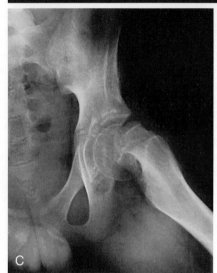

Figure 5–35 ■ Radiographs showing slipped capital femoral epiphysis. *A,* Frog-leg lateral radiograph of a patient with bilateral slipped capital femoral epiphyses: the right is mild; the left is severe. *B,* AP radiograph of the pelvis of a patient with a unilateral slipped capital femoral epiphysis of the left hip that is severe; the right hip is normal as indicated by Klein's line. Klein's line is drawn along the lateral margin of the femoral neck. In the normal right hip the line intersects the lateral portion of the femoral head. In the left hip the line does not intersect the femoral head (indicating displacement between the femoral neck and head) and is diagnostic of a slipped capital femoral epiphysis. *C,* A frog-leg lateral radiograph of the left hip of the patient shown in *B* shows the degree of anterior displacement of the femoral neck on the femoral head through the growth plate. (Courtesy of Joseph J. Gugenheim, MD, and Howard R. Epps, MD, Fondren Orthopedic Group LLP, Texas Orthopedic Hospital, Houston, Texas.)

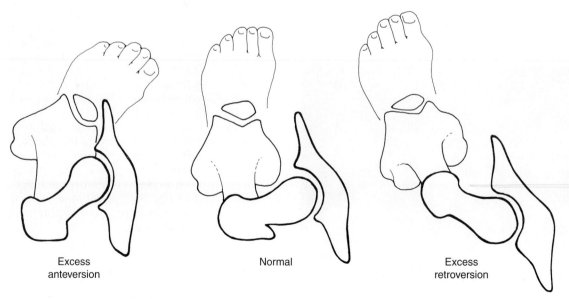

Excess anteversion   Normal   Excess retroversion

Figure 5–36 ■ Excess femoral anteversion and retroversion, as viewed from superior to inferior.

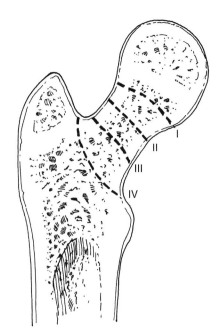

Figure 5–37 ■ Femoral neck fracture classification in children. Type I, transepiphyseal; type II, transcervical; type III, cervical-trochanteric; and type IV, intertrochanteric.

Possibly related to a viral infection, allergic reaction, trauma

Onset can be acute or insidious

ESR typically less than 20

Most commonly affects the hip joint (may also affect other joints such as the knee or shoulder)

Must rule out a septic joint

Diagnosis is made by exclusion of other underlying causes

Treatment—observation

Traumatic injuries of the pediatric hip

Femoral neck fractures

Classification (Fig. 5–37)

Type I—transepiphyseal

Type II—transcervical

Type III—cervical-trochanteric

Type IV—intertrochanteric

Treatment—operative reduction and pinning (except nondisplaced type III and type IV fractures, which can be treated with a spica cast)

Complications—osteonecrosis (increased risk with more proximal and more displaced fractures)

Hip dislocations

Classification—posterior (more common), anterior

Treatment—closed reduction

Complications—greater trochanteric fractures, osteonecrosis of the femoral head

Tumors of the pediatric hip

Osteoid osteoma

Fibrous dysplasia

The Pediatric Thigh

Psoas abscess—from tuberculosis

Traumatic injuries of the pediatric thigh

Femoral shaft fractures (Fig. 5–38)

Treatment—based on age (Fig. 5–39)

0–2 yr	Spica cast
2–10 yr	Traction followed by a spica cast
10–15 yr	90-90 skeletal traction or ORIF versus external fixation, especially for those with polytrauma or closed head injury (who tolerate traction poorly)
>15 yr	Intramedullary nail fixation

Complications—leg length discrepancy, malalignment

Tumors of the pediatric thigh

Osteosarcoma

Aneurysmal bone cyst

Fibrous dysplasia

Eosinophilic granuloma

Ewing's sarcoma

The Pediatric Knee

During normal development there is a progression between the ages of 0 and 2½ years from bow legs (genu varum) to knock knees (genu valgum); between 2½ and 4 years there is a progression from excessive genu valgus to a normal (physiologic) valgus of 5 to 7 degrees (Fig. 5–40)

Genu varum (bow legs) (Fig. 5–41)

Commonly seen in children younger than 2 years of age **(physiologic genu varum)**

Pathologic conditions that cause genu varum (nonphysiologic genu varum) include OI, osteochondromas, bone dysplasias, trauma, and (most commonly) Blount disease

Blount disease (tibia vara) (Fig. 5–42)

Pathologic (nonphysiologic) genu varum

Represents a disorder of the posterior/medial tibial physis

Occurs most commonly in obese African American males

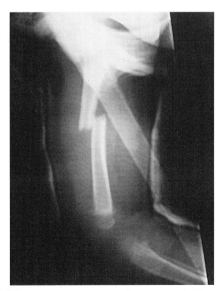

Figure 5–38 ■ Femoral shaft fracture in a child. (Courtesy of Gary T. Brock, MD, Fondren Orthopedic Group LLP, Texas Orthopedic Hospital, Houston, Texas.)

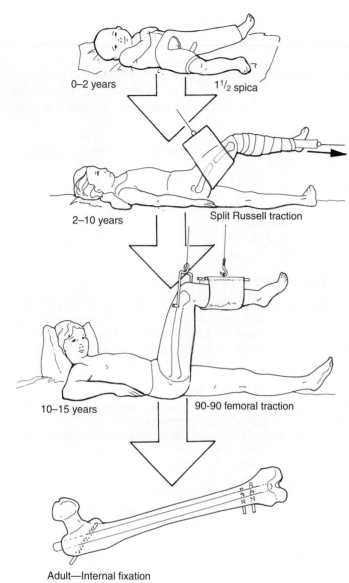

0–2 years   1¹/₂ spica

2–10 years   Split Russell traction

10–15 years   90-90 femoral traction

Adult—Internal fixation

Figure 5–39 ■ The treatment of pediatric femur fractures is based on the age of the patient.

The deformity in Blount disease is progressive and does not correct spontaneously (as compared with physiologic bowing, which does correct with age)

The diagnosis of Blount disease is made based on x-ray measurements

Drennan angle of greater than 11 degrees is abnormal

Tibiofemoral angle of greater than 32 degrees is abnormal

Genu valgum (knock knees)

Up to 15 degrees of knee valgum may be normal in the child of 2 to 6 years of age

Pathologic genu valgum may be associated with renal osteodystrophy, tumors, infections, or trauma

Osteochondritis dissecans (see Chapter 19)

Intra-articular lesion of the knee involving a loose fragment of cartilage and subchondral bone

May affect joints other than the knee, but the knee is the most often affected

Most commonly seen in children 10 to 15 years of age

The lesion is caused by trauma, ischemia, or abnormal epiphyseal ossification

The most common site in the knee is the medial femoral condyle

Symptoms include pain related to activity, with stiffness and swelling and occasional locking and popping

The best radiographic view on which to see the lesion is the **notch view**

Treatment is based on the size and location of the lesion, the age and skeletal maturity of the patient, and the symptoms

Osgood-Schlatter disease

Represents osteochondritis or fatigue failure of the apophysis of the tibial tubercle

Arises from stress on the tibial tubercle apophysis from the extensor mechanism in the rapidly growing adolescent

Discoid meniscus

Abnormal development of the lateral meniscus leads to a disc-shaped (rather than a crescent-shaped) meniscus (see Chapter 19)

Traumatic injuries of the pediatric knee

Distal femoral physeal fractures and proximal tibial physeal fractures

Salter-Harris classification

Treatment

Types I and II—closed reduction and casting

Types III and IV—closed reduction/percutaneous pinning

***Note:* Distal femoral physeal fractures require an absolute anatomic reduction**

Complications—neurovascular (popliteal artery, peroneal nerve), growth plate injury

Tibial tuberosity fractures

Classification—types I, II, and III (Fig. 5–43)

Treatment

Types I and II—closed reduction with the knee in extension

Type III—often requires ORIF

Complications—genu recurvatum, loss of motion, patella alta

Tibial intercondylar eminence fractures (see Chapter 19)

Classification—types I, II, and III

Treatment

Types I and II—closed reduction with the knee in extension

Type III—require ORIF, especially if the fragment is rotated

Complications—loss of full extension, late anterior cruciate ligament (ACL) laxity

Patellar sleeve fractures

Classification—superior or inferior pole (Fig. 5–44)

Treatment

Cylinder cast for nondisplaced fractures

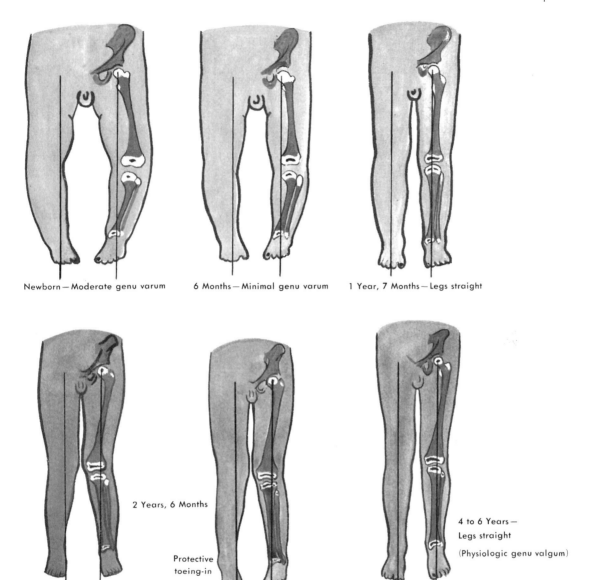

Newborn—Moderate genu varum   6 Months—Minimal genu varum   1 Year, 7 Months—Legs straight

2 Years, 6 Months

Protective toeing-in

4 to 6 Years—
Legs straight

(Physiologic genu valgum)

Figure 5–40 ■ The physiologic evolution of the alignment of the lower limbs at various stages of childhood. (From Tachdjian MO: Pediatric Orthopedics, 2nd ed. Philadelphia, WB Saunders, 1990, vol 4, p 2821.)

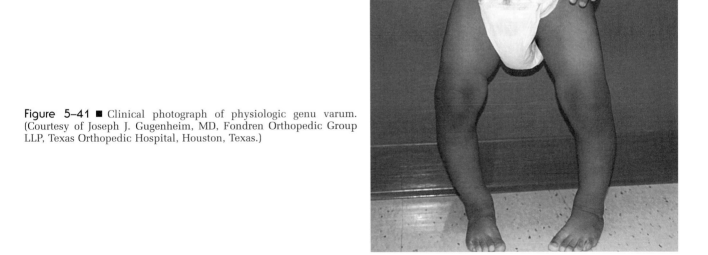

Figure 5–41 ■ Clinical photograph of physiologic genu varum. (Courtesy of Joseph J. Gugenheim, MD, Fondren Orthopedic Group LLP, Texas Orthopedic Hospital, Houston, Texas.)

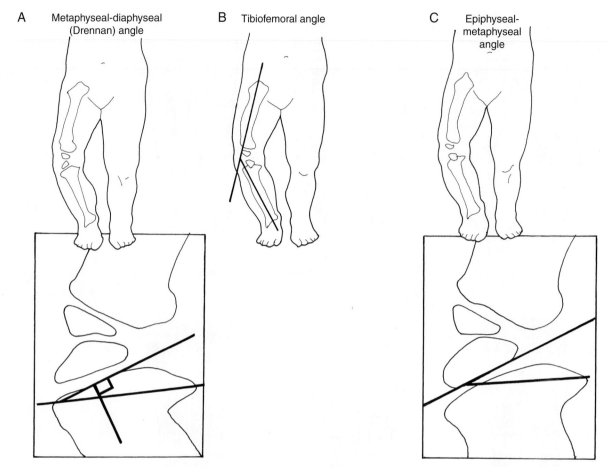

Figure 5–42 ■ Three different methods of measuring genu varum. *A*, Metaphyseal-diaphyseal (Drennan) angle: angle formed by a line drawn perpendicular to the longitudinal axis of the tibia and another drawn through the two beaks of the metaphysis. Normal is ≤11 degrees. *B*, Tibiofemoral angle: angle formed by a line drawn along the longitudinal axis of the tibia and a line drawn along the longitudinal axis of the femur. Normal is ≤32 degrees. *C*, Epiphyseal-metaphyseal angle: angle formed by the intersection of a line drawn through the epiphysis and a line drawn from the midpoint of the epiphysis and the tip of the medial metaphyseal beak.

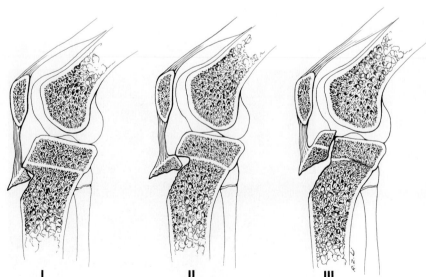

Figure 5–43 ■ Tibial tuberosity fractures. (From Tria AJ, Klein KS: An Illustrated Guide to the Knee. New York, Churchill Livingstone, 1992, p 109.)

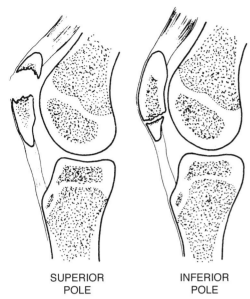

SUPERIOR
POLE

INFERIOR
POLE

Figure 5–44 ■ Patellar sleeve fractures. (From Ogden JA: Skeletal Injury in the Child, 2nd ed. Philadelphia, WB Saunders, 1990, p 762.)

ORIF with tension band wire technique for displaced fractures

Complications

Patella alta, extensor lag (patient cannot fully extend the knee)

Tumors of the pediatric knee

Osteosarcoma

Osteochondroma

Chondroblastoma

Fibrous cortical defect (nonossifying fibroma)

The Pediatric Leg

Tibial torsion

Thought to be rotation of the tibia around the longitudinal axis, but may represent angulation of the tibia in an oblique plane

This is the most common cause of in-toeing in the child

Most commonly presents in the second year of life

Can be associated with metatarsus adductus

Almost always resolves spontaneously with growth

Tibial bowing—three types have been described based on the direction of the apex of the curve

Posteromedial tibial bowing

Represents physiologic bowing

Spontaneous correction almost always occurs, but the patient must be followed to ensure that a leg length discrepancy does not develop

Anteromedial tibial bowing

Most commonly caused by fibula hemimelia (a congenital deficiency of longitudinal growth of the fibula)

Anteromedial tibial bowing is often associated with a significant leg length discrepancy

Anterolateral tibial bowing (Fig. 5–45)

Congenital pseudoarthrosis of the tibia is the most common cause of anterolateral bowing

Congenital pseudoarthrosis of the tibia is very difficult to treat, and the pseudoarthrosis may fail to progress to bony union despite several operative treatments

The classic teaching is that the third operation on individuals with congenital pseudoarthrosis of the tibia should be an amputation (the first two attempts at bony union having failed)

Anterolateral tibial bowing is associated with neurofibromatosis

Tibial hemimelia

Represents a longitudinal deficiency of the tibia

The disorder is inherited through an autosomal dominant pattern

Tibial hemimelia is much less common than fibula hemimelia

Fibula hemimelia

Represents the most common long bone deficiency

Represents the most common skeletal deformity in the leg

Usually associated with anteromedial bowing of the tibia

Commonly associated with ankle instability, equinovarus foot deformities, tarsal coalition, femoral shortening, coxa vara, and proximal femoral focal deficiency

Also commonly associated with a significant leg length discrepancy

Treatment is based on the severity of deformity; treatment options include shoe lifts, bracing, Syme's amputation for severe cases, and lengthening with Ilizarov reconstruction

Traumatic injuries of the pediatric leg

Tibia fractures

Classification

Greenstick, complete, spiral (toddler's fracture), proximal tibial metaphysis (Cozen's fracture)

Treatment—closed reduction and casting

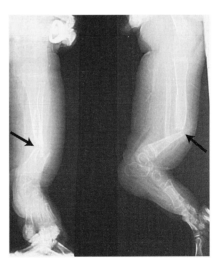

Figure 5–45 ■ AP and lateral radiographs demonstrating anterolateral bowing of the tibia in a child with congenital pseudoarthrosis (*arrow*) of the tibia. (Courtesy of Joseph J. Gugenheim, MD, Fondren Orthopedic Group LLP, Texas Orthopedic Hospital, Houston, Texas.)

Complications
  Valgus deformity is common in proximal tibial metaphyseal (Cozen) fractures; the deformity is usually self-correcting
  Other complications include neurovascular injury, malunion, nonunion
Tumors of the pediatric leg
  Tibia
    Fibrous cortical defect
    Eosinophilic granuloma
    Osteomyelitis
    Ossifying fibroma
    Osteofibrous dysplasia
    Osteoma
    Aneurysmal bone cyst
    Osteosarcoma (periosteal)
    Osteochondroma
    Simple bone cysts
  Fibula
    Ewing's sarcoma
    Ossifying fibroma
    Simple bone cysts
    Osteomyelitis
    Eosinophilic granuloma

The Pediatric Ankle

Ball-and-socket ankle
  Represents abnormal formation of the ankle joint
  Talus is spherical (ball)
  Tibial/fibular articulation is cup-shaped (socket)
  Ball-and-socket ankle deformity usually requires no treatment; however, recognition of the abnormality is important because of its association with tarsal coalition, leg length discrepancies, and ray abnormalities

Traumatic injuries of the pediatric ankle
  Ankle fractures
    Classification (Fig. 5–46) is based on the
      Position of the foot at the time of the injury
      Direction of the force
    Further classification is based on the SH type
    Treatment
      Distal fibula—closed reduction, short-leg walking cast for most injuries
      Distal tibia—SH types I and II injuries are usually treated with closed reduction and immobilization; SH types III and IV injuries require ORIF for displacement of the fragments ≥2 mm
  Other special types of pediatric ankle fractures occur as the child nears maturity (Fig. 5–47)
    Juvenile Tillaux fracture
      SH type III injury of the distal tibial physis usually requires ORIF
    Triplane fracture—three separate bony fragments result from this injury
      Anterolateral physeal fragment
      Major physeal fragment
      Tibial metaphyseal fragment
    These injuries usually require ORIF
Tumors of the pediatric ankle
  Uncommon

The Pediatric Foot

Clubfoot (congenital talipes equinovarus) (Fig. 5–48)
  Foot deformity in the newborn
    Hindfoot deformities of clubfoot
      Inversion
      Equinus (plantar flexion)
    Forefoot deformities of clubfoot

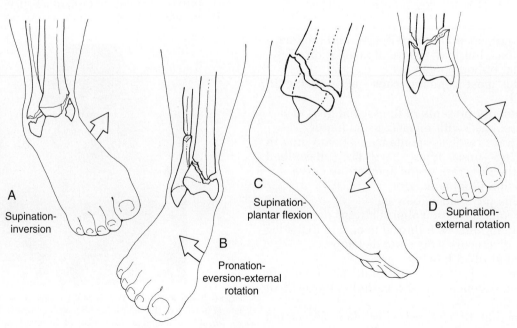

Figure 5–46 ■ Classification of physeal injuries of the distal tibia and fibula. *A*, Supination-inversion. *B*, Pronation-eversion-external rotation. *C*, Supination-plantar flexion. *D*, Supination-external rotation.

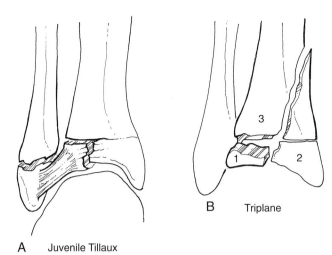

A   Juvenile Tillaux   B   Triplane

Figure 5–47 ■ Special types of ankle fractures that occur in adolescents. *A*, Juvenile Tillaux. *B*, Triplane. Note three fragments involved: 1: anterolateral physis (Salter-Harris type III); 2: remaining physis (Salter-Harris type IV); 3: tibial metaphysis.

Inversion
Adduction
Represents the most common and significant congenital foot disorder
Associated with capsular and ligamentous tightness and bony malformations
Radiographic measurements can be helpful in assessing these foot deformities (Fig. 5–49)
Treatment options
Serial manipulation and casting (successful for lesser deformities)
Operative release

Metatarsus adductus (MTA) (Fig. 5–50)
Adduction of the forefoot in the newborn and child
Can be associated with DDH
Lateral border of the foot does not make a straight line
Treatment options
Serial casting
Successful in most cases
May not be successful for severe cases (especially those associated with a medial skin crease of the foot)
Operative release with or without osteotomies for refractory cases
Pes cavus
Elevated arch and fixed plantar flexion of the forefoot
Associated neurologic disorders are common (Charcot-Marie-Tooth disease, Friedreich's ataxia)
Treatment
Observation if the deformity is flexible (corrects with block placed under the lateral aspect of the foot)
Surgical release for nonflexible or refractory cases
Pes planus
Flatfoot
Can be flexible or rigid
Flexible pes planus
More common (especially in children older than 3 years of age)
Corrects (arch restored) when the foot is not bearing weight
Treatment is observation
Rigid pes planus
Causes

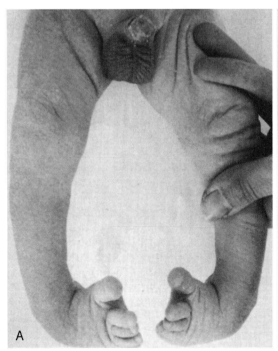
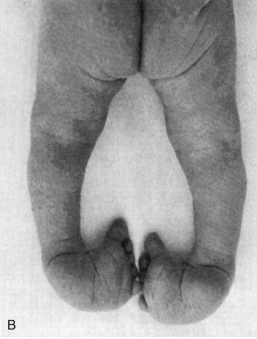

Figure 5–48 ■ Clinical appearance of clubfoot in a newborn. *A*, Front view. *B*, Posterior view. (From Tachdjian MO: Pediatric Orthopedics, 2nd ed. Philadelphia, WB Saunders, 1990, vol 4, p 2449.)

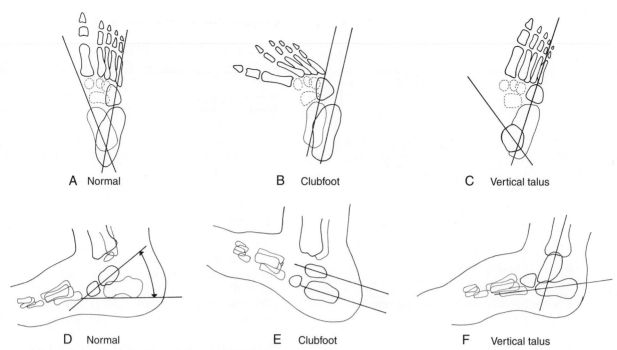

A Normal   B Clubfoot   C Vertical talus

D Normal   E Clubfoot   F Vertical talus

Figure 5–49 ■ Representation of the AP and lateral radiographic appearance of clubfoot and vertical talus. *A*, Normal AP view. *B*, AP view of clubfoot. Note a decreased talocalcaneal angle of less than 20 degrees (0 degrees in this example), with the talus and calcaneal axes parallel. *C*, AP view of congenital vertical talus. Note an increased talocalcaneal angle of greater than 40 degrees. *D*, Normal lateral view. *E*, Dorsiflexed lateral view in clubfoot demonstrates a reduced talocalcaneal angle (the talus and calcaneus are parallel). *F*, Plantarflexed lateral view in vertical talus demonstrates increased tilt to the talus (talus–first metatarsal angle greater than 60 degrees).

Congenital vertical talus
Tarsal coalition
Congenital vertical talus
  Results from an irreducible dorsal dislocation of the navicular on the talus (which locks the talus in a plantarflexed, vertical position) (Fig. 5–51)
  Appearance is that of a "rocker-bottom" foot
  Radiographs may be helpful in making the diagnosis (see Fig. 5–49)
  Treatment
    Corrective casting/manipulative stretching
    Operative soft tissue release/lengthening at 6 to 12 months of age

Tarsal coalition (Fig. 5–52)
  Fibrous, cartilaginous, or bony fusion of two of the tarsal bones
  Calcaneonavicular coalitions are more common than talocalcaneal coalitions

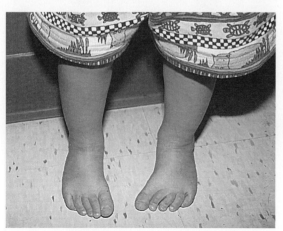

Figure 5–50 ■ Clinical photograph of metatarsus adductus in a 2-year-old child. (Courtesy of Gary T. Brock, MD, Fondren Orthopedic Group LLP, Texas Orthopedic Hospital, Houston, Texas.)

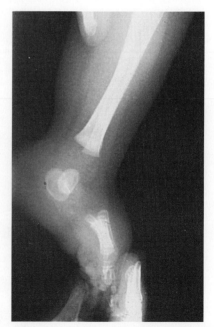

Figure 5–51 ■ Forced plantar flexion radiographic view of a patient with congenital vertical talus. (Courtesy of Joseph J. Gugenheim, MD, Fondren Orthopedic Group LLP, Texas Orthopedic Hospital, Houston, Texas.)

Figure 5–52 ■ Tarsal coalition (calcaneonavicular). *A,* CT scan. *B,* Radiograph, oblique view, demonstrates the coalition (*arrow*). (Courtesy of Gary T. Brock, MD, Fondren Orthopedic Group LLP, Texas Orthopedic Hospital, Houston, Texas.)

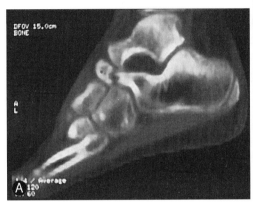

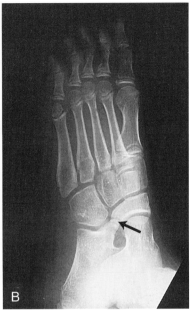

Patient presents with a **rigid flatfoot deformity**
Oblique radiographs are helpful to identify calcaneonavicular coalitions
CT scan is usually needed to diagnose a talocalcaneal coalition
Treatment
    Operative bar resection (early)
    Operative fusion (late)
Juvenile bunions
  Similar to adult bunions
  Higher recurrence rate following surgical correction than for adult bunions
  Delay surgical intervention for as long as possible
Congenital toe disorders
  Similar to the hand
  Surgical release/correction
Toe walkers
  Habitual—typically correct spontaneously 3 to 6 months after onset of childhood walking
  Congenital—can be associated with a tight heel cord or other abnormalities that may require lengthening
Traumatic injuries of the pediatric foot
  Fractures of the talar neck
    Most can be treated with closed reduction (cast in plantar flexion)
    ORIF if the fracture is displaced more than 2 mm or angulated more than 5 degrees
    Osteonecrosis of the talus can occur after fracture because of its tenuous blood supply
  Talar dome osteochondral fractures—ORIF or excise large displaced fragments
  Other foot fractures—treat like adult injuries
Tumors of the pediatric foot
  Enchondroma

CHAPTER 6

Medical Considerations

PERIOPERATIVE PROBLEMS

Pulmonary Problems

General considerations—pulmonary function tests and blood gas measurements are often helpful for evaluating baseline status; thoracic and abdominal surgery can significantly affect these values

Blood gas evaluation—the following is a simple working formula and is useful for evaluating blood gases:

$$Po_2 = 7(Fio_2) - Pco_2$$

where Po_2 is the **anticipated or normal Po_2** for a given Fio_2 in a normal individual; Fio_2 is the percent inspired oxygen; and Pco_2 is the value obtained by the blood gas assay

Example: a 71-year-old woman has acute onset of shortness of breath 12 hours after a total hip arthroplasty. When you arrive at her bed she has a face mask on with an inspired oxygen (Fio_2) of 80%; using our working formula the anticipated, or normal, Po_2 for a normal individual would be

$$Po_2 = 7(80) - Pco_2 = 560 - Pco_2$$

Now let us assume that a blood gas assay (blood obtained 15 minutes after placing the patient on 80% oxygen) reveals the following **observed values:**

$$Po_2 = 130$$
$$Pco_2 = 70$$

With a Pco_2 of 70, the anticipated, or normal, Po_2 would be

$$Po_2 = 560 - 70 = 490$$

Therefore, for the patient on 80% oxygen with a Pco_2 of 70 we would anticipate a Po_2 of 490 if all were normal. Because the observed Po_2 is only 130, there is obviously a problem with this patient's pulmonary status. To quantify the extent of the patient's problem we must next calculate the alveolar-arterial **(Aa) gradient:**

Aa gradient = (anticipated or normal Po_2
                [for a given Fio_2]) − (observed Po_2)

Continuing with the example:

$$\text{Aa gradient} = 490 - 130 = 360$$

Finally, the percent physiologic shunt may be calculated as follows:

Percent physiologic shunt = Aa gradient/20

Continuing with the example:

Percent physiologic shunt = 360/20 = 18%

Thromboembolism—a common problem in orthopaedic patients, especially in those with procedures around the hip

Risk increases with a history of prior thromboembolism, obesity, malignancy, aging, congestive heart failure (CHF), use of birth control pills, varicose veins, smoking, use of general anesthetics (in contrast to continuous epidural anesthesia, which has a lower incidence of thromboemboli), increased blood viscosity, immobilization, paralysis, and pregnancy

Pulmonary embolism (PE)

Pulmonary embolism should be suspected in postoperative patients with acute onset of pleuritic pain, tachypnea (present in 90% of patients with a PE), and tachycardia (present in 60% of patients with a PE)

Initial work-up includes electrocardiogram (ECG) (right bundle-branch block, right axis deviation in 25%; may also show ST depression or T-wave inversion in lead III), chest radiograph (which is often normal), and arterial blood gases (ABGs) (a normal Pao_2 does not exclude a PE)

Nuclear medicine ventilation-perfusion (V/Q) scan may be helpful, but pulmonary angiography (the "gold standard") is required to make the diagnosis if there is any question

Heparin therapy (continuous intravenous [IV] infusion) is initiated for the patient with a documented PE and is monitored by the partial thromboplastin time (PTT); more aggressive therapy (thrombolytic agents, vena cava interruption, and other surgical measures) is usually not required; 7 to 10 days of heparin therapy is followed by 3 months of oral warfarin (Coumadin) (monitored by the prothrombin time [PT])

Approximately 700,000 people in the United States

have an asymptomatic PE each year, of which 200,000 are fatal

The most important factor for survival is early diagnosis with prompt therapy initiation

Coagulation—a cascading sequence of enzymatic reactions that begins with prothrombin-converting activity and concludes with the formation of a **fibrin clot** (as fibrinogen is converted to fibrin); two interconnecting pathways have been described

Intrinsic pathway—monitored by the **PTT**; pathway is activated when factor XII makes contact with the collagen of damaged vessels

Extrinsic pathway—monitored by the **PT**; pathway is activated by release of thromboplastin into the circulation secondary to cellular injury

The **bleeding time test** measures platelet function; the fibrinolytic system is responsible for dissolving clots; plasminogen is converted to plasmin (with the help of tissue activators, factor XIIa, and thrombin); plasmin dissolves the fibrin clot

Adult respiratory distress syndrome (ARDS)

Acute respiratory failure secondary to pulmonary edema after trauma, shock, infection

Etiologies of ARDS include pulmonary infection, sepsis, fat embolism, microembolism, aspiration, fluid overload, atelectasis, oxygen toxicity, pulmonary contusion, and head injury

Tachypnea, dyspnea, hypoxemia, and decreased lung compliance are manifestations of ARDS

The clinical diagnosis of ARDS after a long-bone fracture is best made using ABGs

Normal supportive care is often unsuccessful, and a 50% mortality rate is not uncommon

Ventilation with positive end-expiratory pressure (PEEP) is important; steroids have not been proven to be efficacious

Early stabilization of long-bone fractures (particularly the femur) decreases the risk of pulmonary complications

Fat embolism

Usually seen 24 to 72 hours after trauma (3% to 4% of patients with long-bone fractures)

Fatal in 10% to 15% of cases

Onset may be heralded by tachypnea, tachycardia, mental status changes, and upper-extremity petechiae

May be caused by bone marrow fat (**mechanical theory**), chylomicron changes as a result of stress (**metabolic theory**), or both

Metabolism to free fatty acids, initiation of the clotting cascade, pulmonary capillary leakage, bronchoconstriction, and alveolar collapse result in a **ventilation-perfusion mismatch** (hypoxemia) consistent with ARDS

Treatment includes mechanical ventilation with **high levels of PEEP**; steroids do not appear to have a prophylactic role

Prevention with early fracture stabilization is key

Pneumonia

Postoperative pneumonia is best avoided with early mobilization of the patient (out of bed) and aggressive modalities (incentive spirometry, aerosol

treatments, respiratory therapy, chest percussion, and others) in older, sicker patients

Aspiration pneumonia can occur in patients with decreased mentation, supine positioning, and decreased gastrointestinal (GI) motility; simple preventive measures such as raising the head of the bed and using antacids and metoclopramide (Reglan) can help to avoid problems

Other Medical Problems (Nonpulmonary)

Deep venous thrombosis (DVT)

Clinical suspicion is more helpful than the physical examination findings (pain, swelling, Homans' sign) for making the diagnosis of a DVT

Useful studies include venography (the "gold standard"), which is 97% accurate (70% for iliac veins); indium-labeled fibrinogen (operative site artifact causes false positives); impedance plethysmography (poor sensitivity); duplex ultrasonography (B-mode)—90% accurate for DVT proximal to the trifurcation vessels (popliteal vein and proximal); and Doppler imaging (immediate bedside tool, often best for the first study)

Prophylaxis is the most important factor in decreasing morbidity from a DVT and mortality from thromboemboli (PE) (Table 6–1)

The anticoagulation effects of warfarin can be reversed with vitamin K or more rapidly with fresh frozen plasma

The treatment of DVT postoperatively requires initiation of heparin therapy (followed by later conversion to long-term [3 months] warfarin therapy)

Treatment is recommended for all thigh DVTs; however, treatment of DVTs occurring below the popliteal fossa is controversial

Preoperative identification of a DVT in a patient with lower-extremity trauma is an indication for placement of a **vena cava filter**

Virchow's triad of factors involved in venous thrombosis are **stasis, hypercoagulability, and intimal injury**

Postoperative fever

Fever in the postoperative patient is most commonly the result of one of the **five Ws**

Wind—atelectasis or pneumonia—most commonly seen on postoperative days 1 to 3

Water—urinary tract infection—most commonly seen on postoperative days 3 to 5

Wound—surgical wound infection—most commonly seen on postoperative days 5 to 7

Wonder drugs—a thorough review of all medications should be undertaken in the patient who continues to have a fever 1 week postoperatively without an obvious source; the fever might be the result of a drug reaction

Walking—fever from a DVT can occur at any time after surgery

Nutrition—adequate nutrition should be ensured before elective surgery

Malnutrition may be present in 50% of patients on a surgical ward; several indicators of nutritional

Table 6–1
THROMBOEMBOLISM PROPHYLAXIS

Method	Effect	Advantages	Disadvantages
Heparin			
Intravenous	Coagulation cascade—antithrombin III	Reversible, effective	Control, embolization
Subcutaneous	Antithrombin III inhibitor	Reversible	No effect in extremity surgery
Warfarin	Coagulation cascade—vitamin K	Most effective, oral	3–5 days to full effect; control-limited efficacy
Aspirin	Inhibits platelet aggregation	Easy, no monitoring	Limited efficacy
Dextran	Dilutional	Effective	Fluid overload, bleeding
Pneumatic compression (and foot pumps)	Mechanical	Inexpensive, no bleeding	Bulky
Enoxaparin (Lovenox), a low-molecular-weight heparin	Inhibits clotting—forms complexes between antithrombin III and factors IIa and Xa	Fixed dose, no monitoring	Bleeding

status exist (e.g., anergy panels, albumin levels, transferrin level); **arm muscle circumference measurement is the best indicator of nutritional status**

Wound dehiscence and infection, pneumonia, and sepsis can result from poor nutrition

Nutritional requirements are significantly elevated as a result of stress, such as in patients with musculoskeletal injuries and those undergoing an operative procedure

Myocardial infarction (MI)

Acute chest pain, radiation of pain, and ECG changes are classic and warrant monitoring in an appropriate critical care environment where cardiac enzymes and the ECG can be monitored on a continuous basis

Risk factors of MI include increased age, smoking, elevated cholesterol, hypertension, aortic stenosis, a history of coronary artery disease, and a variety of other factors

GI complications

Can range from ileus (treated with nasogastric suction [NG tube] and antacids) to upper GI bleeding

Postoperative ileus is common in diabetic patients with neuropathy

Upper GI bleeding is more likely in patients with a history of ulcers, nonsteroidal anti-inflammatory drug (NSAID) use, and smoking; treatment includes lavage, antacids, and histamine$_2$-blockers

Decubitus ulcers

Associated with advanced age, critical illness, and neurologic impairment

Common sites include the sacrum, heels, and buttocks, which may be a source of infection and increased morbidity

Prevention, with constant changing of position, special mattresses, and treatment of systemic illness and malnutrition, is essential

Once a decubitus ulcer is established, débridement and sometimes soft tissue flaps are required for treatment

Urinary tract

Urine output is normally ≥30 cc/hr

Decreased urine output (oliguria) can result from

Urinary retention

Urethral strictures

Prostatic obstruction

Conditions that lead to decreased production of urine

Hypovolemia

Acute tubular necrosis

Narcotic overdose (such as postoperative pain medication)

Congestive heart failure

Others

Polyuria (urine output >3000 cc/day)

Differential diagnosis

Diabetes mellitus

Overhydration

Syndrome of inappropriate antidiuretic hormone secretion (SIADH)—occurs most commonly after major surgery with significant blood loss

Urinary tract infection (UTI)

Most common nosocomial infection (6% to 8%)

Causes increased risk for joint sepsis after total joint arthroplasty

Established UTIs should be adequately treated preoperatively

Prostatic hypertrophy

Causes postoperative urinary retention

If the history, physical examination (prostate), and urine flow studies (<17 cc/sec peak flow rate) are suggestive, urologic referral should be accomplished preoperatively

Acute tubular necrosis—can cause renal failure in trauma patients; alkalization of the urine is important during the early treatment of this disorder

Genitourinary injury

NSAIDs can affect the kidney, and appropriate screening laboratory tests are required at regular intervals

Shock—capillary blood flow is insufficient for the perfusion of vital tissues and organs

There are four types of shock

Hypovolemic shock (volume loss)—decreased cardiac output (CO), increased peripheral vascular resistance (PVR), venous constriction

Cardiogenic shock (ineffective pumping)—decreased CO, increased PVR, venous dilation

Vasogenic shock (PE or pericardial tamponade)—arteriolar constriction, venous dilation

Neurogenic shock/septic shock (blood pooling)—arteriolar, capillary, and venous dilation

The preferred initial fluid for hypovolemic shock is Ringer's lactate; for patients in shock with a suboptimal response to Ringer's lactate, add blood transfusion; massive blood replacement requires concomitant fresh frozen plasma and platelets

The best indicator of the adequacy of fluid resuscitation is urine output

Patients with inadequate fluid resuscitation show decreased urine output as well as metabolic acidosis on ABGs

Transfusion—because of the possibility of disease transmission, transfusion has become an important issue

Transfusion reactions—include allergic, febrile, and hemolytic reactions

Allergic reactions—most common; occur toward the end of transfusions; symptoms include chills, pruritus, erythema, and urticaria; symptoms usually subside spontaneously; pretreatment with diphenhydramine (Benadryl) and hydrocortisone may be appropriate in patients with a history of allergic reactions

Febrile reactions—also common; occur after the initial 100 to 300 cc of packed red blood cells (RBCs) have been transfused; chills and fever are caused by antibodies to foreign white blood cells (WBCs); treatment is similar to that for an allergic reaction

Hemolytic reactions—less common but most serious; they occur early in the transfusion with symptoms that include chills, fever, tachycardia, chest tightness, and flank pain; treatment includes stopping the transfusion, administering IV fluids, performing appropriate laboratory studies; and monitoring in an intensive care setting

Transfusion risks—include transmission of hepatitis (hepatitis C [2% to 3%] and hepatitis B [<1%]); cytomegalovirus (highest incidence but not clinically important); human T-cell lymphotropic virus type I and human immunodeficiency virus; donor deferral for high-risk individuals and more effective screening methods are decreasing these risks

Alternatives to homologous blood transfusion

Autologous deposition—requires a hemoglobin level of approximately 11 (and a hematocrit of 33%) and some lead time; iron supplementation during donation is routine; allows storage of several units before elective procedures when significant blood loss is anticipated; most donations significantly reduce the risk of developing hepatitis C

Cell-saver—intraoperative autotransfusion; usually requires 400 cc of blood loss to recover 1 unit (250 cc)

Autotranfusion—allows postoperative drainage recovery and use

Acute preoperative normovolemic hemodilution—allows storage of autologous blood (replace with crystalloid) immediately preoperatively for use intraoperatively and postoperatively

Pharmacologic intervention—alternatives including desmopressin (antidiuretic hormone [ADH] analogue that increases levels of plasma factor VIII), recombinant erythropoietin (stimulates erythrogenesis), and synthetic erythrocyte substitutes

Judicious use of blood products—**platelet transfusion** with massive bleeding or coagulopathies is performed based on clinical parameters rather than set platelet thresholds; **fresh frozen plasma** is reserved for patients with massive bleeding and significantly abnormal coagulation tests; **cryoprecipitate** is used for hemophilia (with less exposure than factor concentrates) and as a source of fibrinogen for consumptive coagulopathies

DIFFERENTIAL DIAGNOSIS OF COMMON SIGNS AND SYMPTOMS

Fever

Atelectasis
Pneumonia
UTI
Wound infection
Cellulitis
Drug reaction
Sepsis
DVT

Chest Pain

Referred from the abdomen
PE
MI
Pneumothorax
Pneumonia

Shortness of Breath/Tachypnea

Atelectasis
PE
MI
Pneumothorax
Pneumonia
Fat embolism
ARDS
CHF (from myocardial dysfunction or fluid overload)
Postoperative pain/anxiety

Tachycardia

Postoperative fever
Atelectasis

MI
PE
Fat embolism
Atrial arrhythmias (such as supraventricular tachy-
    cardia)

Bradycardia

MI
Vasovagal reaction
Electrolyte abnormalities
Drug toxicity (such as β-blockers, digitalis, or calcium
    channel blockers)
Pericardial tamponade
Cerebrovascular accident
Pacemaker failure

Elevated Blood Pressure

Postoperative pain
Essential hypertension
Pheochromocytoma
Cushing's syndrome
Multiple endocrine neoplasias (MENs)
Renal artery thrombosis
Unknown coarctation of the aorta

Low Blood Pressure

Bleeding
Hypovolemia
Shock
Sepsis
MI
Pneumothorax
Drug toxicity (such as overdose of anesthesia or pain
    medications)
Fat embolism
Supraventricular tachycardia
Adrenal crisis

Decreased Urinary Output

Hypovolemia
MI
Pericardial tamponade
Acute tubular necrosis
CHF
Fat embolism

Urinary Retention

Narcotic overdose
Urethral stricture
Prostatic obstruction

Pedal Edema

CHF (from myocardial dysfunction)
Fluid overload
DVT
Postoperative swelling
Compartment syndrome
Venous or arterial obstruction

Altered Mental Status/Sensorium

Overdose of pain medications
Cerebrovascular accident
PE
Fat embolism
Any other causes of hypoxia or hypercarbia
Acidosis (metabolic or respiratory)
Drug overdose
Intensive care unit psychosis (sundowner's syn-
    drome)
Elevated ammonia levels
Electrolyte disorders
Increased intracranial pressure (arterial bleed, sub-
    dural hematoma)
Meningitis
Encephalitis

Constipation

Narcotic overdose
Fecal impaction
Bowel obstruction
Dehydration

Extremity Pain (Postoperative)

Muscle spasm
DVT (more common in the lower extremity)
Compartment syndrome
Infection
Loss of reduction (of the fracture fragments)
Hardware failure
Ischemia
Nerve injury/impingement
Electrolyte disturbances (such as calcium)

CHAPTER 7

Orthopaedic Devices and Implants

ORTHOPAEDIC IMPLANTS

Screws (Fig. 7–1)

Available in various sizes (less than 2 mm to greater than 7 mm in diameter)

May be cortical or cancellous screws

Available in various lengths

Often used in conjunction with plates or other fixation devices

Can be cannulated (so that they can be placed over a guide wire)

Can be fully or partially threaded

Screw nomenclature (see Fig. 7–1)

Pitch—distance between threads

Lead—distance advanced with one revolution of the screw

Root diameter (inner diameter)—proportional to tensile strength

Outer diameter—proportional to pull-out strength

Special screws

Lag screws (Fig. 7–2)—provide interfragmentary compression of fracture fragments; the near (or gliding) hole is overdrilled with a larger drill bit, and a smaller drill bit is used to drill the far (or thread) hole; placement of a screw in this fashion causes the far fragment to be pulled toward the near fragment during tightening of the screw ("the lag effect"), resulting in interfragmentary compression

Dynamic compression screws (Fig. 7–3)—large sliding screw used in conjunction with a side plate

Most commonly used for compression of hip (intertrochanteric or femoral neck) fractures and supracondylar femur fractures

Herbert screws—these screws have different pitches on each end to allow for compression across a fracture site

Most commonly used for fixation of scaphoid fractures

Plates

A method of stabilizing a fracture

May be used in conjunction with screws (most commonly) or cables, bands, or wires

Plates are most effective when placed on the tension side of a fracture

Types of plates

Dynamic compression plates (Fig. 7–4)

Allow for compression across a fracture site as a result of specially contoured plate holes and an offset drill guide

Used for long bone fractures requiring rigid fixation

Neutralization plates (Fig. 7–5)

Serve to protect the lag screw fixation of a diaphyseal fracture (where the lag screw fixation alone is not strong enough to withstand the loading)

Neutralize a fracture against displacing forces and prevent shortening, rotation, and angulation

The neutralization plate provides no true compression across a fracture site

Buttress plates (Fig. 7–6)

Provide support to a fracture site

Are most commonly used for fixation of metaphyseal fractures (such as the tibial plateau or the tibial plafond)

A variety of buttress plates are available (T plates, L plates, spoon plates, cloverleaf plates, plateau plates, condylar plates, and others)

Condylar blade plates (Fig. 7–7)

Most commonly used to fix supracondylar or proximal femur fractures

Pins and Wires

Steinmann pins (Fig. 7–8)—threaded or smooth pins that can be placed (usually temporarily) through bone to allow for skeletal traction

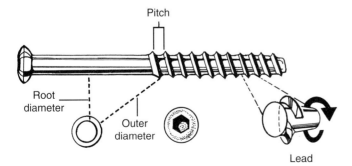

Figure 7–1 ■ Screw nomenclature. Pitch is the distance between threads. Lead is the distance traveled with one revolution of the screw. The inner, or root, diameter is proportional to the tensile strength; the outer diameter is proportional to the pull-out strength.

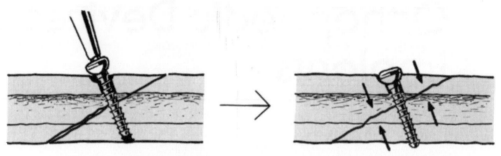

Figure 7–2 ■ Lag screw. Note that the proximal hole is overdrilled to allow compression across the fracture site. (From Muller ME, Allgower M, Schneider R, et al: Manual of Internal Fixation. New York, Springer-Verlag, 1991, p 189.)

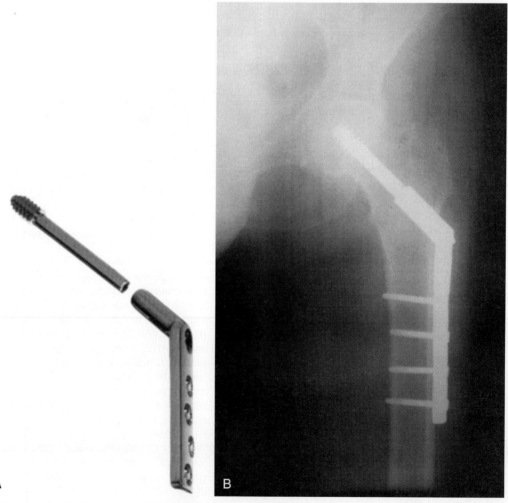

A   B

Figure 7–3 ■ Dynamic compression screw. *A,* Photograph of the implant. *B,* AP radiograph of a dynamic hip screw used in the treatment of an intertrochanteric hip fracture. (*A* from Muller ME, Allgower M, Schneider R, et al: Manual of Internal Fixation. New York, Springer-Verlag, 1991, p 271. *B* from Kenmore PI, Attinger C: Fractures. *In* Wiesel SW, Delahay JN, Connell MC [eds]: Essentials of Orthopaedic Surgery. Philadelphia, WB Saunders, 1993, p 75.)

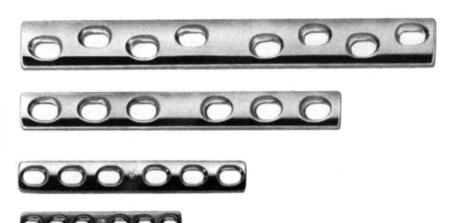

Figure 7–4 ■ Dynamic compression plates of various sizes. (From Muller ME, Allgower M, Schneider R, et al: Manual of Internal Fixation. New York, Springer-Verlag, 1991, p 235.)

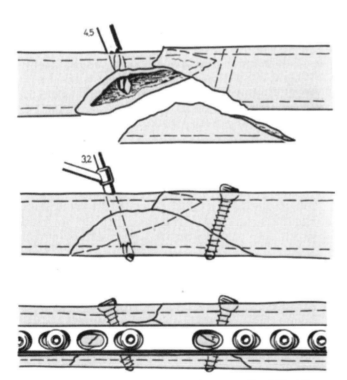

Figure 7–5 ■ Neutralization plate. (From Muller ME, Allgower M, Schneider R, et al: Manual of Internal Fixation. New York, Springer-Verlag, 1991, p 201.)

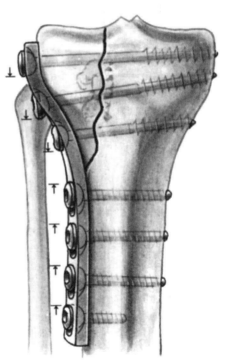

Figure 7–6 ■ Buttress plate. (From Muller ME, Allgower M, Schneider R, et al: Manual of Internal Fixation. New York, Springer-Verlag, 1991, p 209.)

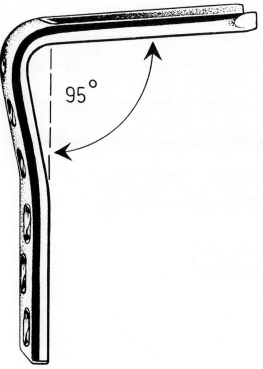

Figure 7–7 ■ Condylar blade plate. (From Muller ME, Allgower M, Schneider R, et al: Manual of Internal Fixation. New York, Springer-Verlag, 1991, p 255.)

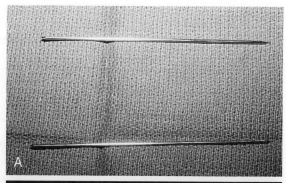

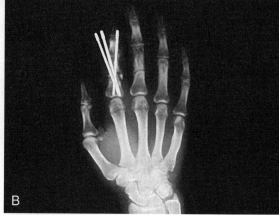

Figure 7–9 ■ A, Kirschner wires. B, Radiograph of Kirschner wires used to stabilize a proximal phalanx fracture.

K wires (Kirschner wires)

Threaded or smooth metallic wires of a small diameter

Can be used percutaneously to fix fractures in smaller bones (such as the hand) (Fig. 7–9)

Can also be used in conjunction with a malleable wire to perform the technique of **tension band wiring** (which is most commonly used for olecranon or patella fractures); tension band wiring allows for pure compression at a fracture site (the malleable wire absorbs all tensile forces) during active joint range of motion (Fig. 7–10)

Intramedullary Nails (Rods) (Fig. 7–11)

Metallic implant placed down the medullary canal of a long bone to stabilize a fracture

Most commonly used to fix diaphyseal fractures of the femur and tibia

Other applications include fixation of fractures of the supracondylar femur, humerus, fibula, radius, and ulna

Types of intramedullary nails and nailing techniques

Reamed—the canal is widened via serial reaming before insertion of the rod; the rod is most commonly cannulated and is placed over a guide wire

Unreamed—the rod is generally of a smaller diameter to allow for passage down the medullary canal without reaming

Slotted (flexible)—the cross-section of the rod is interrupted with a longitudinal groove or slot

Unslotted—the cross-section is not interrupted; these nails are generally stronger than slotted nails

Locked versus unlocked—screws can be placed from the cortices through preplaced holes in the rod proximally and distally; locking screws offer enhanced stability by not allowing **rotation** of the fracture fragments about the longitudinal axis of the rod

Fractures most commonly treated with intramedullary nails (Fig. 7–12)

Femoral shaft

Supracondylar femur

Tibial shaft

Fibula

Humeral shaft

Proximal humerus

External Fixators

Wires, pins, or screws are placed through a bone proximal and distal to a fracture and fixed to an

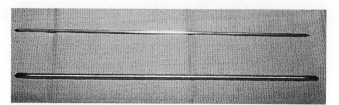

Figure 7–8 ■ Steinmann pins. *Top,* A small, smooth Steinmann pin. *Bottom,* A larger, threaded Steinmann pin. Threaded pins are generally used when it is anticipated that the pin will be in place for an extended period of time.

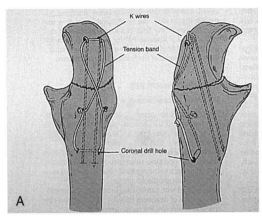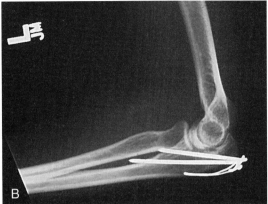

Figure 7-10 ■ *A*, Technique used for tension band wiring. *B*, Radiograph of fixation of a displaced olecranon fracture using the tension band wire technique. (*A* from Jupiter JB, Menhe DK: Trauma to the adult elbow and fractures of the distal humerus. *In* Browner BD, Jupiter JB, Levine AM, et al [eds]: Skeletal Trauma. Philadelphia, WB Saunders, 1992, p 1138. *B* courtesy of Fondren Orthopedic Group LLP, Texas Orthopedic Hospital, Houston, Texas.)

external device to allow fracture stabilization; allow for access to the extremity for wound care in cases of an open fracture

Used for the treatment of open fractures, severely comminuted fractures, and periarticular and intra-articular fractures

Types (Fig. 7–13)

   Unilateral frames

      One plane

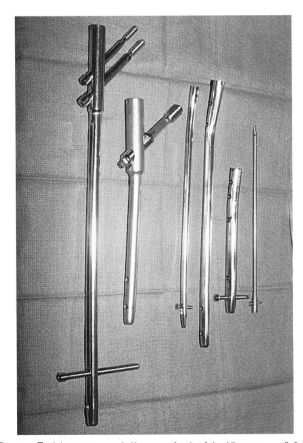

Figure 7-11 ■ Intramedullary nails (rods). (Courtesy of John Ozyp, Dusty Sullivan Corporation, Houston, Texas.)

      Two planes (delta configuration)

   Bilateral frames

      One plane

      Two planes (delta configuration)

   Hybrid frames

   Thin wire circular frames (Ilizarov)

   Others

Joint Replacement Arthroplasty

Used to replace a joint that has become painful or is no longer functional (because of degenerative arthritis, post-traumatic arthritis, or an injury so severe that the joint cannot be repaired)

A joint arthroplasty can replace the entire joint (total joint arthroplasty) or only a portion of the joint

Types of joint replacement arthroplasty

   Hip arthroplasty—useful for hip arthritis or after certain hip fractures that are not amenable to internal fixation

      Total hip arthroplasty (Fig. 7–14)

         A metal ball (head) and stem (femoral component) are used to replace the proximal femur

         The acetabulum is resurfaced and replaced with a polyethylene cup with or without a metal backing (acetabular component)

         The femoral and acetabular components can be fixed with bone cement (PMMA) or without cement (Press-Fit)

         Hybrid fixation refers to cement fixation of one component and noncemented fixation of the other

         The femoral component can have a fixed or modular head (sizes range from 26 to 32 mm)

         The acetabular component is usually modular with metal backing and a snap-in polyethylene cup; the acetabular component should be placed in 45 degrees of abduction and 15 degrees of anteversion

   Hip hemiarthroplasty—most commonly used for displaced hip fractures in the elderly; two types of hip hemiarthroplasty are available

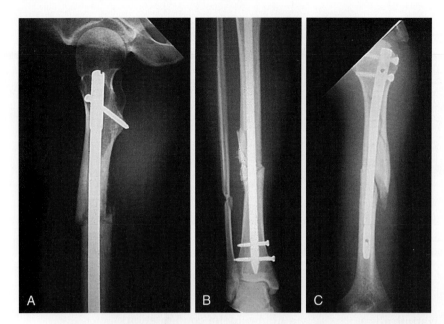

Figure 7–12 ■ Radiographs showing examples of intramedullary nail fixation for fractures of various long bones. *A*, Femoral shaft. *B*, Tibial shaft. *C*, Humeral shaft.

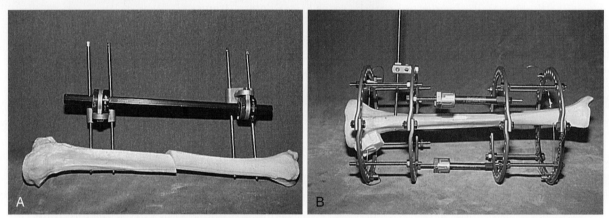

Figure 7–13 ■ External fixators. *A*, Unilateral external fixator. *B*, Circular external fixator.

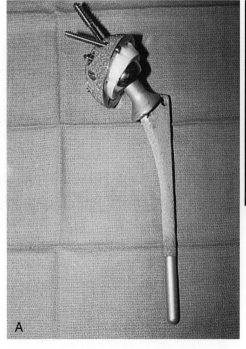

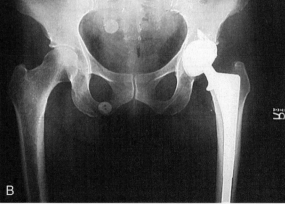

Figure 7–14 ■ Total hip arthroplasty. *A*, Photograph of the implant. *B*, Radiograph of a patient who has undergone a total hip arthroplasty because of debilitating arthritis. (Courtesy of Richard J. Kearns, MD, Fondren Orthopedic Group LLP, Texas Orthopedic Hospital, Houston, Texas.)

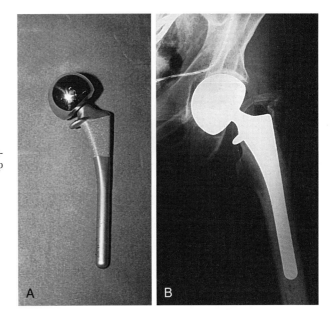

Figure 7–15 ■ Unipolar hip arthroplasty. *A,* Photograph of the implant. *B,* Radiograph of a patient who has undergone a unipolar hip arthroplasty because of a severe hip fracture.

Unipolar hip arthroplasty (Fig. 7–15)—femoral component with a head sized to match the amputated femoral head (this head size is much larger than those used for total hip arthroplasty)

Bipolar hip arthroplasty (Fig. 7–16)—femoral component has what is best described as a head-within-a-head configuration; the outer head articulates with the acetabulum and there is motion at this interface; the inner head articulates with the outer head; there are two instant centers of rotation, and this type of hip arthroplasty is very stable (least likely to be complicated by a postoperative hip dislocation)

Knee arthroplasty (Fig. 7–17)—useful for knee arthritis or after certain knee fractures that are not amenable to internal fixation

Total knee arthroplasty—the articular surfaces of the knee are resurfaced using prosthetic components

The femur is resurfaced using a metal femoral component

The tibia is resurfaced using a polyethylene component with or without a metal tibial tray (metal backing)

The patella is sometimes resurfaced with a polyethylene patella button

Total knee arthroplasty components can be cemented, noncemented, or hybrid

Unicondylar knee arthroplasty—only one compartment of the knee is resurfaced (femur and tibia) when the degenerative process is primarily confined to one compartment (medial or lateral)

Shoulder arthroplasty (Fig. 7–18)—similar to total hip arthroplasty except the socket (glenoid) is more shallow and flat

Can be a total shoulder arthroplasty (replacement of the proximal humerus and glenoid) or a hemiarthroplasty (replacement of the proximal humerus only)

Fixation may be cemented or noncemented

Glenoid component loosening can be a problem

Total elbow arthroplasty (Fig. 7–19)—elbow resurfacing usually with "hinged" components

Used primarily in patients with rheumatoid arthritis

Also useful for traumatic injuries in elderly patients where fixation of a comminuted fracture is often not possible (the bone is too soft to hold screws)

Suture Anchors (Fig. 7–20)

Deployable devices that take advantage of the different densities of cortical and cancellous bone and have hooks or threads that anchor a suture within a bone

Useful for attaching soft tissue to bone (such as in a rotator cuff repair)

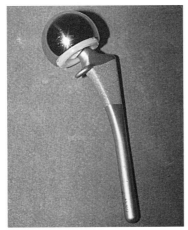

Figure 7–16 ■ Implant used for bipolar hip arthroplasty. Note the head-within-a-head configuration.

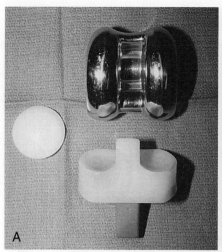
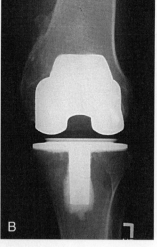

Figure 7–17 ■ Total knee arthroplasty. *A*, Photograph of the implant. *B*, Radiograph of a patient who has undergone a total knee arthroplasty because of debilitating arthritis. (Courtesy of Richard J. Kearns, MD, Fondren Orthopedic Group LLP, Texas Orthopedic Hospital, Houston, Texas.)

Spinal Implants

Pedicle screws—designed to allow fixation of implants in the lower spine by gaining purchase in the thick pedicles of the vertebrae
  Use is controversial
  Risk of neurovascular injury because of the narrow pedicle diameter
Segmental rods—bridge different spinal levels to stabilize and correct deformities (e.g., scoliosis)
  Used for structural deformities (e.g., scoliosis)
  Types of segmental rods
    Cotrel-Dubousset
    Harrington
    Scottish Rite

Other spinal implants
  Segmental (laminar) hooks
  Sublaminar wires
  Various spinal plate and screw systems
  Cages (interbody, for fusions)

Hand and Foot Implants

Silicone implants ("rubber knuckles")
  Best in patients with rheumatoid arthritis
  Wear particles from the implant can lead to synovitis

OPERATING ROOM EQUIPMENT

Protective gear
Surgical instruments
Special tables
Fluoroscopy
Operating microscope
Intraoperative autotransfusion ("cell-saver")
Others

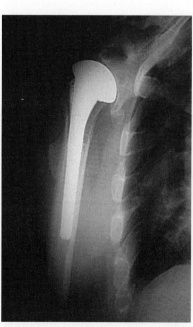

Figure 7–18 ■ Total shoulder arthroplasty. Radiograph of a patient who has undergone a total shoulder arthroplasty because of debilitating arthritis. (Courtesy of Gary M. Gartsman, MD, Fondren Orthopedic Group LLP, Texas Orthopedic Hospital, Houston, Texas.)

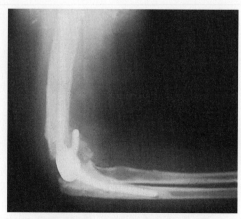

Figure 7–19 ■ Total elbow arthroplasty. Radiograph (lateral view) of a patient who has undergone a total elbow arthroplasty because of debilitating rheumatoid arthritis. (Courtesy of James B. Bennett, MD, Fondren Orthopedic Group LLP, Texas Orthopedic Hospital, Houston, Texas.)

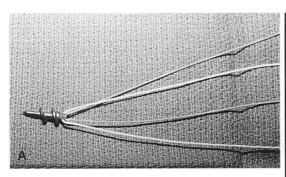

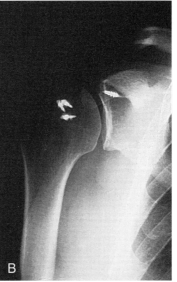

Figure 7–20 ■ One type of suture anchor. *A*, Photograph of the implant. *B*, Radiograph of a patient who has undergone a rotator cuff repair with stabilization of the soft tissues to bone using suture anchors.

SPLINTS, BRACES, CASTS, ASSISTIVE DEVICES, AND PROSTHETIC LIMBS

Definitions

Splint—a rigid support that maintains a body part in a fixed position
Brace—a device that limits unwanted joint motion
Support—a nonrigid device that maintains a body part in a position
Orthosis—a supportive device that serves to correct and prevent deformities by imposing counterforce on a limb or the spine

Types of Splints and Braces

Shoulder (Fig. 7–21)
Elbow/forearm (Fig. 7–22)
Wrist/hand (Fig. 7–23)
Cervical spine (Fig. 7–24)
Thoracolumbar spine (Fig. 7–25)
Pelvis/hip

Knee (Fig. 7–26)
Leg (Fig. 7–27)
Ankle (Fig. 7–28)
Foot (Fig. 7–29)

Types of Casts

Upper extremity (Fig. 7–30)
Spine (Fig. 7–31)
Lower extremity (Fig. 7–32)

Assistive Devices

Canes
Crutches
Walkers
Wheelchairs

Prosthetic Limbs

Upper extremity
Lower extremity

Text continued on page 117

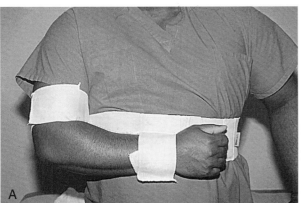

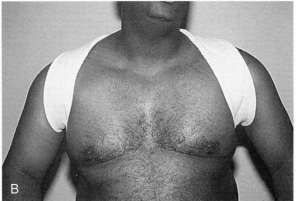

Figure 7–21 ■ Shoulder braces (and some common indications). *A*, Shoulder immobilizer (postoperative). *B*, Figure-of-8 clavicle splint (clavicle fracture).

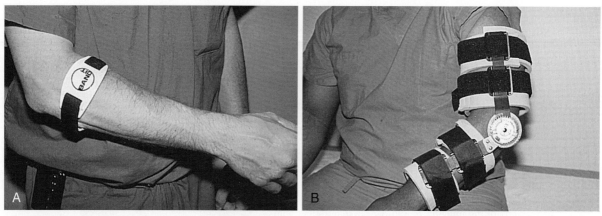

Figure 7–22 ■ Elbow braces (and some common indications). *A*, Tennis elbow strap (tennis elbow). *B*, Hinged elbow brace (elbow fractures or ligament injuries).

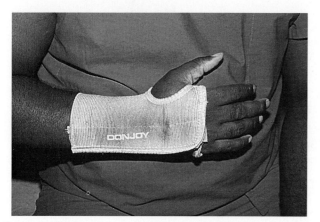

Figure 7–23 ■ Wrist brace (and some common indications). Wrist splint (carpal tunnel syndrome, strains, sprains).

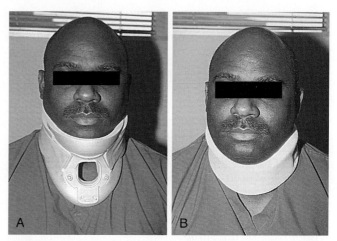

Figure 7–24 ■ Cervical spine braces (and some common indications). *A*, Philadelphia collar (cervical fractures or immobilization after an emergency). *B*, Soft cervical collar (sprains and strains).

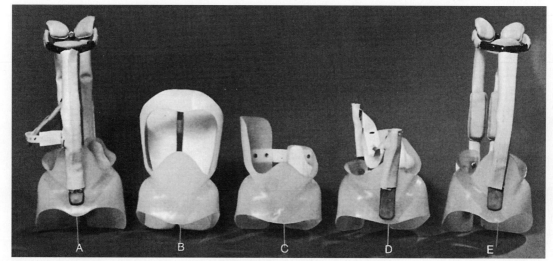

Figure 7–25 ■ Five basic spinal orthoses. *A*, Cervicothoracolumbosacral orthosis (CTLSO), commonly known as a Milwaukee brace. *B*, Thoracolumbosacral orthosis (TLSO). *C*, Modified TLSO. *D*, Modified TLSO with extension. *E*, CTLSO for kyphosis. (From Ogilvie JY: Orthotics. *In* Bradford DS, Lonstein JE, Moe JH, et al [eds]: Moe's Textbook of Scoliosis and Other Spinal Deformities, 2nd ed. Philadelphia, WB Saunders, 1987, p 106.)

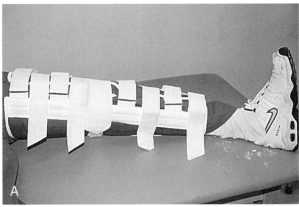

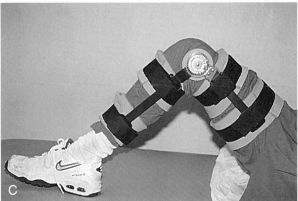

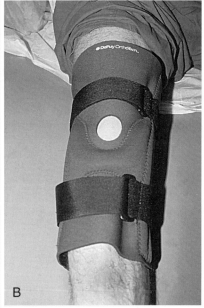

Figure 7–26 ■ Knee braces (and some common indications). *A,* Knee immobilizer (postoperative, after trauma). *B,* Knee sleeve (patella subluxation). *C,* Hinged knee brace (postoperative, ligament injuries [most commonly the medial collateral ligament]).

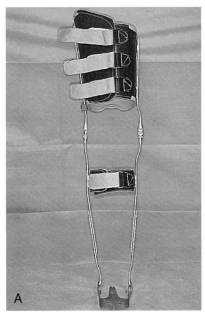

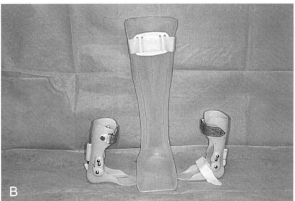

Figure 7–27 ■ *A,* Knee-ankle-foot orthosis. *B,* Ankle-foot orthoses.

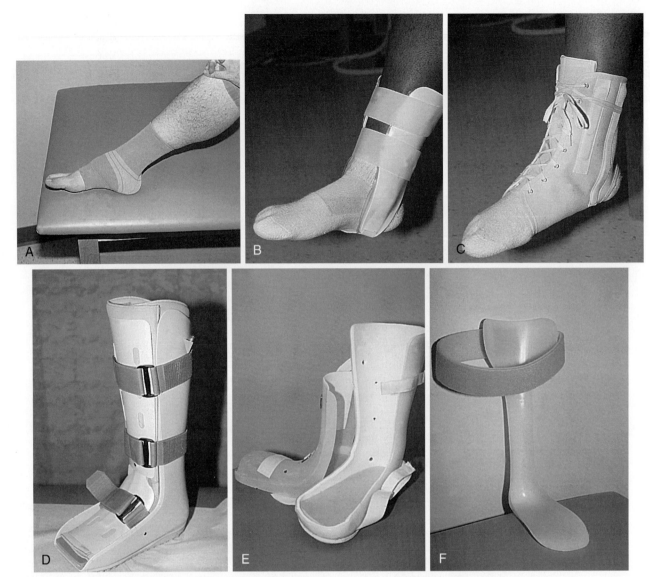

Figure 7–28 ■ Ankle braces (and some common indications). *A,* Ankle wraps (chronic ankle sprains). *B,* Ankle aircast stirrup (mild acute sprains, recovery after a higher level of immobilization). *C,* Lace-up splints (athletes with chronic ankle instability, patients with significant ankle instability who are poor surgical candidates). *D,* Walking boot (severe sprains, nondisplaced fractures, recovery after a higher level of immobilization [such as a cast]). *E,* Pressure-relief orthosis (diabetic foot ulcers). *F,* Ankle-foot orthosis (paralytic disorders, peroneal nerve injury [resulting in footdrop]).

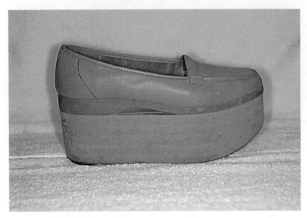

Figure 7–29 ■ Shoe modification to correct for leg length discrepancy. Note that various other shoe modifications and orthoses are also available.

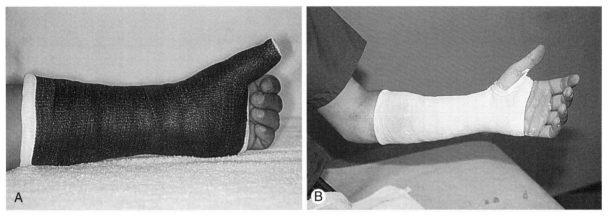

Figure 7–30 ■ *A*, Thumb spica cast commonly used in the treatment of a scaphoid fracture. *B*, Standard short arm cast. Note that both of these casts can be made as a long arm cast by simply extending the cast material proximal to the elbow (the elbow is typically placed in the neutral position and is flexed 90 degrees).

Figure 7–31 ■ *A*, Halo cast used in the treatment of cervical spine injuries. *B*, Underarm cast with right leg extension used for spondylolysis or spondylolisthesis. (From Lonstein JE, Winter RB, Bradford DS, et al [eds]: Moe's Textbook of Scoliosis and Other Spinal Deformities, 3rd ed. Philadelphia, WB Saunders, 1995, pp 127 and 129.)

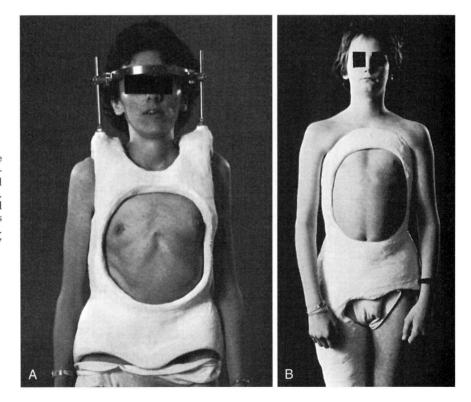

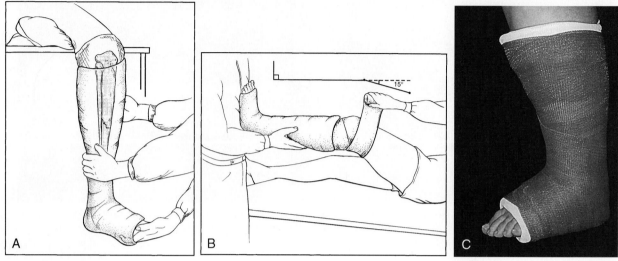

Figure 7–32 ■ Treatment of an acute tibial shaft fracture with a long leg cast. *A*, After reducing the fracture over the end of a table, padding and cast material are applied and molded. *B*, Once the lower portion of the cast is firm, and adequate reduction is confirmed radiographically, the long leg portion of the cast is applied with the knee flexed approximately 15 degrees. Alignment and rotation are controlled during cast application. *C*, Short leg cast used for the treatment of foot and ankle injuries. (*A* and *B* from Trafton PG: Tibial shaft fractures. *In* Browner BD, Jupiter JB, Levine AM, et al [eds]: Skeletal Trauma, 2nd ed. Philadelphia, WB Saunders, 1998, p 2221.)

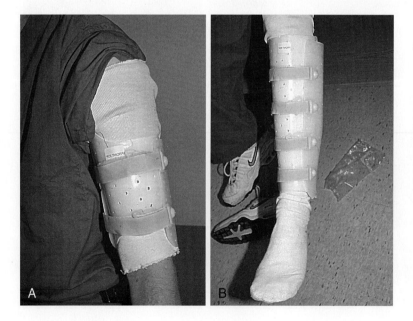

Figure 7–33 ■ Fracture cuffs. *A*, Humeral. *B*, Tibial.

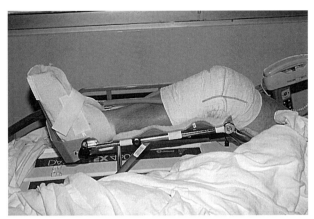

Figure 7–34 ■ Continuous passive motion (CPM) machine. The most common type, shown here, is a knee CPM machine. The machine gently brings the joint through a passive range of motion that can be adjusted.

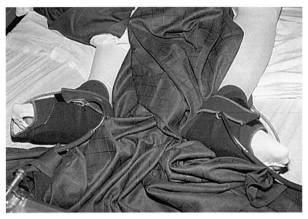

Figure 7–35 ■ Sequential compression devices (SCDs). Useful to prevent deep venous thrombosis. The device shown is one example of a SCD known as a foot pump. The device intermittently squeezes the plantar venous plexus and promotes flow through the deep veins.

Fracture Cuffs (Fig. 7–33)

Humeral
Tibial

OTHER DEVICES

Continuous Passive Motion Devices
(Fig. 7–34)

Allow for passive joint range of motion through a preset arc and speed with the goal of preventing joint stiffness after injury or surgery
Useful after surgery to the knee, elbow, shoulder, and other joints

Sequential Compression Devices
(Fig. 7–35)

Mechanical devices that apply external force to the venous system of the lower extremity in an effort to prevent deep venous thrombosis

Cold Therapy Devices

Help in decreasing pain and swelling after injury or surgery

Bone Stimulators

A variety of technologies have been used to promote fracture or fracture nonunion healing; the technologies include
Direct current
Alternating current
Pulsed electromagnetic fields
Combined electromagnetic fields
Low-intensity pulsed ultrasound

Transcutaneous Electrical Nerve Stimulation (TENS) Unit

Low-amperage alternating current applied using skin electrodes (noninvasive) for the treatment of acute or chronic pain

CHAPTER 8

The Adult Shoulder

SHOULDER ANATOMY

Bones (Fig. 8–1)

Scapula
  Spans ribs 2 to 7
  Three main processes
    Spine
    Acromion
    Coracoid
Clavicle
  Connects the sternum to the acromion
  "S" shaped
Proximal humerus (parts)
  Head
  Anatomic neck
  Surgical neck (distal to the anatomic neck)
  Greater tuberosity (rotator cuff insertion—supraspinatus, infraspinatus, teres minor)
  Lesser tuberosity (rotator cuff insertion—subscapularis)

Joints (Fig. 8–2)

Glenohumeral joint
  Ball (humeral head) and socket (glenoid)
  Ligaments—glenohumeral (inferior glenohumeral is the most important), coracohumeral, capsular
Sternoclavicular joint
  Gliding joint
  Articular disc interspaced between surfaces
  Rotates 30 degrees with glenohumeral motion
  Ligaments—anterior and posterior sternoclavicular, capsular
Acromioclavicular joint
  Gliding joint
  Disc interspaced between surfaces
  Anchors the lateral clavicle
  Ligaments—acromioclavicular, coracoclavicular
Scapulothoracic joint

Muscles (Fig. 8–3)

Spine connectors
  Trapezius
  Latissimus dorsi
  Rhomboids
  Levator scapulae
Thoracic connectors
  Pectoralis major
  Pectoralis minor

Subclavius
Serratus anterior
Shoulder movers
  Deltoid (abduction)
  Teres major (adduction, internal rotation)
  Supraspinatus (abduction, external rotation)
  Infraspinatus (external rotation)
  Teres minor (external rotation)
  Subscapularis (internal rotation)
Rotator cuff muscles ("SITS")—movers and dynamic stabilizers
  Supraspinatus
  Infraspinatus
  Teres minor
  Subscapularis

Nerves

Brachial plexus (Fig. 8–4)
  Organization: **R**oots → **T**runks → **D**ivisions → **C**ords → **B**ranches (remember: **R**obert **T**aylor **D**rinks **C**old **B**eer)

Vessels (see Fig. 8–4)

Subclavian artery
Axillary artery (divided in thirds by the pectoralis minor)
Anterior humeral circumflex artery—primary blood supply to the humeral head

SURGICAL APPROACHES TO THE SHOULDER

Anterior (Deltopectoral)

Used for anterior capsulolabral repairs (recurrent anterior glenohumeral instability), shoulder arthroplasty (arthritis), and others
Approach
  Between the deltoid (axillary nerve) and pectoralis major (pectoral nerves)
  Cephalic vein defines the interval
  Subscapularis muscle (deep) is split or reflected
  Capsule is visualized and an arthrotomy exposes the joint

Lateral

Used for open acromioplasty and rotator cuff repairs
Approach
  Horizontal or vertical incision

Deltoid split (not more than 5 cm distal to the lateral edge of the acromion because of the risk of axillary nerve injury) or subperiosteal dissection of the deltoid off the acromion
Underlying cuff (supraspinatus tendon) is exposed

Posterior

Used for posterior capsular shift and posterior pathology
Approach
Deltoid split or detached from the scapular spine
Interval is between the infraspinatus muscle (suprascapular nerve) and teres minor (axillary nerve)
Stay above the teres minor (axillary nerve at risk!)

HISTORY AND PHYSICAL EXAMINATION OF THE SHOULDER

History

Age is a key factor
Younger patients tend to have
Instability
Acromioclavicular injuries
Distal clavicle osteolysis (especially weight lifters)
Older patients tend to have
Rotator cuff injuries
Degenerative joint disease
Mechanism of injury
Abduction-external rotation
Anterior glenohumeral instability
Direct fall onto the shoulder
Acromioclavicular injuries
Chronic pain with overhead activity/night pain
Rotator cuff tears

Physical Examination

Observation
Asymmetry
Muscle wasting
Deformities
Swelling
Skin changes
Abnormal contours
Popeye muscle (proximal biceps tendon rupture)
Prominent distal clavicle (acromioclavicular separation)
Scapular winging (long thoracic nerve injury)
Shoulder dislocation
Acromioclavicular/sternoclavicular dislocation
Scapular asymmetry (Sprengel's deformity)
Palpation
Bones
Clavicle
Scapula
Acromion
Coracoid process
Spine (of scapula)
Vertebral border

Humerus
Greater tuberosity
Bicipital groove
Joints
Sternoclavicular
Acromioclavicular
Glenohumeral
Scapulothoracic
Soft tissues
Rotator cuff muscles
Subacromial bursa
Axilla
Supporting muscles
Sternocleidomastoid
Pectoralis major
Biceps
Deltoid
Trapezius
Rhomboids
Latissimus dorsi
Serratus anterior
Hyperlaxity
Motion (Fig. 8–5)
Forward flexion (elevation)
Normal, 150 to 180 degrees
Extension
Abduction
Normal, 150 to 180 degrees
Adduction
External rotation
Normal, 30 to 60 degrees with elbow at side
Normal, 70 to 90 degrees with arm abducted
Internal rotation (behind the back)
Normal, T4-8 vertebral level
Neurovascular examination
Sensation (see Fig. 2–5)
Axillary nerve (C5) lateral arm
Reflexes
Biceps (C5-6)
Triceps (C7)
Strength testing (Table 8–1)
Forward flexion (anterior deltoid, coracobrachialis)
Extension (latissimus dorsi, teres major, posterior deltoid)
Abduction (deltoid, supraspinatus)
Adduction (pectoralis major, latissimus dorsi)
External rotation (teres minor, infraspinatus)
Internal rotation (subscapularis, pectoralis major, latissimus dorsi)
Scapular elevation (trapezius, levator scapulae)
Scapular retraction (rhomboideus major and minor)
Scapular protraction (serratus anterior)
Special testing (condition-specific)
Anterior glenohumeral instability (Fig. 8–6)
Apprehension (fulcrum) test (see Fig. 8–6)—shoulder abduction to 90 degrees with external rotation to 90 degrees causes apprehension in the patient because this position tends to push the humeral head anteriorly and recreate the sensation of anterior glenohumeral instability

Text continued on page 127

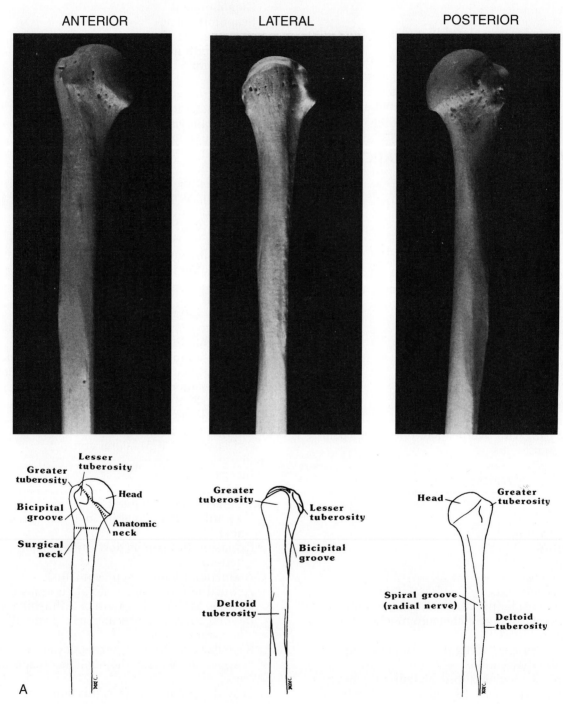

Figure 8–1 ■ Bones of the shoulder. *A,* Anterior, lateral, and posterior views of the humerus.

ANTERIOR   POSTERIOR   LATERAL

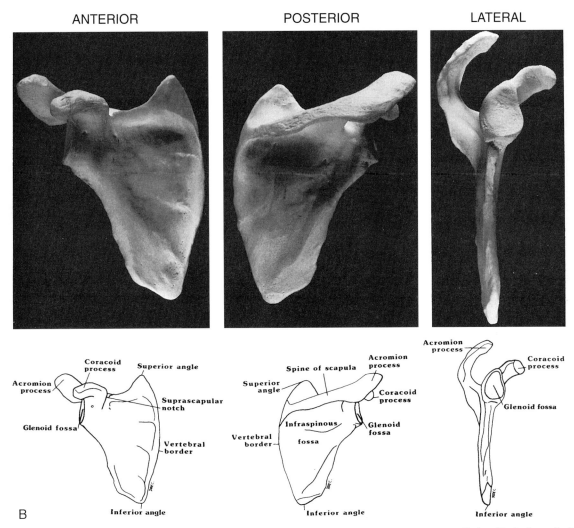

B

Figure 8–1 ■ *Continued. B,* Anterior, posterior, and lateral views of the scapula. (From Weissman BNW, Sledge CB: Orthopedic Radiology. Philadelphia, WB Saunders, 1986, pp 216, 217.)

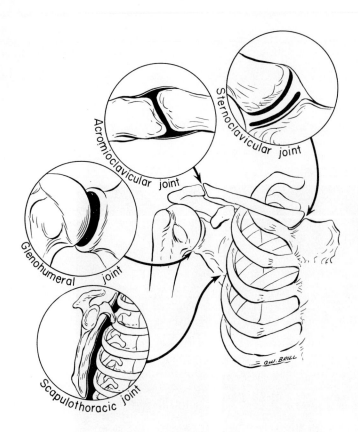

Figure 8–2 ■ Shoulder joints: sternoclavicular, acromioclavicular, glenohumeral, and scapulothoracic. (From DePalma AF: Surgery of the Shoulder, 2nd ed. Philadelphia, JB Lippincott, 1973.)

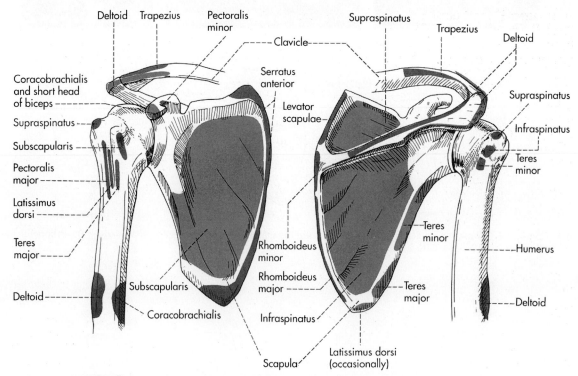

Figure 8–3 ■ Origins (light color) and insertions (dark color) of the shoulder girdle muscles. (From Jenkins DB: Hollinshead's Functional Anatomy of the Limbs and Back, 6th ed. Philadelphia, WB Saunders, 1991.)

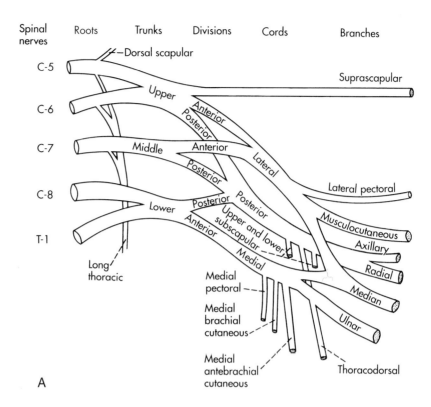

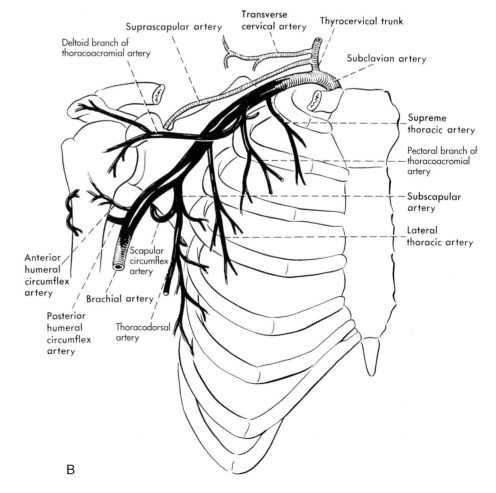

Figure 8–4 ■ *A,* Organization of the brachial plexus. *B,* Axillary artery (shown in solid black) and its branches (also in solid black). (From Jenkins DB: Hollinshead's Functional Anatomy of the Limbs and Back, 6th ed. Philadelphia, WB Saunders, 1991.)

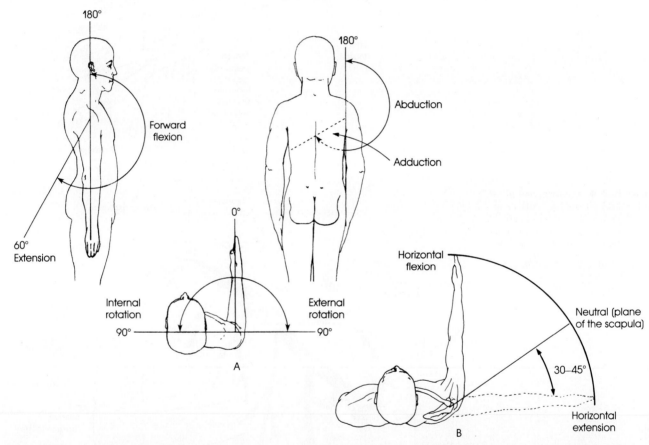

Figure 8–5 ■ Shoulder motion. (From Magee DJ: Orthopedic Physical Assessment, 2nd ed. Philadelphia, WB Saunders, 1992, p 98. Adapted from Perry J: Clin Sports Med 2:255, 1983.)

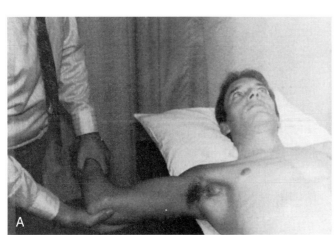

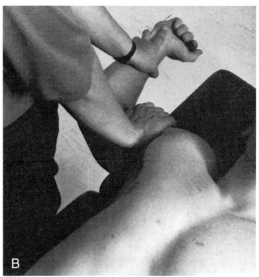

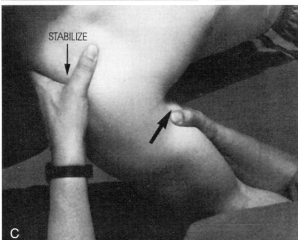

Figure 8–6 ■ Tests for anterior instability. *A*, Apprehension test. *B*, Relocation test. *C*, Anterior draw test. (From Magee DJ: Orthopedic Physical Assessment, 2nd ed. Philadelphia, WB Saunders, 1992, pp 107, 110, 111.)

Table 8–1
MUSCLES ABOUT THE SHOULDER: THEIR ACTIONS AND NERVE SUPPLY (INCLUDING NERVE ROOT DERIVATION)

Action	Muscles Performing Action	Nerve Supply	Nerve Root Derivation
Forward flexion	1. Deltoid (anterior fibers)	Axillary	C5-6 (posterior cord)
	2. Pectoralis major (clavicular fibers)	Medial and lateral pectoral	C5-6 (lateral cord)
	3. Coracobrachialis	Musculocutaneous	C5-7 (lateral cord)
	4. Biceps (when strong contraction required)	Musculocutaneous	C5-7 (lateral cord)
Extension	1. Deltoid (posterior fibers)	Axillary	C5-6 (posterior cord)
	2. Teres major	Lower subscapular	C5-6 (posterior cord)
	3. Teres minor	Axillary	C5-6 (posterior cord)
	4. Latissimus dorsi	Thoracodorsal	C6-8 (posterior cord)
	5. Pectoralis major (sternocostal fibers)	Medial and lateral pectoral	C5-6 (lateral cord)
	6. Triceps (long head)	Radial	C6-8 (posterior cord)
Horizontal adduction	1. Pectoralis major	Medial and lateral pectoral	C5-6 (lateral cord)
	2. Deltoid (anterior fibers)	Axillary	C5-6 (posterior cord)
Horizontal abduction	1. Deltoid (posterior fibers)	Axillary	C5-6 (posterior cord)
	2. Teres major	Lower subscapular	C5-6 (posterior cord)
	3. Teres minor	Axillary	C5-6 (brachial plexus trunk)
	4. Infraspinatus	Suprascapular	C5-6 (brachial plexus trunk)
Abduction	1. Deltoid	Axillary	C5-6 (posterior cord)
	2. Supraspinatus	Suprascapular	C5-6 (brachial plexus trunk)
	3. Infraspinatus	Suprascapular	C5-6 (brachial plexus trunk)
	4. Subscapularis	Upper and lower subscapular	C5-6 (posterior cord)
	5. Teres minor	Axillary	C5-6 (posterior cord)
	6. Long head of biceps (if arm externally rotated first, trick movement)	Musculocutaneous	C5-7 (lateral cord)
Adduction	1. Pectoralis major	Medial and lateral pectoral	C5-6 (lateral cord)
	2. Latissimus dorsi	Thoracodorsal	C5-6 (posterior cord)
	3. Teres major	Lower subscapular	C5-6 (posterior cord)
	4. Subscapularis	Upper and lower subscapular	C5-6 (posterior cord)
Internal rotation	1. Pectoralis major	Medial and lateral pectoral	C5-6 (lateral cord)
	2. Deltoid (anterior fibers)	Axillary	C5-6 (posterior cord)
	3. Latissimus dorsi	Thoracodorsal	C6-8 (posterior cord)
	4. Teres major	Lower subscapular	C5-6 (posterior cord)
	5. Subscapularis (when arm is by side)	Upper and lower subscapular	C5-6 (posterior cord)
External rotation	1. Infraspinatus	Suprascapular	C5-6 (brachial plexus trunk)
	2. Deltoid (posterior fibers)	Axillary	C5-6 (posterior cord)
	3. Teres minor	Axillary	C5-6 (posterior cord)
Elevation of scapula	1. Trapezius (upper fibers)	Accessory	Cranial nerve XI
		C3-4 nerve roots	C3-4
	2. Levator scapulae	C3-4 nerve roots	C3-4
		Dorsal scapular	C5
	3. Rhomboideus major	Dorsal scapular	(C4), C5
	4. Rhomboideus minor	Dorsal scapular	(C4), C5
Depression of scapula	1. Serratus anterior	Long thoracic	C5-6 (C7)
	2. Pectoralis major	Medial and lateral pectoral	C5-6 (lateral cord)
	3. Pectoralis minor	Medial pectoral	C8, T1 (medial cord)
	4. Latissimus dorsi	Thoracodorsal	C6-8 (posterior cord)
	5. Trapezius (lower fibers)	Accessory	Cranial nerve XI
		C3-4 nerve roots	C3-4
Protraction (forward movement) of scapula	1. Serratus anterior	Long thoracic	C5-6 (C7)
	2. Pectoralis major	Medial and lateral pectoral	C5-6 (lateral cord)
	3. Pectoralis minor	Medial pectoral	C8, T1 (medial cord)
	4. Latissimus dorsi	Thoracodorsal	C6-8 (posterior cord)
Retraction (backward movement) of scapula	1. Trapezius	Accessory	Cranial nerve XI
		C3-4 nerve roots	C3-4
	2. Rhomboideus major	Dorsal scapular	(C4), C5
	3. Rhomboideus minor	Dorsal scapular	(C4), C5
Lateral (upward) rotation of inferior angle of scapula	1. Trapezius (upper and lower fibers)	Accessory	Cranial nerve XI
		C3-4 nerve roots	C3-4
	2. Serratus anterior	Long thoracic	C5-6 (C7)
Medial (downward) rotation of inferior angle of scapula	1. Levator scapulae	C3-4 nerve roots	C3-4
		Dorsal scapular	C5
	2. Rhomboideus major	Dorsal scapular	(C4), C5
	3. Rhomboideus minor	Dorsal scapular	(C4), C5
	4. Pectoralis minor	Medial pectoral	C8, T1 (medial cord)

Modified from Magee DJ: Orthopedic Physical Assessment, 2nd ed. Philadelphia, WB Saunders, 1992, p 104.

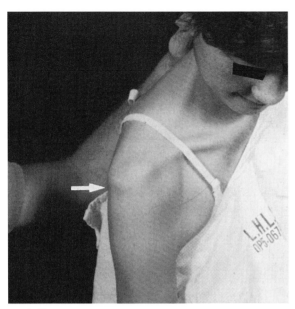

Figure 8–7 ■ Sulcus test. Note dimpling of the skin (*arrow*) distal to the acromion. (From Magee DJ: Orthopedic Physical Assessment. Philadelphia, WB Saunders, 1992, p 115. Adapted from Hawkins RJ, Bokor DJ: Clinical evaluation of shoulder problems. *In* Rockwood CA, Matson RA [eds]: The Shoulder. Philadelphia, WB Saunders, 1990, p 169.)

(subluxation) in patients with anterior instability

Relocation test (see Fig. 8–6)—supine apprehension test with posteriorly directed force relieves apprehension because the posteriorly directed force does not allow anterior subluxation

Anterior draw (load and shift) test (see Fig. 8–6)—passive anterior displacement of the humeral head; best done with the patient under anesthesia; translation of the humeral on the glenoid is graded

Inferior (and multidirectional) glenohumeral instability (Fig. 8–7)

Sulcus test (see Fig. 8–7)—traction on the adducted arm causes abnormal inferior displace-

ment of the humeral head, which manifests on examination as dimpling of the skin distal to the acromion

Posterior glenohumeral instability (Fig. 8–8)

Jerk test (see Fig. 8–8)—axially load the humerus and passively move the arm horizontally across the body (adduction) with the shoulder held in 90 degrees of abduction and 90 degrees of internal rotation; the arm will "jerk" posteriorly with posterior displacement of the humeral head as the arm nears the midline

Posterior draw (load and shift) test (see Fig. 8–8)—passive posterior displacement of the humeral head

Impingement syndrome (Fig. 8–9)

Impingement *sign* (see Fig. 8–9)—passive forward flexion of the arm greater than 90 degrees causes impingement-related pain

Impingement *test*—subacromial injection of lidocaine into the subacromial bursa relieves the pain of impingement

Hawkins' (impingement reinforcement) test (see Fig. 8–9)—90 degrees of forward flexion, adduction, and passive internal rotation causes impingement-related pain

Rotator cuff disease (Fig. 8–10)

Drop arm test (see Fig. 8–10)—the patient is unable to oppose even gentle downward force on the arm held in 90 degrees of abduction; the arm "drops" to the side

Supraspinatus test (see Fig. 8–10)—resistance is applied with the patient's arms abducted 90 degrees, forward flexed 30 degrees, and pronated (the thumbs of the patient point toward the ground); this position helps isolate the supraspinatus muscle; muscle strength (of the supraspinatus) is graded for both extremities

Lift-off sign—the arm is placed behind the back and the hand is passively positioned away from the body; patients with a subscapularis injury are unable to maintain this position

Biceps tendon pathology (Fig. 8–11)

Yergason's test (see Fig. 8–11)—elbow is flexed 90

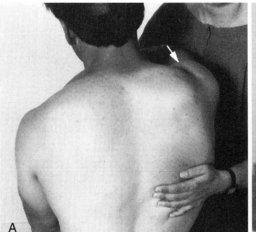
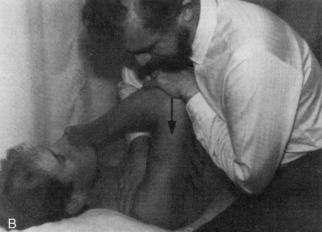

Figure 8–8 ■ Tests for posterior instability. *A,* Jerk test. *Arrow* indicates posterior displacement of the humeral head. *B,* Load and shift test. (From Magee DJ: Orthopedic Physical Assessment, 2nd ed. Philadelphia, WB Saunders, 1992, pp 113, 114.)

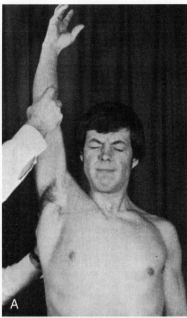

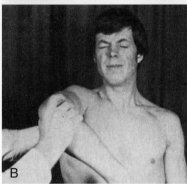

Figure 8–9 ■ Tests for impingement syndrome. *A*, Impingement sign. *B*, Hawkins' (impingement reinforcement) test. (From Hawkins RJ, Kennedy JC: Impingement syndrome in athletics. Am J Sports Med 8:151–158, 1980.)

degrees and the forearm is placed in the pronated position; resisted supination (the examiner resists against the patient's attempt to supinate the forearm) causes bicipital groove tenderness

Speed's test (see Fig. 8–11)—the elbow is extended and the forearm is placed in the supinated position; resisted forward flexion of the humerus (the examiner resists against the patient's attempt to forward flex the humerus) past 60 degrees causes bicipital groove tenderness

Axial compression/rotation test—rotation and loading of the glenohumeral joint may cause pain/clicking in patients with SLAP (**s**uperior glenoid **l**abral tear in the **a**nterior to **p**osterior direction) lesions

Acromioclavicular joint pathology (Fig. 8–12)

Cross-chest adduction (see Fig. 8–12)—passive adduction of the arm across the midline causes acromioclavicular joint pain

Thoracic outlet syndrome (Fig. 8–13)

Adson's maneuver (see Fig. 8–13)—shoulder ex-

tension and head rotation to the ipsilateral side while holding a breath leads to loss of the radial pulse

Modified Adson's (Wright's) test—shoulder extension, abduction to 90 degrees, and external rotation with the head rotated to the contralateral side leads to loss of the radial pulse

Hyperabduction syndrome test—radial pulse is reduced with hyperabduction of the shoulder; "flapping" of the arms can also exacerbate symptoms

Halstead's test (see Fig. 8–13)—the neck is extended, the head is turned to the opposite shoulder; traction on the affected arm obliterates pulses

Provocative elevation test—the arms elevated past 90 degrees and the hands opened and closed rapidly 15 times leads to cramping/tingling of the hands (claudication)

Cervical spine pathology (Fig. 8–14)

Spurling's test (see Fig. 8–14)—lateral flexion and rotation with compression causes nerve root encroachment and pain on the ipsilateral side

DIAGNOSTIC TESTS FOR THE SHOULDER

Radiographic Evaluation of the Shoulder

Standard radiographs (Fig. 8–15)

Routine anteroposterior (AP) (see Fig. 8–15)

True AP in the plane of the glenoid (see Figure 8–15) allows best visualization of the glenohumeral joint

Scapular Y view (see Fig. 8–15)

True lateral view of the scapula

Normally the humeral head is centered over the glenoid

Axillary lateral/modified axillary lateral

The axillary lateral is the key to avoid missing a glenohumeral dislocation (especially posterior dislocations); it should be performed on every trauma patient with shoulder symptoms (Fig. 8–16)

Special radiographs

Anterior instability (Fig. 8–17)

West Point axillary lateral (see Fig. 8–17)—prone axillary lateral with the x-ray beam angled 25 degrees downward and medially; visualizes a bony Bankart lesion (fracture at the anterior inferior aspect of the glenoid that occurs with anterior glenohumeral instability [from a dislocation or repetitive subluxation])

Stryker notch view (see Fig. 8–17)—10-degree cephalic tilt with the arm held overhead; visualizes a Hill-Sachs defect (bony defect in the posterolateral aspect of the humeral head caused by contact of this area of the humeral head with the glenoid during anterior shoulder dislocation/subluxation)

Impingement syndrome/rotator cuff disease (Fig. 8–18)

AP—cystic changes in the greater tuberosity and

Text continued on page 135

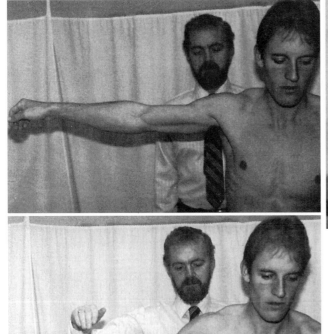

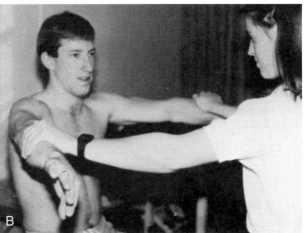

Figure 8–10 ■ Tests for rotator cuff disease. *A*, Drop arm test. *B*, Supraspinatus test. (From Magee DJ: Orthopedic Physical Assessment, 2nd ed. Philadelphia, WB Saunders, 1992, pp 118, 119.)

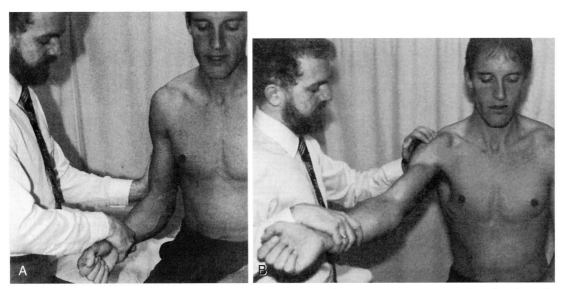

Figure 8–11 ■ Tests for biceps tendon pathology. *A*, Yergason's test. *B*, Speed's test. (From Magee DJ: Orthopedic Physical Assessment, 2nd ed. Philadelphia, WB Saunders, 1992, p 117.)

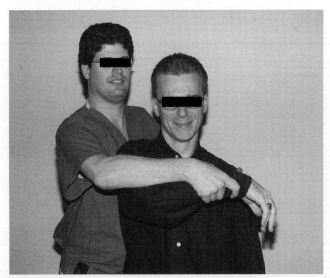

Figure 8–12 ■ Test for acromioclavicular joint pathology. Symptoms are exacerbated by cross-chest adduction.

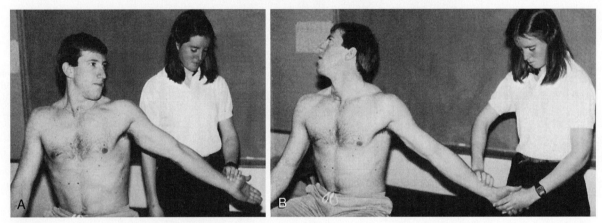

Figure 8–13 ■ Tests for thoracic outlet syndrome. *A*, Adson's maneuver. *B*, Halstead's test. (From Magee DJ: Orthopedic Physical Assessment, 2nd ed. Philadelphia, WB Saunders, 1992, p 122.)

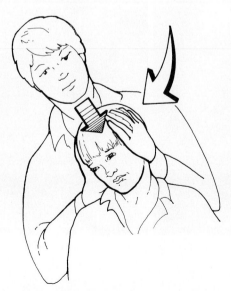

Figure 8–14 ■ Spurling's test. Lateral flexion and rotation with compression may cause nerve root encroachment and pain on the ipsilateral side in patients with cervical root impingement. (From Miller MD, Cooper DE, Warner JJP: Review of Sports Medicine and Arthroscopy. Philadelphia, WB Saunders, 1995, p 129.)

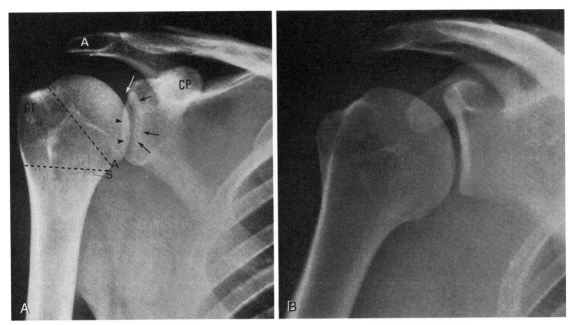

ROUTINE AP SHOULDER   TRUE AP SHOULDER

ROUTINE AP SHOULDER

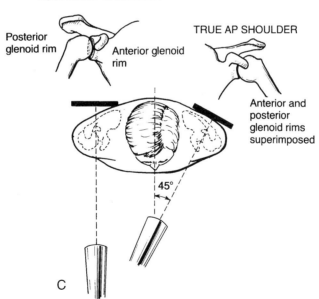

Posterior glenoid rim   Anterior glenoid rim

TRUE AP SHOULDER

Anterior and posterior glenoid rims superimposed

45°

C

Figure 8–15 ■ Standard shoulder radiographs. *A*, Routine AP radiograph. Note that the greater tuberosity (GT) is seen in profile and that the humeral head and glenoid normally overlap on this view. Anatomic (A) and surgical (S) necks of the humerus are indicated with dotted lines. The coracoid process (CP) and acromion (white A) are also labeled. *Dark arrows* and *arrowheads* outline the glenoid. The *white arrow* outlines air within the joint (vacuum phenomenon). *B*, True AP radiograph. Note that the humerus and glenoid do not overlap. *C*, Positioning for the routine and true AP views of the shoulder.

Illustration continued on following page

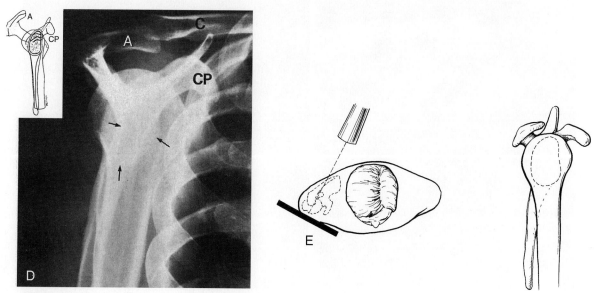

Figure 8–15 ■ *Continued. D,* Scapular Y radiographic view and schematic (*inset*). A, acromion, C, clavicle; CP, coracoid process. *E,* Positioning for the scapular Y view. (*A, B,* and *D* from Weissman BNW, Sledge CB: Orthopedic Radiology. Philadelphia, WB Saunders, 1986, p 219. *C* and *E* from Warner JJP, Caborn DN: Overview of shoulder instability. Crit Rev Phys Rehabil Med 4:145–198, 1992.)

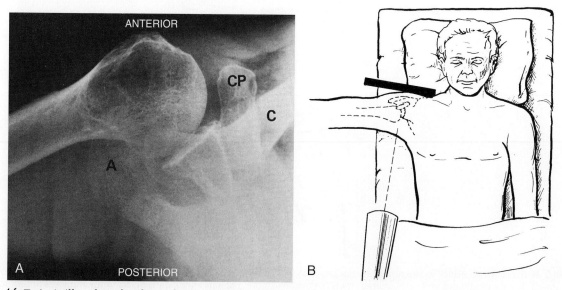

Figure 8–16 ■ *A,* Axillary lateral radiograph. A, acromion; CP, coracoid process; C, clavicle. *B,* Positioning for the axillary lateral radiograph. (*A* from Weissman BNW, Sledge CB: Orthopedic Radiology. Philadelphia, WB Saunders, 1986, pp 219, 220. *B* from Warner JJP, Caborn DN: Overview of shoulder instability. Crit Rev Phys Rehabil Med 4:145–198, 1992.)

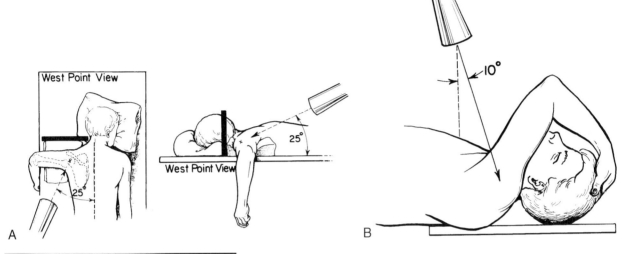

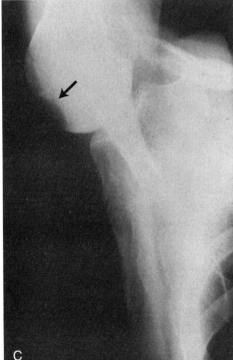

Figure 8–17 ▪ *A*, Positioning for the West Point axillary lateral radiograph (for detecting bony Bankart lesions). *B*, Positioning for the Stryker notch view (for detecting Hill-Sachs impression fractures). *C*, Example of a Hill-Sachs defect (*arrow*) using the Stryker notch view. (*A* and *B* from Warner JJP, Caborn DN: Overview of shoulder instability. Crit Rev Phys Rehabil Med 4:145–198, 1992. *C* from Miller MD, Cooper DE, Warner JJP: Review of Sports Medicine and Arthroscopy. Philadelphia, WB Saunders, 1995, p 131.)

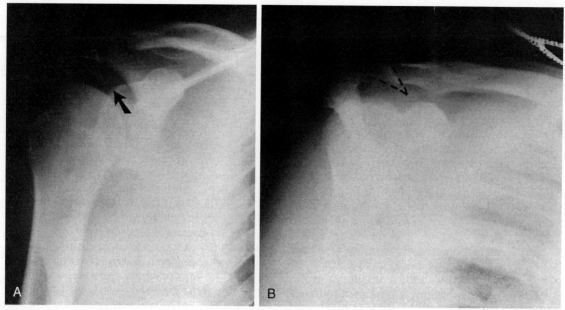

Figure 8–18 ■ *A*, Thirty-degree caudal tilt view demonstrating large subacromial spur and spike (*arrow*). B, Supraspinatus outlet view showing a type III (hooked) acromion (outlined). (From Miller MD, Cooper DE, Warner JJP: Review of Sports Medicine and Arthroscopy. Philadelphia, WB Saunders, 1995, p 134.)

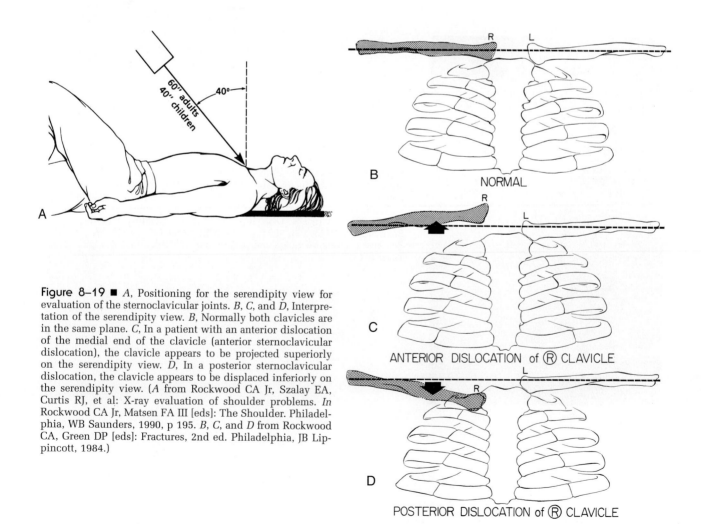

Figure 8–19 ■ *A*, Positioning for the serendipity view for evaluation of the sternoclavicular joints. *B, C,* and *D,* Interpretation of the serendipity view. *B,* Normally both clavicles are in the same plane. *C,* In a patient with an anterior dislocation of the medial end of the clavicle (anterior sternoclavicular dislocation), the clavicle appears to be projected superiorly on the serendipity view. *D,* In a posterior sternoclavicular dislocation, the clavicle appears to be displaced inferiorly on the serendipity view. (*A* from Rockwood CA Jr, Szalay EA, Curtis RJ, et al: X-ray evaluation of shoulder problems. *In* Rockwood CA Jr, Matsen FA III [eds]: The Shoulder. Philadelphia, WB Saunders, 1990, p 195. *B, C,* and *D* from Rockwood CA, Green DP [eds]: Fractures, 2nd ed. Philadelphia, JB Lippincott, 1984.)

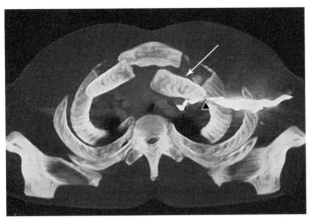

Figure 8–20 ■ CT scan showing a posterior sternoclavicular dislocation (*arrow*) with compression of the subclavian artery (*arrowhead*). (Courtesy of Fondren Orthopedic Group LLP, Texas Orthopedic Hospital, Houston, Texas.)

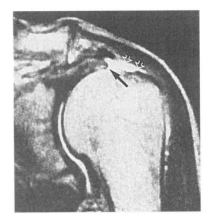

Figure 8–21 ■ MRI demonstrating a rotator cuff tear. Note retracted tendon (*closed arrow*) and void where tendon should occupy (*open arrows*).

superior displacement of the proximal humerus are seen with long-standing rotator cuff disease

30-degree caudal tilt (Rockwood)—subacromial spurs visualized (see Fig. 8–18)

Supraspinatus outlet (Y) view (see Fig. 8–18)—acromial morphology (for bony impingement) characterized

Acromioclavicular pathology

10-degree cephalic tilt (or Zanca) view—visualizes acromioclavicular arthritis, distal clavicle osteolysis

Bilateral acromioclavicular (stress) views with 10 pounds of hanging weights—detects subtle acromioclavicular separations

Sternoclavicular pathology (Fig. 8–19)

Hobbs' view—PA view with the patient slumped over the x-ray cassette

Serendipity view (see Fig. 8–19)—supine 40-degree cephalic tilt

Computed Tomography (CT) (Fig. 8–20)

Can be helpful for evaluation of sternoclavicular dislocations, proximal humerus fractures (especially with 3-D reconstructions), and glenoid version (anteversion versus retroversion)

Magnetic Resonance Imaging (MRI)
(Fig. 8–21)

Can be useful in the diagnosis of rotator cuff tears, other tendon ruptures (pectoralis major, biceps), labral tears (with contrast), and other disorders

Arthrography (Fig. 8–22)

Helpful in the diagnosis of adhesive capsulitis and rotator cuff tears

Diagnostic Injections

Subacromial injection—can relieve impingement pain

Acromioclavicular injection—relieves pain associated with acromioclavicular arthritis and distal clavicle osteolysis

Arthroscopy (Fig. 8–23)

Rarely used for purely diagnostic purposes but can confirm or clarify a diagnosis

COMMON ADULT CONDITIONS OF THE SHOULDER

Shoulder (Glenohumeral) Instability

Glenohumeral instability can result in subluxation or dislocation

The instability can be anterior, posterior, or multidirectional

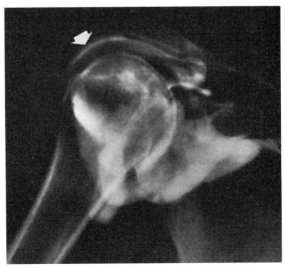

Figure 8–22 ■ Single contrast arthrogram of the shoulder shows abnormal leakage of contrast into the subacromial bursa (*arrow*), indicating a full-thickness rotator cuff tear. (From Weissman BNW, Sledge CB: Orthopedic Radiology: Philadelphia, WB Saunders, 1986, p 233.)

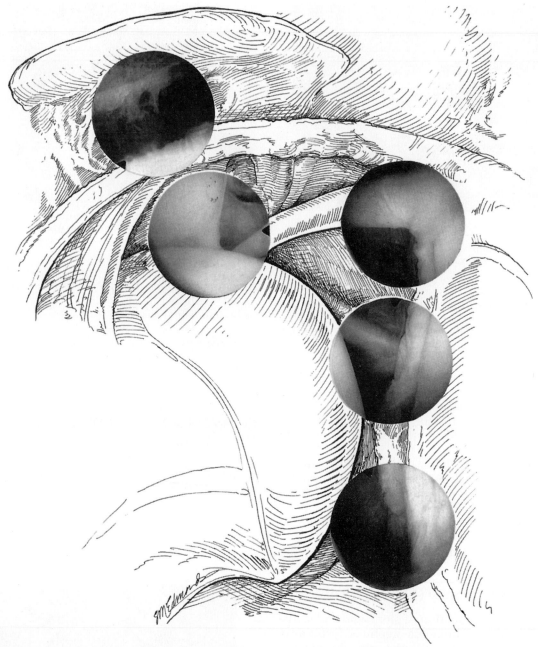

Figure 8–23 ■ Arthroscopic anatomy of the shoulder. (From Miller MD, Osborne JR, Warner JJP, et al: MRI-Arthroscopy Correlative Atlas. Philadelphia, WB Saunders, 1997, p 160.)

Two specific instability patterns have been described
    TUBS—**T**raumatic **u**nilateral dislocations with a **B**ankart lesion that can be successfully treated with **s**urgery
    AMBRI—**A**traumatic **m**ultidirectional instability that is commonly **b**ilateral and is often successfully treated with **r**ehabilitation and occasionally an **i**nferior capsular shift (surgery)
Anterior glenohumeral instability—much more common than posterior instability; may be traumatic (dislocation) or chronic/stretching (subluxation)
Occurs more commonly in younger patients
High recurrence rate

Associated fractures (Fig. 8–24)
    Hill-Sachs defect—impression fracture in the posterolateral humeral head
    Bony Bankart lesion—anterior inferior glenoid rim injury
    Greater tuberosity fracture—especially in older patients
Classification
    Dislocation
        High recurrence rate, especially in young patients
        Patients present with the arm abducted and externally rotated (Fig. 8–25)

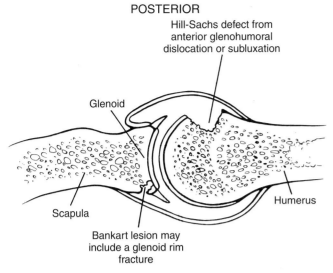

POSTERIOR

Hill-Sachs defect from anterior glenohumoral dislocation or subluxation

Glenoid

Scapula

Bankart lesion may include a glenoid rim fracture

Humerus

ANTERIOR

Figure 8–24 ■ Schematic drawing (axillary view) demonstrating lesions associated with anterior glenohumeral instability. (Adapted from Connell MD, Kenmore PI: The shoulder. *In* Wiesel SW, Delahay JN, Connell MC [eds]: Essentials of Orthopaedic Surgery. Philadelphia, WB Saunders, 1993, p 207.)

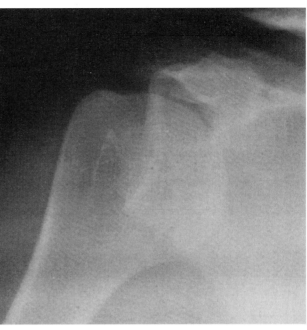

Figure 8–26 ■ AP radiograph of the right shoulder demonstrating an anterior glenohumeral dislocation. (From Matsen FA III, Thomas SC, Rockwood CA Jr: Glenohumeral instability. *In* Rockwood CA Jr, Matsen FA III [eds]: The Shoulder. Philadelphia, WB Saunders, 1990, p 554.)

X-rays are diagnostic (Fig. 8–26)
Reduction of an anterior shoulder dislocation—traction with countertraction (Fig. 8–27)
Subluxation usually responds to physical therapy (rotator cuff strengthening exercises)
Posterior glenohumeral instability
Less common than anterior glenohumeral instability
Classification
Dislocation

Can be caused by seizure/shock—internal rotators of the shoulder overpower the external rotators and lead to posterior dislocation
Patients present with the arm adducted and internally rotated (Fig. 8–28)
Patients have limited external rotation and forward flexion

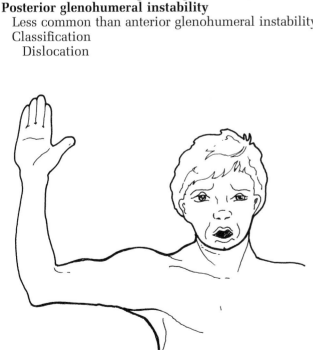

Figure 8–25 ■ Anterior shoulder dislocation. The patient presents with the upper extremity held in abduction and external rotation.

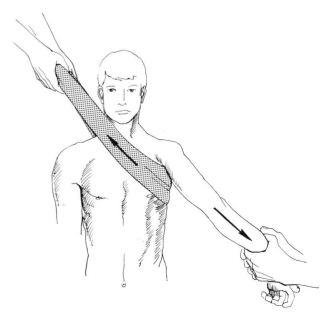

Figure 8–27 ■ Closed reduction for anterior shoulder dislocation with traction–counter traction. (From Rockwood CA, Green DP [eds]: Fractures, 2nd ed. Philadelphia, JB Lippincott, 1984.)

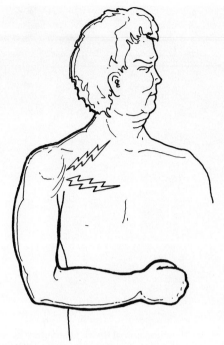

Figure 8–28 ■ Posterior shoulder dislocation. The patient presents with the upper extremity held in adduction and internal rotation.

Axillary radiograph is diagnostic, and without it a posterior dislocation can be missed (**CATASTROPHIC!**) (see Fig. 8–16)

Associated fractures (Fig. 8–29)—reverse Hill-Sachs defect (hatchet-shaped anterior humeral head impression fracture); reverse Bankart lesion (posterior glenoid rim); lesser tuberosity fracture

Reduction of a posterior shoulder dislocation—distal and lateral traction, avoid external rotation; defect in the humeral head (reverse Hill-Sachs defect) may require operative treatment; recurrent dislocations require operative intervention

Missed dislocation (CATASTROPHIC!)

Chronic traumatic (missed)—more commonly seen in alcoholics

Subluxation

Habitual (voluntary with pyschiatric overlay)

Voluntary (intentional)

Involuntary (unintentional)

Multidirectional glenohumeral instability

Shoulder examination shows instability in multiple directions

Patients often display hyperelasticity of several joints (metacarpophalangeal, elbow, knee, and others)

Nonoperative treatment favored

Impingement/Rotator Cuff Disease

Common condition in middle-aged patients; usually associated with "pinching" or impingement of the rotator cuff tendon(s) (especially supraspinatus) by a subacromial spur; the most common cause of shoulder bursitis

Three stages of disease are commonly recognized (Table 8–2)

A rotator cuff tear is the end stage of impingement; it can be a result of a traumatic injury or, more frequently, the final erosion of the cuff from chronic impingement

Physical examination is helpful (impingement sign/test, Hawkins' test, weakness, drop arm test) (see Figs. 8–9 and 8–10)

Impingement sign—passive forward flexion to 130 to 170 degrees results in pain

Impingement test—subacromial lidocaine administration relieves pain of impingement

Hawkins' test—forward flexion with passive internal rotation leads to impingement pain

Type III ("hooked") acromion and/or a large subacromial spur are common in patients with impingement/rotator cuff disease (see Fig. 8–18)

Treatment options

Nonoperative

Activity modification

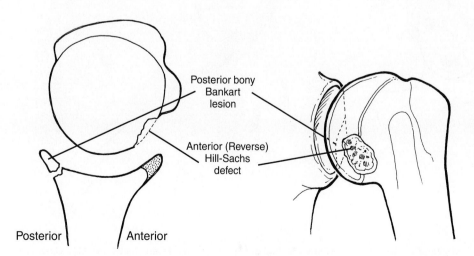

Posterior bony Bankart lesion

Anterior (Reverse) Hill-Sachs defect

Posterior   Anterior

Figure 8–29 ■ Schematic drawings (axillary view on the left and AP view on the right) demonstrating lesions associated with posterior glenohumeral instability.

Table 8–2
STAGES OF SUBACROMIAL IMPINGEMENT SYNDROME

Stage	Age (yr)	Rotator Cuff Pathology	Clinical Course	Treatment
I	<25	Edema and hemorrhage	Reversible	Conservative
II	25–40	Fibrosis and tendinitis	Activity-related pain	Therapy/operative
III	>40	Acromioclavicular spur and cuff tear	Progressive disability	Operative

Modalities (ultrasound, iontophoresis)
Subacromial injection (lidocaine with or without steroids)
Rotator cuff strengthening
Operative
Acromioplasty (open versus arthroscopic)
Rotator cuff repair
Rotator cuff "salvage" operations (débridement, subscapularis transfer, pectoralis transfer, latissimus transfer, hemiarthroplasty)

Biceps Tendon Injuries

The biceps can be injured proximally (described here) or distally (described in Chapter 10); proximal ruptures are more common than distal ruptures and are often associated with impingement
Biceps tendinitis/injury
Physical examination
"Popeye" muscle (for ruptures) (Fig. 8–30)
Localized tenderness
Positive Speed's or Yergason's test (see Fig. 8–11)
Nonoperative treatment
Strengthening
Modalities
Injection (into the tendon sheath, not into the tendon!)
Operative treatment
Decompression/acromioplasty
Biceps tenodesis

SLAP lesions—disruption of the long head of the biceps tendon at its origin can cause shoulder pain, clicking, and difficulty throwing

Acromioclavicular Problems

Acromioclavicular separation
Results from an injury to the acromioclavicular ligament with or without an injury to the coracoclavicular ligaments
Commonly known as a "shoulder separation"
Mechanism of injury—direct trauma
Treatment based on classification (degree of injury) (see Fractures and Dislocations section of this chapter)
Acromioclavicular degenerative joint disease—arthritis of this joint is common; patients may complain of pain with cross-chest adduction (see Fig. 8–12) and may get relief with a diagnostic (lidocaine) injection
Symptoms may include painful thickening and swelling or a "lump" over the acromioclavicular joint
Nonoperative treatment—injections, nonsteroidal anti-inflammatory drugs (NSAIDs), activity modification
Operative treatment—distal clavicle resection (Mumford procedure)
Distal clavicle osteolysis (Fig. 8–31)—degeneration of the distal clavicle with associated osteopenia and/or cystic changes—seen in weight lifters

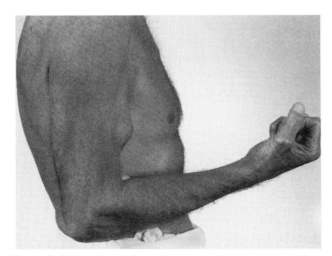

Figure 8–30 ■ "Popeye" muscle associated with proximal biceps tendon rupture. (From Burkhead WZ Jr: The biceps tendon. *In* Rockwood CA Jr, Matsen FA III [eds]: The Shoulder. Philadelphia, WB Saunders, 1990, p 815.)

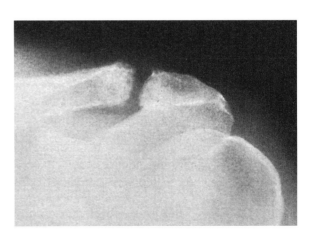

Figure 8–31 ■ Distal clavicle osteolysis in a 35-year-old weight lifter. (From Lyons FR, Rockwood CA Jr: Osteolysis of the clavicle. *In* DeLee JC, Drez D Jr [eds]: Orthopaedic Sports Medicine: Principles and Practice. Philadelphia, WB Saunders, 1994, p 544.)

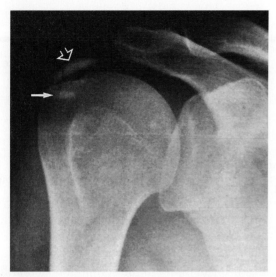

Figure 8–32 ■ Calcific tendinitis. AP radiograph of the shoulder shows calcification at the base of the greater tuberosity (*closed arrow*) and in the supraspinatus tendon (*open arrow*). (From Weissman BNW, Sledge CB: Orthopedic Radiology. Philadelphia, WB Saunders, 1986, p 277.)

Treatment—activity modification, injection, occasionally distal clavicle resection

Muscle/Tendon Ruptures

More common in weight lifters (pectoralis major) and steroid users
Biceps tendon ruptures (can occur proximally [at the origin] or distally [at the insertion]) (see Fig. 8–30)
Direct immediate surgical repair is the best treatment

Calcific Tendinitis

Deposition of calcium, usually in the supraspinatus tendon
Tendon degeneration or autoimmune phenomenon
Supraspinatus tendon is most commonly involved
Radiographic diagnosis (Fig. 8–32)
Nonoperative treatment
  Physical therapy
  Needling calcification with local anesthetic
  Radiotherapy
Operative treatment
  Surgical excision

Bursitis

Bursitis of the shoulder most commonly occurs in the subacromial bursa in the patient with impingement syndrome
True isolated bursitis of the shoulder is very uncommon and is seen primarily in cases of septic bursitis or crystal deposition disease

Adhesive Capsulitis ("Frozen Shoulder")

Pain and restricted glenohumeral motion
Etiology
  Autoimmune?
  Trauma?
  Inflammatory?
Associated risk factors for developing adhesive capsulitis
  Diabetes
  Chest or breast surgery
  Prolonged immobilization
  Medical disease (thyroid, pulmonary, cardiac)
Clinical stages
  Painful phase
  Stiffening phase
  Thawing phase
Imaging
  Radiography—osteopenic appearance of bone
  Arthrography—reduced size of the capsular axillary fold (caused by scarring of the capsule) is visualized
Treatment
  Observation/home therapy ("orthotherapy")
  Manipulation (risk of fracture, etc.)
  Arthroscopic débridement (investigational)

Glenohumeral Degenerative Joint Disease

Loss of articular cartilage of the humeral head/glenoid

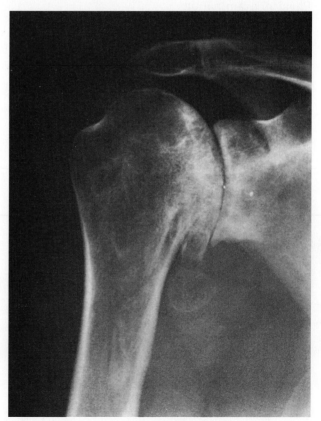

Figure 8–33 ■ AP radiograph demonstrating advanced degenerative joint disease of the glenohumeral joint. Note joint space narrowing, sclerosis, and a large inferior osteophyte. (From Cofield RH: Degenerative and arthritic problems of the glenohumeral joint. *In* Rockwood CA Jr, Matsen FA III [eds]: The Shoulder. Philadelphia, WB Saunders, 1990, p 687.)

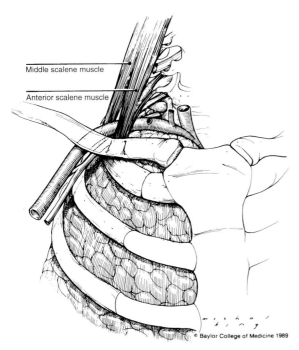

Figure 8-34 ■ Thoracic outlet anatomy. Note that the axillary vessels and the brachial plexus can be compressed by the scalene muscles, first rib, cervical rib (not shown), and other anomalous structures. (From Bennett JB, Mehlhoff TL: Thoracic outlet syndrome. *In* DeLee JC, Drez D Jr [eds]: Orthopaedic Sports Medicine: Principles and Practice. Philadelphia, WB Saunders, 1994, p 795.)

Diagnosis
  Progressive pain
  Decreased range of motion
  Radiographic findings (Fig. 8-33)
    Loss of joint space
    Osteophytes
Treatment options
  Activity modification
  Arthroscopic débridement
  Arthroplasty (see Fig. 7-18)
    Humeral component—placed in 30 to 40 degrees of retroversion
    Glenoid component—loosening is the most common complication

Snapping Scapula

Can be caused by irritation of the scapulothoracic bursa or by an exostosis (bony projection) that catches between the scapula and the rib cage
Presents with scapulothoracic pain, crepitus, and a sensation of snapping
Pain is exacerbated by manipulation of the scapula
This is a difficult diagnosis to make
CT scan can be useful in imaging the exostosis
Treatment is supportive; rarely is surgical treatment required

Nerve Disorders

Brachial plexus injury
  Mechanism of injury
    Traction
    Compression (Erb's point)

Most injuries are transient
  Stinger/burner—transient brachial plexopathy (traction or compression) commonly seen in football players; return to play after resolution of a stinger/burner is allowed unless recurrent episodes occur
Thoracic outlet syndrome—compression of a portion of the brachial plexus (most commonly the lower portion [C8, T1]) and the axillary artery
  Etiology
    Compression by the scalene muscles/first rib on the lateral cord of the brachial plexus and the subclavian artery (Fig. 8-34)
  Diagnosis (see Fig. 8-13)—Adson's maneuver, Wright's test, hyperabduction syndrome test, Halstead's test
  Treatment options
    Nonoperative—physical therapy, postural training
    Operative—first rib resection, others
Long thoracic nerve palsy
  Causes serratus anterior muscle dysfunction
  Etiology often unclear
  Diagnosis made by recognition of scapular winging (Fig. 8-35)
  Treatment options
    Nonoperative—orthoses/observation
    Operative—pectoralis major transfer
Suprascapular nerve compression
  Often compressed at the supraglenoid notch by a ganglion or other soft tissue lesions
  Diagnosis
    Weakness, atrophy of the supraspinatus/infraspinatus muscles
    EMG
    MRI
  Treatment
    Surgical decompression

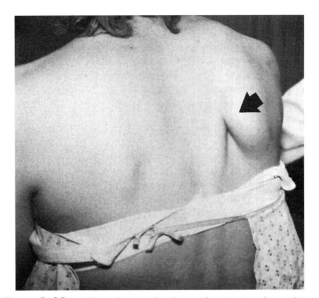

Figure 8-35 ■ Clinical example of scapular winging (*arrow*) in a patient with a long thoracic nerve palsy. (From Miller MD, Cooper DE, Warner JJP: Review of Sports Medicine and Arthroscopy. Philadelphia, WB Saunders, 1996, p 124.)

Table 8–3
FRACTURES OF THE ADULT SHOULDER

Fracture	Eponym or Other Name	Classification	Treatment	Most Common Complications of the Injury
Proximal humerus (see Fig. 8–36)		Neer (4-part classification) Parts are 1. Humeral head 2. Greater tuberosity 3. Lesser tuberosity 4. Humeral shaft *Note:* Fragments are only counted as a separate part if they are displaced by >1 cm or angulated >45 degrees; therefore, a comminuted fracture that is in 5 pieces would still be classified as a one-part fracture if none of the pieces were displaced or angulated		Missed dislocation, adhesive capsulitis, malunion, avascular necrosis, nonunion, rotator cuff tear
		1st part	Early ROM	
		2nd part (3 types) Humeral head	Closed treatment if stable fracture pattern, otherwise operative treatment	
		Greater tuberosity	Operative treatment	
		Lesser tuberosity	Generally closed treatment	
		3rd part (3 types)	ORIF in younger patients; arthroplasty in older patients	
		4th part (1 type)	Arthroplasty	
Special types of proximal humerus fractures	Head splitting		Arthroplasty	Avascular necrosis, post-traumatic arthritis
	Impression (Hill-Sachs defect)	Stable (<20% of articular surface involved)	Closed treatment	
		Unstable (≥20% of articular surface involved)	Operative treatment	
Fracture-dislocation of the proximal humerus *Note:* Fracture-dislocations of the shoulder are generally *more* stable after healing than a simple shoulder dislocation. In a simple shoulder dislocation, all of the energy of the injury is used to tear the capsular and ligamentous structures of the shoulder that are so important in maintaining shoulder stability. In a fracture-dislocation of the shoulder, some of the energy of the injury is dissipated by the bone (fracture) so that there is less of a ligamentous injury and therefore fewer long-term problems with shoulder instability.		Anterior dislocation (greater tuberosity may be fractured and displaced)	Closed reduction of shoulder dislocation; operative repair of greater tuberosity if greater tuberosity remains displaced following reduction of shoulder dislocation	Missed dislocation, adhesive capsulitis, malunion, avascular necrosis, nonunion, rotator cuff tear, axillary nerve injury, brachial plexus injury, hetertopic ossification
		Posterior dislocation (lesser tuberosity may be fractured and displaced)	Closed reduction of shoulder dislocation; operative reduction for a 3- or 4-part fracture-dislocation	
Clavicle (see Fig. 8–37)		Middle third	Figure-of-8 sling	Vascular injury, pneumothorax, other thoracic injuries, malunion, nonunion, thoracic outlet syndrome
		Distal third	Figure-of-8 sling if minimally displaced; operative treatment if fracture has occurred medial to coracoclavicular ligaments and the proximal clavicle is displaced superiorly (Neer types IIA and IIB)	
		Proximal third	Figure-of-8 sling	
Scapula		Body	Closed treatment	Associated injuries (clavicle and rib fractures), pneumothorax, axillary artery injury, brachial plexus injury
		Coracoid and acromion	Closed treatment; ORIF for large, displaced fragment	
		Neck and glenoid (Ideberg I–V)	Closed treatment; ORIF for 1. Large, displaced fragment 2. Intra-articular glenoid fracture that is displaced 3. Subluxation of the humeral head	

ROM, range of motion; ORIF, open reduction with internal fixation.

FRACTURES AND DISLOCATIONS
(Tables 8–3 and 8–4)

Overview

Fractures of the adult shoulder include proximal humerus fractures, special types of proximal humerus fractures (head splitting and Hill-Sachs defect), and fracture-dislocations; other injuries include fractures of the clavicle and scapula

Dislocations and ligamentous injuries include anterior and posterior dislocations and subluxations that can be isolated or recurrent

Other injuries include injuries to the acromioclavicular joint, sternoclavicular joint, and scapulothoracic joint

The treatment of proximal humerus fractures is based on the anatomic region of the fracture lines and the degree of displacement (Fig. 8–36)

Most clavicle and scapular fractures can be treated conservatively, but operative intervention is occasionally necessary (Fig. 8–37)

Dislocations and subluxations of the glenohumeral joint are typically managed with rehabilitation early on, with a small percentage of patients requiring operative reconstructions

Acromioclavicular injuries (the so-called separated shoulder) can be classified into six types, and treatment is based on the specific type (Fig. 8–38)

Sternoclavicular injuries include anterior and posterior dislocations; a posterior dislocation must be reduced because of its displaced position within the mediastinum and the potential for catastrophic neurovascular injuries (see Fig. 8–20)

Scapulothoracic dissociation is an uncommon but catastrophic entity (Fig. 8–39)

TUMORS OF THE SHOULDER

Bone

Periosteal chondroma
Chondrosarcoma

Soft Tissues

Lipoma
Synovial chondromatosis
Liposarcoma
Synovial sarcoma

DIFFERENTIAL DIAGNOSIS OF COMMON SHOULDER COMPLAINTS

Pain

Fractures (and fracture nonunions)
Dislocations (any joint)
Rotator cuff tear (night pain)

Displaced Fractures

Figure 8–36 ■ Neer four-part classification of proximal humerus fractures. Note that displacement of more than 1 cm or angulation greater than 45 degrees is required to designate a "part." (From Bigliani LU: Fractures of the proximal humerus. In Rockwood CA Jr, Matsen FA III [eds]: The Shoulder. Philadelphia, WB Saunders, 1990, p 282. Adapted from Neer CS: Displaced proximal humeral fractures. Part I. Classification and evaluation. J Bone Joint Surg 52A:1077–1089, 1970.)

Impingement (with overhead activities)
Referred pain (cervical spine, radicular)
Rheumatologic conditions
Soft tissue contusions/ruptures
Arthritis (glenohumeral, acromioclavicular, sternoclavicular)
Glenohumeral instability
Bursitis (scapulothoracic, subdeltoid)
Calcific tendinitis
Adhesive capsulitis
Thoracic outlet syndrome
Tumors (also with systemic symptoms)
Infection
Referred pain from the mediastinum

Instability

Glenohumeral dislocation (any direction)
Glenohumeral subluxation (any direction)

Table 8–4
DISLOCATIONS AND LIGAMENTOUS INJURIES OF THE ADULT SHOULDER

Dislocation	Eponym or Other Name	Classification	Treatment	Most Common Complications of the Injury
Anterior glenohumeral dislocation (see Fig. 8–26)		Subcoracoid (most common), infraclavicular, intrathoracic	Closed reduction; shoulder immobilizer (× 2 weeks in younger patients and 5–7 days in older patients); later, rehabilitation/physical therapy	Axillary nerve neuropraxis, axillary artery injury, rotator cuff injury (most common in patients over 40 years of age), recurrent dislocation (most common in patients younger than 20 years of age), associated fractures (Hill-Sachs defect [compression fracture of posterolateral humeral head that occurs during dislocation], Bankart lesion [avulsion fracture of anterior inferior glenoid labrum])
Anterior glenohumeral subluxation		Atraumatic	Rehabilitation	Recurrent subluxation, nerve impingement
		Traumatic	Rehabilitation	
Recurrent anterior glenohumeral dislocation or subluxation			Rehabilitation; requires operative treatment if 6–12 months of rehabilitation fails	
Posterior glenohumeral dislocation (much less common than anterior; etiology—trauma, seizures, and electrocution) (see Fig. 8–28)			Closed reduction; immobilize for 2–4 weeks; recurrent dislocations require operative treatment	Late recognition of dislocation, missed lesser tuberosity fracture
Inferior glenohumeral dislocation	Luxatio erecta		Closed reduction and immobilization	Neurovascular injuries, axillary artery thrombosis
Acromioclavicular (see Fig. 8–38)		Neer and Rockwood (I–VI)		Joint stiffness, deformity, post-traumatic arthritis of acromioclavicular joint, associated fractures, distal clavicle osteolysis
		I. Acromioclavicular ligament sprain	1–2 weeks of rest	
		II. Acromioclavicular ligament tear with coracoclavicular ligament sprain	Sling × 2 weeks	
		III. Acromioclavicular ligament tear with coracoclavicular ligament tear	May require operative stabilization	
		IV. Complete ligament tears with clavicle displaced posteriorly through the trapezius muscle	Closed reduction; may require operative stabilization	
		V. Complete ligament tears with clavicle elevated superiorly (in base of neck) >100% as compared to opposite side (measure distances between coracoid tip and inferior border of clavicle on injured and normal sides)	ORIF	
		VI. Complete ligament tears with clavicle displaced inferior to coracoid	Closed reduction; may require operative stabilization	
Sternoclavicular injuries		Anterior dislocation	Closed reduction, okay to leave unreducible injuries alone	Bump (cosmetic), post-traumatic arthritis
		Posterior dislocation (see Fig. 8–20)	Closed reduction (must be performed in the operating room with chest prepped and draped and a thoracic surgeon on standby); unreducible injuries require ORIF	Impingement on mediastinal structures, injuries to great vessels and other thoracic structures, dysphagia, dyspnea
Scapulothoracic dissociation (diagnosis made on AP chest radiograph; distance from medial border of the scapula to spinous process on the injured side is increased ≥50% as compared to the uninjured side) (see Fig. 8–39)	Closed traumatic "amputation" of the upper limb		Closed reduction, complex reconstruction later	Vascular and brachial plexus/cervical root injuries in *all* of these patients

ORIF, open reduction with internal fixation.

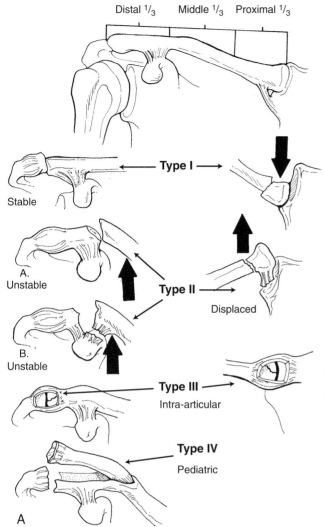

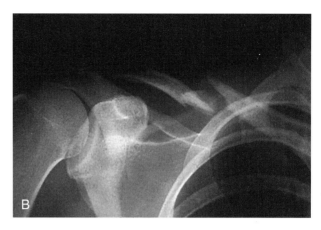

Figure 8 37 ■ *A*, Classification of clavicle fractures with a detailed description of distal third and proximal third types. *B*, Radiograph of a displaced middle third clavicle fracture. (Courtesy of Fondren Orthopedic Group LLP, Texas Orthopedic Hospital, Houston, Texas.)

Weakness

Rotator cuff tear
Neuromuscular abnormalities
Nerve entrapment (cervical roots, brachial plexus, peripheral nerves [long thoracic nerve, suprascapular nerve])
Traumatic nerve injuries
Fractures
Tumors

Tingling/Loss of Sensation

Brachial plexopathy (stingers/burners)
Anterior shoulder instability ("dead arm syndrome")
Traumatic nerve injuries

Deformity

Fractures (and fracture malunions)
Dislocations (any joint)
Soft tissue ruptures (such as the proximal biceps)
Sprengel's deformity
Long thoracic nerve injury (scapula winging)

Tumors/cysts
Neuromuscular disorders (muscle wasting)

Catching/Locking

Glenoid labrum tear
Loose bodies (in the glenohumeral joint)
SLAP lesions

Loss of Motion

Adhesive capsulitis
Fractures
Dislocations
Rheumatologic conditions
Infection
Impingement (from pain)
Rotator cuff tear (passive range of motion is normal; active range of motion is decreased because of weakness)
Tumors
Nerve injuries (active range of motion decreased)
Chronic/missed posterior glenohumeral dislocation

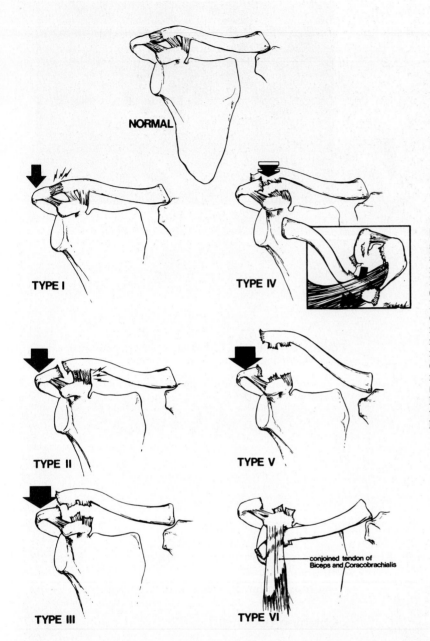

NORMAL

TYPE I

TYPE IV

TYPE II

TYPE V

TYPE III

TYPE VI

conjoined tendon of Biceps and Coracobrachialis

Figure 8–38 ■ Acromioclavicular joint injury classification. Type I—Acromioclavicular (AC) ligament sprain; AC and coracoclavicular (CC) ligaments remain intact. Type II—AC ligament disrupted; CC ligament intact (usually sprained). Type III—AC and CC ligaments are disrupted. Type IV—AC and CC ligaments are disrupted and the distal (lateral) clavicle is displaced posteriorly through the trapezius muscle. Type V—AC and CC ligaments are disrupted; attachments of the deltoid and trapezius muscles on the clavicle are disrupted and the clavicle displaces superiorly. Type VI—AC and CC ligaments are disrupted, the clavicle displaces inferiorly (subcoracoid). (From Rockwood CA Jr, Young DC: Disorders of the acromioclavicular joint. *In* Rockwood CA Jr, Matsen FA III [eds]: The Shoulder. Philadelphia, WB Saunders, 1990, p 423.)

Figure 8–39 ■ Scapulothoracic dissociation demonstrating lateral displacement ≥50% on the injured left side as compared to the normal right side. (From Butters KP: The scapula. *In* Rockwood CA Jr, Matsen FA III [eds]: The Shoulder. Philadelphia, WB Saunders, 1990, p 362.)

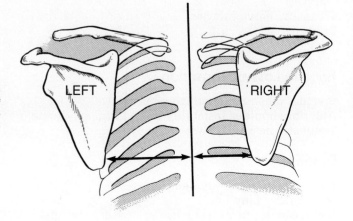

LEFT

RIGHT

PEARLS AND PITFALLS

The glenohumeral joint has the greatest range of motion and the least stability of any joint in the body

Age is an important factor in making the correct diagnosis in the patient with shoulder complaints; younger patients tend to present with glenohumeral instability and acromioclavicular injuries; older patients present with rotator cuff tears, glenohumeral arthritis, or fractures of the proximal humerus

Every traumatic shoulder injury should be evaluated using three x-rays, including an AP view, a transscapular lateral view, and an axillary lateral view; without an axillary view, glenohumeral dislocations (especially posterior dislocations) can be missed!

Sternoclavicular joint injuries are commonly missed and are difficult to evaluate on x-ray; any suspicion of a sternoclavicular joint injury requires a CT scan

MRIs should not be used routinely for the evaluation of shoulder symptoms and complaints; an MRI should never replace a thorough physical examination

Prolonged (several weeks) immobilization of the shoulder, particularly in the elderly, should be avoided and can lead to adhesive capsulitis

Axillary nerve injuries and rotator cuff tears can occur at the time of an anterior glenohumeral dislocation (especially in the elderly) and should not be missed

Anterior glenohumeral dislocations are commonly associated with greater tuberosity fractures, and posterior glenohumeral dislocations are commonly associated with lesser tuberosity fractures

Most clavicle fractures (even displaced or segmental fractures) will heal; clavicle fractures with evidence of neurovascular injuries, open fractures, those with bony fragments tenting the skin, or those who have shown poor early callus formation (delayed union) should be referred to an orthopaedic specialist

A scapular fracture is usually the result of a high-energy injury, and these patients require close observation and are best evaluated by a trauma surgeon with expertise in thoracic surgery

CHAPTER 9

The Adult Arm

ARM ANATOMY

Bone

Humerus (Fig. 9–1)
  Intertubercular groove for biceps tendon
  Groove for radial nerve (posteriorly in the middle
    third of the humerus)

Muscles (Fig. 9–2)

Coracobrachialis (shoulder flexion)
Biceps (supination, elbow flexion)
Brachialis (elbow flexion)
Triceps (elbow extension)

Nerves (Fig. 9–3)

Musculocutaneous
  Supplies coracobrachialis, biceps (short head), bra-
    chialis
  Becomes lateral antebrachial cutaneous nerve of
    the forearm
Radial
  Spirals around humerus posteriorly from medial
    to lateral
  Supplies triceps and wrist extensors
Median
  Runs anteriorly
  Supplies wrist and hand flexors

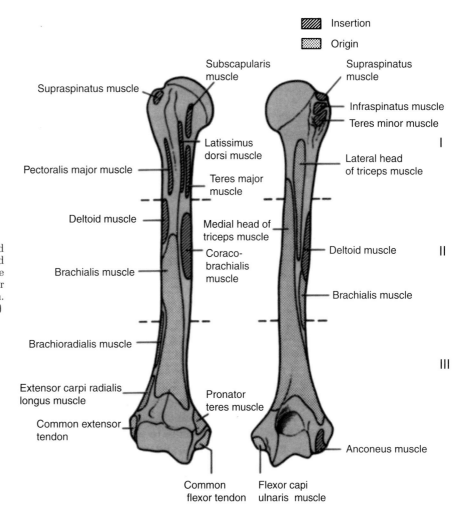

Figure 9–1 ■ Humerus with origins and insertions of muscles. (Modified from Ward EF, Savoie FH, Hughes JL: Fractures of the diaphyseal humerus. *In* Browner BD, Jupiter JB, Levine AM, et al [eds]: Skeletal Trauma. Philadelphia, WB Saunders, 1992, p 1178.)

149

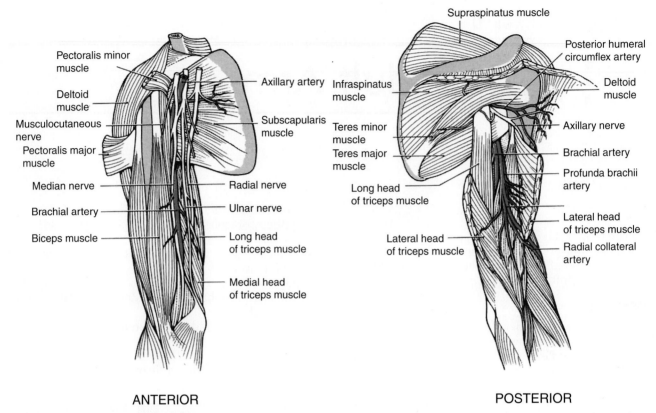

ANTERIOR   **POSTERIOR**

Figure 9–2 ■ Major muscles of the arm and associated neurovascular structures. (Modified from Ward EF, Savoie FH, Hughes JL: Fractures of the diaphyseal humerus. *In* Browner BD, Jupiter JB, Levine AM, et al [eds]: Skeletal Trauma. Philadelphia, WB Saunders, 1992, p 1179.)

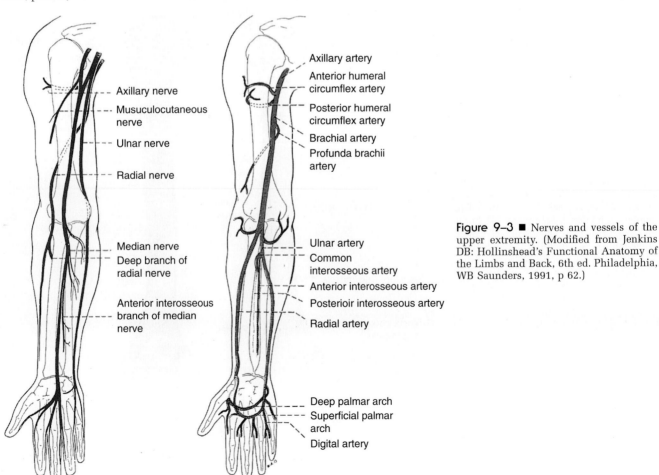

Figure 9–3 ■ Nerves and vessels of the upper extremity. (Modified from Jenkins DB: Hollinshead's Functional Anatomy of the Limbs and Back, 6th ed. Philadelphia, WB Saunders, 1991, p 62.)

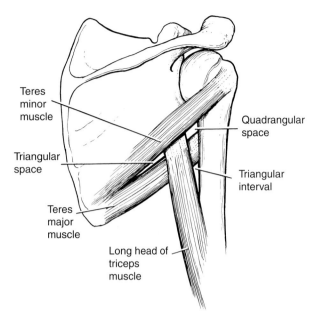

Figure 9–4 ■ Important anatomic relationships. The quadrangular space is bordered by the teres minor (superiorly), the teres major (inferiorly), the long head of the triceps (medially), and the proximal humerus (laterally). The posterior humeral circumflex vessels and axillary nerve pass through this space. The triangular space is bordered by the teres minor (superiorly), the teres major (inferiorly), and the long head of the triceps (laterally). It contains the circumflex scapular vessels. The triangular interval, bordered by the teres major (superiorly), the long head of the triceps (medially), and the humerus (laterally), allows visualization of the profunda brachii artery and radial nerve. (Modified from Kaplan EB: Surgical Approaches to the Neck, Cervical Spine, and Upper Extremity. Philadelphia, WB Saunders, 1966, p. 81.)

Ulnar
  Runs anterior and medial
  Supplies ulnar muscles and intrinsics

Vessels (see Fig. 9–3)

Brachial artery gives
off the radial and ulnar arteries at the elbow

Important Anatomic Relationships
(Fig. 9–4)
SURGICAL APPROACHES TO THE ARM

Anterolateral

Proximal—extended deltopectoral
Distal—brachialis splitting (radial and musculocutaneous nerves)
More distal—between brachialis and brachioradialis (radial nerve)

Posterior

Between lateral and long head of triceps
Deep (medial) head of the triceps is split

Lateral

Between triceps and brachioradialis (below common extensor)

HISTORY AND PHYSICAL EXAMINATION OF THE ARM

History

Injury

Referred pain
Chronicity

Physical Examination

Observation
  Abnormal contours ("Popeye" muscle, atrophy, swelling, skin changes)
Palpation
  Humerus
  Muscles (deltoid, biceps, coracobrachialis, triceps)
  Crepitus/pseudomotion
Neurovascular examination
  Distal muscle function
  Brachial pulse
  Sensation (see Fig. 2–5)
  Strength testing (elbow flexors and extensors)

DIAGNOSTIC TESTS FOR THE ARM

Radiographs

Anteroposterior
Lateral

COMMON ADULT CONDITIONS OF THE ARM

Muscle Contusions

Triceps
Deltoid

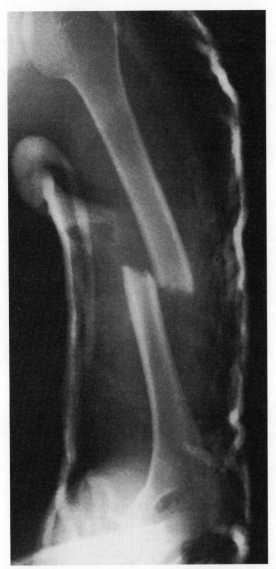

Figure 9–5 ■ Typical humeral shaft fracture. This radiograph demonstrates a humeral shaft fracture in a coaptation splint. (From Ward EF, Savoie FH, Hughes JL: Fractures of the diaphyseal humerus. *In* Browner BD, Jupiter JB, Levine AM, et al [ed]: Skeletal Trauma. Philadelphia, WB Saunders, 1992, p 1184.)

Nerve Entrapment/Injury

Radial nerve

FRACTURES AND DISLOCATIONS OF THE ARM

Overview

Humeral shaft fractures (Fig. 9–5) are classified based on a description of their fracture fragments; treatment of most humeral shaft fractures is nonoperative, with immobilization initially in a sling and swath followed by treatment in a fracture brace approximately 2 weeks after injury; most humeral shaft fractures heal uneventfully; those with poor early callus formation (6 to 8 weeks) or evidence of a radial nerve injury should be referred to an orthopaedic specialist

A floating elbow injury is one in which there is a fracture of the humerus and the forearm—this is a highly unstable situation and requires open reduction and internal fixation

For specific indications for operative treatment of humeral shaft fractures, see Table 9–1

TUMORS OF THE ARM

Bone

Chondrosarcoma
Fibrosarcoma
Angiosarcoma

Soft Tissue

Fibrosarcoma

Table 9–1
FRACTURES OF THE ADULT ARM

Fracture	Classification	Treatment	Most Common Complications of the Injury
Humeral shaft (see Fig. 9–5)	Descriptive	Cast brace/fracture brace, coaptation splint Indications for operative treatment 1. Open fractures 2. Pathologic fractures 3. Segmental fractures 4. Unstable fracture patterns 5. Extension of fracture into (or very close to) shoulder or elbow joint 6. Floating elbow injury (fracture of the humerus and forearm) 7. Polytraumatized patients 8. Distal spiral fractures with radial nerve injury (Holstein-Lewis) 9. Large arm or breasts that will hamper controlling the fracture in a splint or brace 10. Fracture associated with a vascular injury	Malunion, radial nerve injury, vascular injury, nonunion

CHAPTER 10

The Adult Elbow

ELBOW ANATOMY

Bones (Fig. 10–1)

Distal humerus
  Trochlea (articulates with the ulna)
  Capitellum (articulates with the radial head)
  Medial epicondyle (common flexor origin)
  Lateral epicondyle (common extensor origin)
Proximal ulna
  Olecranon (posterior)
  Coronoid process (anterior)

Proximal radius
  Head
  Neck
  Radial (bicipital) tuberosity (biceps insertion)

Joints (Fig. 10–2)
Humeroulnar
  Hinge joint
  Ligaments
    **Medial (ulnar) collateral ligament (MCL) is the
    key stabilizer of the elbow joint** (especially the
    anterior band)

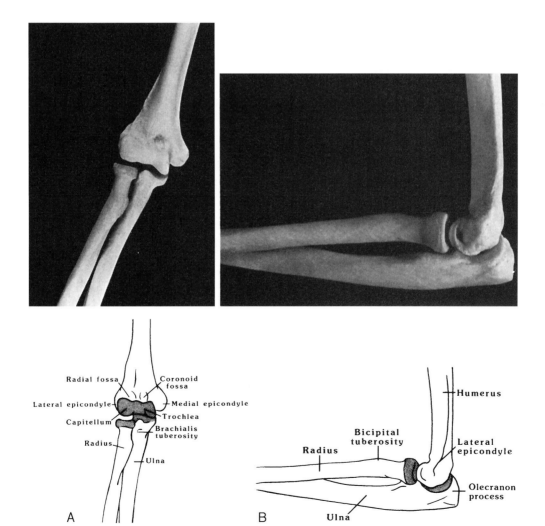

Figure 10–1 ■ Bones of the elbow. *A,* Anterior view of the bones of the elbow. *B,* Lateral view. (From Weissman BNW, Sledge CB: Orthopedic Radiology. Philadelphia, WB Saunders, 1986, pp 170–171.)

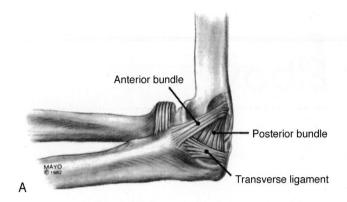

A

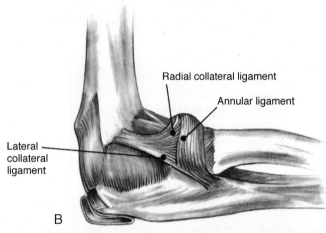

B

Figure 10–2 ■ Elbow joint. *A*, Note the medial collateral ligament with its important anterior bundle. *B*, The lateral collateral ligament. (With permission of the Mayo Foundation. From Morrey BF: Biomechanics of the elbow and forearm. *In* DeLee JC, Drez D Jr [eds]: Orthopaedic Sports Medicine: Principles and Practice. Philadelphia, WB Saunders, 1994, pp 818–819.)

Lateral (radial) collateral ligament (LCL)—originates on the lateral epicondyle and inserts on the radial side of the proximal ulna and on the annular ligament

Humeroradial

  Pivot joint (between the capitellum and the radial head)

  Ligaments

    LCL—inserts onto the radial neck via the annular ligament

Proximal radioulnar

  Allows rotation of the radius around the ulna for (forearm) pronation and supination

  Ligaments

    Annular ligament—originates on the proximal ulna, encircles the radial neck, and then inserts on the proximal ulna

Muscles (Fig. 10–3)

Coracobrachialis (arm flexion)
Biceps (supination, forearm flexion)
Brachialis (forearm flexion)
Triceps (forearm extension)

Nerves (Fig. 10–4)

Radial—lies between the brachioradialis and the brachialis at the medial elbow
Median—lies on the ulnar side of the brachial artery, lateral to the biceps
Ulnar—runs behind the medial epicondyle

Vessels (see Fig. 10–4)

Brachial artery gives off the radial and ulnar arteries at the elbow (cubital fossa)

SURGICAL APPROACHES TO THE ELBOW

Posterior

Olecranon osteotomy gives direct access to the elbow

Medial

Between brachialis (musculocutaneous nerve) and triceps (radial nerve) or brachialis and pronator teres (median nerve) more distally

Anterolateral (Henry)

Between pronator teres and brachioradialis

Posterolateral (Kocher)

Between anconeus (radial nerve) and extensor origin (posterior interosseous nerve)

HISTORY AND PHYSICAL EXAMINATION OF THE ELBOW

History

Mechanism of injury
Aggravating motions
Onset of symptoms
  Acute (such as with a distal biceps avulsion or a MCL injury)
  Chronic (such as lateral epicondylitis or arthritis)
Occupation/activities
  Baseball pitcher—MCL injury
  Tennis player—lateral epicondylitis
  Golfer—medial epicondylitis
  Factory worker—compression neuropathy
Age
  Little League pitcher—medial epicondyle stress fracture and osteochondritis dissecans (capitellum)
  Major League pitcher—MCL injury and ulnohumeral arthritis

Physical Examination

Observation
  Carrying angle (Fig. 10–5)

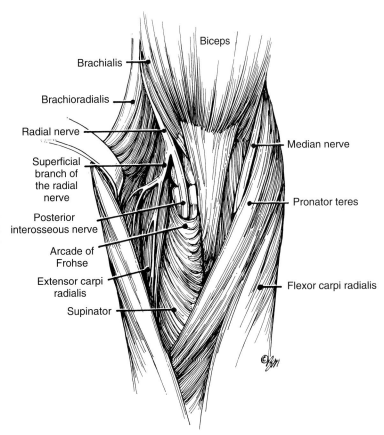

Figure 10–3 ■ Important muscles around the elbow. Note that the triceps is not shown. (Modified from Eversman WW: Entrapment and compression neuropathies. *In* Green DP [ed]: Operative Hand Surgery. New York, Churchill Livingstone, 1988, p 1458.)

Males—normal, 5 degrees of valgus
Females—normal, 10 to 15 degrees of valgus
Swelling
  Intra-articular (hemarthrosis, synovitis)
  Extra-articular (bursitis)
Contour
  Malunited fractures
  Other deformities
Palpation
  Bones
    Humerus (medial epicondyle, olecranon fossa, lateral epicondyle)
    Olecranon
    Radial head
  Soft tissues
    Medial—ulnar nerve, common flexor origin, MCL
    Posterior—olecranon bursa, triceps insertion
    Lateral—common extensor origin, brachioradialis, extensor carpi radialis longus and brevis, LCL, annular ligament
    Anterior—cubital fossa, biceps insertion, brachial artery, median nerve, musculocutaneous nerve
Motion (Fig. 10–6) (Table 10–1)
  Flexion (normal, 135 degrees)
  Extension (normal, 0 to −5 degrees)
  Supination (normal, 90 degrees)
  Pronation (normal, 90 degrees)
Neurovascular exam
  Sensation (see Fig. 2–5)
  Reflexes
    Brachioradialis (C6)

    Triceps (C7)
  Strength testing
    Flexion (brachialis, biceps)
    Extension (triceps)
    Supination (biceps, supinator)
    Pronation (pronator teres, pronator quadratus)
Special testing (condition specific)
  Instability
    Varus/valgus stress test—stress elbow (in both full extension and 30 degrees of flexion) to test the MCL and LCL
    Lateral pivot shift test—tests the LCL and tests for posterolateral instability (the lateral pivot shift test of the elbow must be learned with experience)
  Cubital tunnel syndrome (ulnar nerve entrapment at the elbow)
    Tinel's sign (Fig. 10–7)—tapping over the ulnar nerve at the elbow produces radicular symptoms (tingling sensation) to the volar aspect of the small and ring fingers consistent with ulnar nerve entrapment
    Hyperflexion stress test
  Lateral epicondylitis
    Pain with resisted wrist extension

DIAGNOSTIC TESTS FOR THE ELBOW

Plain Radiographs

Anteroposterior (forearm supinated)
Lateral (forearm neutral, elbow flexed 90 degrees)

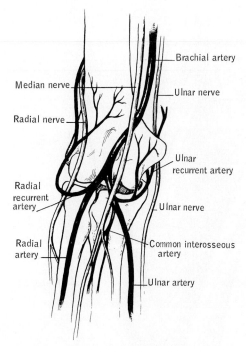

Figure 10–4 ■ Nerves (*white*) and arteries (*black*) of the elbow region. (From Hume EL: The upper extremity. *In* Gartland JJ [ed]: Fundamentals of Orthopaedics. Philadelphia, WB Saunders, 1986, p 243.)

Presence of a fat pad on the lateral radiograph is often associated with an elbow fracture (see Fig. 5–15)

Special Radiographs

Medial oblique view (forearm and arm internally rotated 45 degrees)
    Allows better visualization of the trochlea, olecranon, coronoid

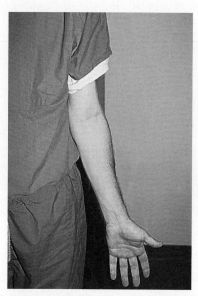

Figure 10–5 ■ Carrying angle of the elbow. Note the valgus positioning of the normal elbow.

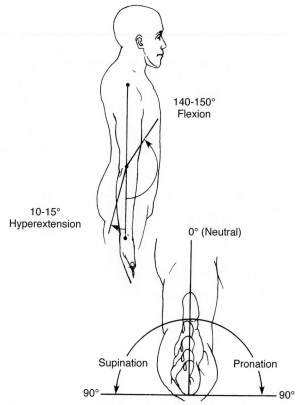

Figure 10–6 ■ Elbow motion. (Modified from Magee DJ: Orthopedic Physical Assessment, 2nd ed. Philadelphia, WB Saunders, 1992, p 147.)

Lateral oblique view (external rotation of the forearm and arm)
    Radiocapitellar joint, medial epicondyle, radioulnar joint, and coronoid tubercle seen well
Radial head view (45 degree caudal tilt lateral)
    Evaluation of radial head fractures

Stress Radiographs

An increase in the lateral or medial joint space of more than 2 mm to varus or valgus stress, respectively, is abnormal and suggests a collateral ligament injury
    Positive lateral side joint opening to varus stress = LCL injury
    Positive medial side joint opening to valgus stress = MCL injury
Gravity valgus stress test to evaluate MCL laxity (Fig. 10–8)

Tomography/Computed Tomography

Complex fractures/loose bodies

Magnetic Resonance Imaging

Collateral ligament injury
Tendon ruptures

Table 10-1
MUSCLES OF THE ELBOW: THEIR ACTIONS AND NERVE SUPPLY, INCLUDING ROOT DERIVATIONS

Action	Muscles Involved	Nerve Supply	Nerve Root Derivation
Flexion of elbow	1. Brachialis	Musculocutaneous	C5-6 (C7)
	2. Biceps brachii	Musculocutaneous	C5-6
	3. Brachioradialis	Radial	C5-6 (C7)
	4. Pronator teres	Median	C6-7
	5. Flexor carpi ulnaris	Ulnar	C7-8
Extension of elbow	1. Triceps	Radial	C6-8
	2. Anconeus	Radial	C7-8 (T1)
Supination of forearm	1. Supinator	Posterior interosseous (radial)	C5-6
	2. Biceps brachii	Musculocutaneous	C5-6
Pronation of forearm	1. Pronator quadratus	Anterior interosseous (median)	C8, T1
	2. Pronator teres	Median	C6-7
	3. Flexor carpi radialis	Median	C6-7
Flexion of wrist	1. Flexor carpi radialis	Median	C6-7
	2. Flexor carpi ulnaris	Ulnar	C7-8
Extension of wrist	1. Extensor carpi radialis longus	Radial	C6-7
	2. Extensor carpi radialis brevis	Posterior interosseous (radial)	C7-8
	3. Extensor carpi ulnaris	Posterior interosseous (radial)	C7-8

From Magee DJ: Orthopedic Physical Assessment, 2nd ed. Philadelphia, WB Saunders, 1992, p 149.

Diagnostic Injection

Intra-articular injection can help differentiate intra-
versus extra-articular pathology
  Aspiration/injection in the anconeus triangle (Fig.
  10–9)

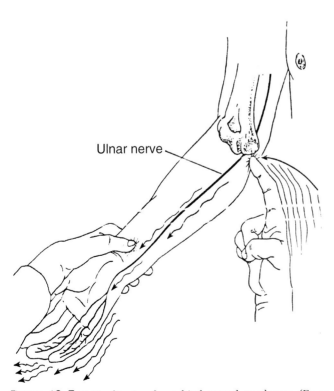

Ulnar nerve

Figure 10–7 ■ Tinel's sign for cubital tunnel syndrome. (From Magee DJ: Orthopedic Physical Assessment, 2nd ed. Philadelphia, WB Saunders, 1992, p 154.)

Arthroscopy

COMMON ADULT CONDITIONS OF THE ELBOW

Compression Neuropathies

Cubital tunnel syndrome
  Compression of the ulnar nerve at the medial epi-
    condyle
  Symptoms—paresthesia (tingling sensation) in the
    ring and small fingers
    Aggravated by elbow flexion
    Can awaken the patient at night
  Findings
    Pain/symptoms with elbow hyperflexion
    Sensory loss (ulnar side of the hand)
    Positive Tinel's sign at the medial elbow (over the
      ulnar nerve) (Fig. 10–7)
    Ulnar claw deformity (late)—caused by motor in-
      jury to the ulnar nerve
    Electromyogram/nerve conduction study abnor-
      malities

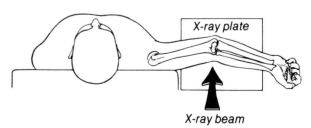

X-ray plate

X-ray beam

Figure 10–8 ■ Gravity valgus stress test demonstrates medial collateral ligament insufficiency. (Modified from Schwab GH, Bennett JB, Woods GW: Biomechanics of elbow instability. Clin Orthop 146:42, 1980.)

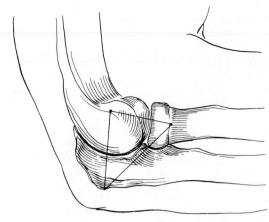

Figure 10–9 ■ Aspiration or injection of the elbow joint is best done in the anconeus triangle outlined by the radial head, lateral epicondyle, and olecranon. (From Magee DJ: Orthopedic Physical Assessment, 2nd ed. Philadelphia, WB Saunders, 1992, p 146.)

Treatment options
    Extension splinting of the elbow (at night)
    Operative—ulnar nerve transposition

Tendon Injuries

Lateral epicondylitis (tennis elbow)
    Etiology
        Caused by chronic degeneration of the extensor carpi radialis brevis (ECRB) at the common extensor origin
        Related to poor technique in racket sports (backhand)
    Symptoms/diagnosis
        Tenderness at the extensor origin
        Pain exacerbated by resisted wrist extension (patient extends the wrist, and the examiner attempts to flex the wrist while the patient resists)
        Relieved by injection of local anesthetic in the area of the ECRB origin
    Treatment options
        Nonoperative—rest, activity modifications, stretching, electrical stimulation, ultrasound, iontophoresis, injection, counterforce bracing (tennis-elbow strap [see Fig. 7–22])
        Operative—ECRB débridement
Medial epicondylitis (golfer's elbow)
    Etiology—degeneration/tear at pronator teres/flexor carpi radialis interface
    Treatment—similar to that for lateral epicondylitis
Distal biceps avulsion
    Etiology—sudden force overload with the elbow in the midflexed position
    Middle-aged males most commonly affected
    Diagnosis
        Acute onset of pain in the antecubital fossa
        Swelling, ecchymosis
        Weakness of elbow flexion and especially forearm supination
    Treatment—operative reattachment
Distal triceps avulsion

Etiology—decelerating counterforce during active elbow extension
Diagnosis—sudden total loss of elbow extension, palpable defect in the triceps tendon
Treatment—operative reattachment

Elbow Instability

Ulnar collateral ligament injury
    Etiology
        Repetitive valgus stress with throwing
        Injury to **the anterior band of the ulnar collateral ligament**
    Symptoms/diagnosis
        Localized medial elbow pain (at the insertion site on the ulnar)
        Valgus instability
        Magnetic resonance imaging (MRI) sometimes helpful
    Treatment options
        Nonoperative—rest, activity modification, bracing
        Operative—reconstruction of the anterior band of the ulnar collateral ligament
Radial collateral ligament injury
    Etiology—elbow dislocation/subluxation
    Symptoms/diagnosis
        Recurrent clicking and/or locking of the elbow with extension and supination
        Positive varus stress test—lateral joint side opens to varus stress
        Lateral pivot shift test may be positive
    Treatment—similar to ulnar collateral ligament injury

Periarticular Injuries of the Elbow

Medial epicondyle injury
    Etiology—repetitive valgus stress (throwers)
    Diagnosis—pain, radiographic changes to the medial epicondyle
    Treatment—activity modification, ice, splinting; operative for a displaced bony fragment
Osteochondritis dissecans
    Osteochondral (bone and cartilage) defect resulting from repetitive microtrauma or a vascular insult
    Most commonly involves the capitellum (Panner's disease)
    Diagnosis—capitellar changes seen on radiographs (Fig. 10–10)
    Treatment—similar to that for a medial epicondyle injury

Other Conditions of the Elbow

Arthritis
    Etiology
        Overuse (degenerative, post-traumatic)
        Rheumatoid arthritis (RA) (Fig. 10–11)
    Diagnosis—radiographs, loss of motion, crepitus
    Treatment options
        Nonoperative—symptomatic, nonsteroidal anti-inflammatory drugs (NSAIDs), other medications for RA patients

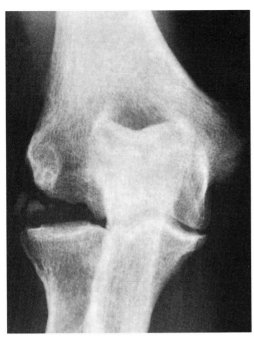

Figure 10–10 ■ Osteochondritis dissecans of the capitellum (Panner's disease). Note that the capitellum is small and irregular, with multiple loose bodies present. (From Weissman BNW, Sledge CB: Orthopedic Radiology. Philadelphia, WB Saunders, 1986, p 207.)

Operative—débridement, synovectomy (for RA patients), total elbow arthroplasty
Olecranon bursitis (Fig. 10–12)
  Inflammation of the soft tissues (bursa) overlying the olecranon process
  Can be septic or nonseptic (more common)

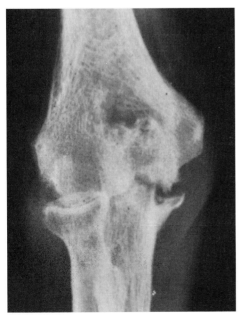

Figure 10–11 ■ Rheumatoid arthritis of the elbow. The AP view demonstrates erosion of the coranoid process and distal humerus and radiocapitellar cartilage space narrowing. (From Weissman BNW, Sledge CB: Orthopedic Radiology. Philadelphia, WB Saunders, 1986, p 183.)

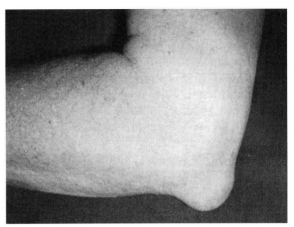

Figure 10–12 ■ Olecranon bursitis. Note enlargement of the olecranon bursa that can become reddened and inflamed, making the differentiation from septic bursitis difficult. (From Singer KM, Butters KP: Olecranon bursitis. In DeLee JC, Drez D Jr [eds]: Orthopaedic Sports Medicine: Principles and Practice. Philadelphia, WB Saunders, 1994, p 892.)

Patient presents with a swollen, painful posterior elbow
Treatment—rest, NSAIDs, elbow padding or immobilization; operative excision rarely required
When a septic bursitis is suspected, aspiration of the bursa (using sterile technique) with fluid sent for culture is indicated

FRACTURES AND DISLOCATIONS OF THE ELBOW

Overview (Tables 10–2 and 10–3)

Injuries to the elbow include fractures of the distal humerus, fractures of the proximal ulna, fractures of the radial head, and dislocations of the proximal radius and/or ulna
Distal humerus fractures (Fig. 10–13) include supracondylar humerus fractures, transcondylar fractures, intercondylar fractures, condylar fractures, capitellar fractures, and epicondylar fractures; because of the complex bony architecture of the distal humerus, anatomic reduction of these fractures (especially those with intra-articular extension) is mandatory, and these injuries must be referred to an orthopaedic specialist
Displaced olecranon fractures and coronoid fragments involving more than 50% of the bony coronoid require operative fixation (Figs. 10–14 and 10–15)
Radial head injuries involve the proximal articulation of the radius at the elbow and are probably best treated by an orthopedic specialist (Fig. 10–16)
Elbow dislocations (Fig. 10–17) are typically high-energy injuries and are treated initially with closed reduction

Table 10–2
FRACTURES OF THE ADULT ELBOW

Fracture	Eponym or Other Name	Classification	Treatment	Most Common Complications of the Injury
Supracondylar humerus (see Fig. 10–13)		Extension (proximal fragment anterior to distal fragment) Undisplaced Displaced Flexion (proximal fragment posterior to distal fragment)	Immobilization ORIF Closed reduction (reduce in flexion) vs. operative treatment	Neurovascular injury, nonunion, malunion, elbow contracture, pain, decreased ROM
Transcondylar (see Fig. 10–13)	Kocher; Posadas		ORIF	Decreased ROM
Intercondylar (see Fig. 10–13)	"T" or "Y" fracture	Riseborough and Radin Undisplaced Displaced or comminuted in younger patients Severely comminuted in older patients	Immobilization ORIF Traction and early motion ("bag of bones" technique) or total joint arthroplasty	Stiffness, decreased ROM, heterotopic ossification, ulnar neuropathy
Condylar (see Fig. 10–13)	Milch		ORIF	Cubitus varus or valgus, ulnar nerve neuropathy, post-traumatic arthritis
Capitellar	Hahn-Steinthal; Kocher-Lorenz	Nondisplaced Displaced	Immobilization Operative treatment	
Epicondylar		Undisplaced Displaced	Immobilization Operative treatment	Pain, poor cosmetic results, ulnar nerve symptoms
Olecranon (see Fig. 10–14)		Undisplaced Displaced	Immobilize for 3 weeks Operative treatment	Decreased ROM, post-traumatic arthritis, ulnar neuropraxia, elbow instability
Coronoid (see Fig. 10–15)		<50% involvement ≥50% involvement	Early ROM Operative fixation	Elbow instability, post-traumatic arthritis
Radial head (see Fig. 10–16)		Mason (and Johnston) (I–IV) I. Undisplaced II. Marginal fracture, displaced	Early ROM Operative treatment for 1. Angulation of ≥30 degrees 2. Involvement of one third or more of the radial head 3. ≥3 mm of joint incongruity	Injury to posterior interosseous nerve, distal radioulnar joint disruption (Essex Lopresti injury)
		III. Comminuted IV. Radial head fracture with elbow dislocation	Radial head excision Operative treatment	
Highly comminuted, high-energy elbow fracture	Sideswipe		Traction vs. operative treatment	

ORIF, open reduction with internal fixation; ROM, range of motion.

Table 10–3
DISLOCATIONS OF THE ADULT ELBOW

Dislocation	Classification	Treatment	Most Common Complications of the Injury
Both radius and ulna (see Fig. 10–17)	Anterior Posterior Medial Lateral	Closed reduction, splint 3–5 days, then gentle, active ROM Open reduction for irreducible dislocation and reduced but unstable elbows	Irreducibility, injury to median and ulnar nerves, brachial artery injury, flexion contractures, heterotopic ossification, unrecognized
Radius alone	Anterior Posterior Lateral	Closed reduction under general anesthesia with early, gentle active ROM; open reduction may be necessary	Irreducibility, injury to median and ulnar nerves, brachial artery injury, flexion contractures, heterotopic ossification, unrecognized
Ulna alone	Anterior Posterior	Closed reduction, splint 3–5 days, then gentle, active ROM Open reduction for irreducible dislocation and reduced but unstable elbows	Irreducibility, injury to median and ulnar nerves, brachial artery injury, flexion contractures, heterotopic ossification, unrecognized

ROM, range of motion.

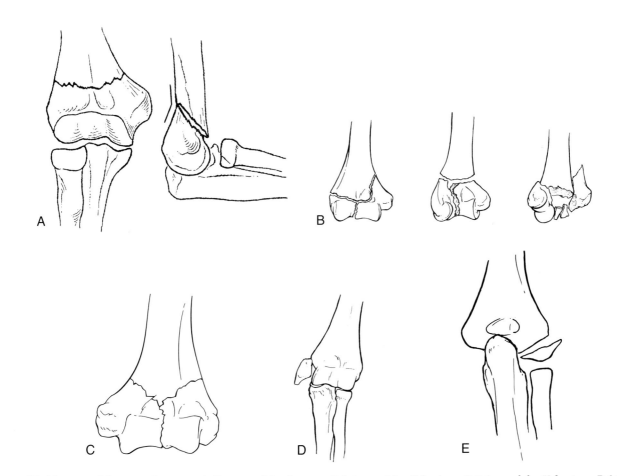

Figure 10–13 ■ Distal humerus fractures. *A,* Supracondylar fracture. *B,* Intercondylar T fracture. *C,* Intercondylar Y fracture. *D,* Medial condylar fracture. *E,* Lateral condylar fracture. (Modified from Connolly JF: DePalma's The Management of Fractures and Dislocations: An Atlas, 3rd ed. Philadelphia, WB Saunders, 1981, pp 765, 772, 775, 782, 789.)

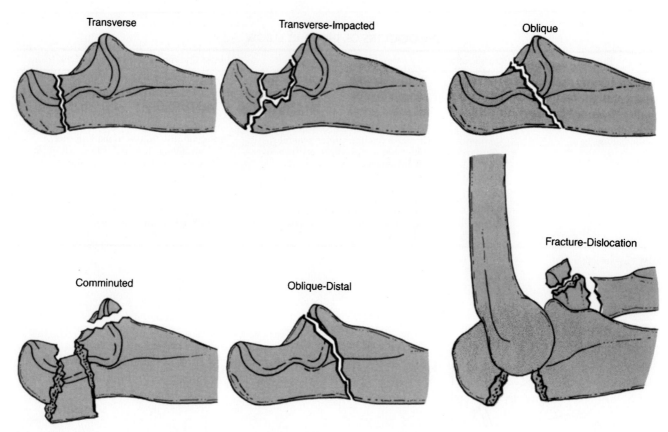

Figure 10–14 ■ Olecranon fracture classification. (Modified from Jupiter JB: Trauma to the adult elbow. *In* Browner BD, Jupiter JB, Levine AM, et al [eds]: Skeletal Trauma. Philadelphia, WB Saunders, 1992, p 1137.)

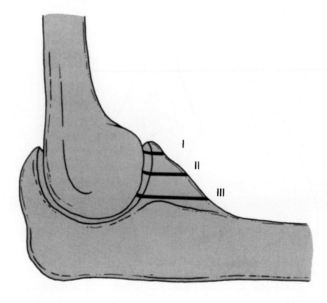

Figure 10–15 ■ Coronoid fracture classification. Note that types I and II fractures involve less than 50% of the coronoid and are usually amenable to nonoperative treatment, whereas type III fractures involve 50% or more of the coronoid and usually require operative stabilization. (From Jupiter JB: Trauma to the adult elbow. *In* Browner BD, Jupiter JB, Levine AM, et al [eds]: Skeletal Trauma. Philadelphia, WB Saunders, 1992, p 1145.)

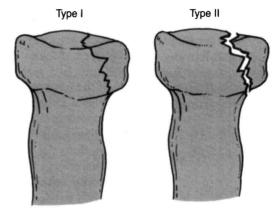

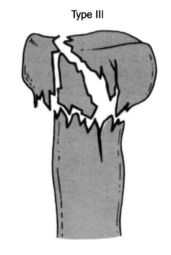

Figure 10–16 ■ Radial head fractures (a type IV–radial head fracture with an elbow dislocation is not shown). (From Jupiter JB: Trauma to the adult elbow. *In* Browner BD, Jupiter JB, Levine AM, et al [eds]: Skeletal Trauma. Philadelphia, WB Saunders, 1992, p 1128.)

TUMORS OF THE ELBOW

Soft Tissue

Synovial chondromatosis
Synovial sarcoma

DIFFERENTIAL DIAGNOSIS OF COMMON ELBOW COMPLAINTS

Pain

Lateral elbow
  Lateral epicondylitis
  Osteochondritis dissecans of the capitellum
  Fractures (radial head, capitellum)
  Nerve entrapments
Medial elbow
  Medial epicondylitis
  Fractures
Diffuse
  Biceps tendon rupture
  Tumor
  Referred pain
  Rheumatologic conditions
  Soft tissue contusions
  Arthritis
  Synovitis

Olecranon bursitis
Infection
Fracture

Instability

Dislocation
Collateral ligament injury
Fracture

Weakness

Biceps tendon rupture
Neuromuscular abnormalities
Nerve entrapments
Traumatic nerve injuries
Fractures
Tumors

Catching/Locking

Loose bodies
Osteochondritis dissecans

Loss of Motion

Arthritis
Rheumatologic conditions
Loose bodies
Synovitis

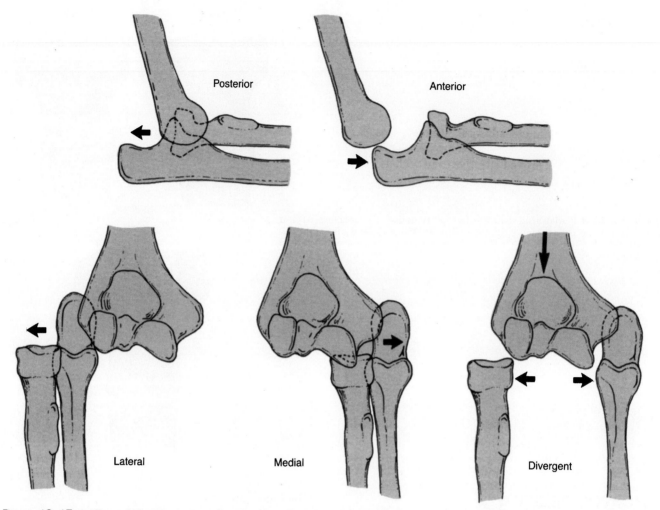

Figure 10–17 ■ Elbow dislocations. Note classification is based on the direction of displacement of the forearm bones. (From Jupiter JB: Trauma to the adult elbow. *In* Browner BD, Jupiter JB, Levine AM, et al [eds]: Skeletal Trauma. Philadelphia, WB Saunders, 1992, p 1142.)

Heterotopic ossifications
Osteochondritis dissecans
Infection
Nerve injuries
Fractures
Chronic missed dislocations (such as of the radial
  head)

PEARLS AND PITFALLS

An adult elbow should never be immobilized in a
  cast or a splint for more than 3 weeks; the elbow
becomes stiff and loses its motion very rapidly, and
  this motion is very difficult, if not impossible, to
  regain even with long-term physical therapy
A thorough search for a fat-pad sign should be made
  when evaluating the radiographs of a patient sus-
  taining elbow trauma; a posterior fat pad is almost
  always diagnostic of an intra-articular fracture of
  the elbow
Posterior dislocations of the elbow are far more common than anterior dislocations
Fractures near or into (intra-articular) the elbow joint
  require anatomic reduction and most commonly require operative stabilization

CHAPTER 11

The Adult Forearm

FOREARM ANATOMY

Bones (Fig. 11–1)

Radius—increases in size distally
Ulna—decreases in size distally

Muscles (Fig. 11–2)

Superficial flexors
  Pronator teres (PT) (median nerve)
  Flexor carpi radialis (FCR) (median nerve)
  Palmaris longus (PL) (median nerve)
  Flexor carpi ulnaris (FCU) (median and ulnar nerves)
  Flexor digitorum superficialis (FDS) (median nerve)
Deep flexors
  Flexor digitorum profundus (FDP) (median and ulnar nerves)
  Flexor pollicis longus (FPL) (median nerve)
  Pronator quadratus (PQ) (median nerve)
Superficial extensors
  Brachioradialis (BR) (radial nerve)
  Extensor carpi radialis longus (ECRL) (radial nerve)
  Extensor carpi radialis brevis (ECRB) (radial nerve)
  Anconeus (radial nerve)
  Extensor digitorum communis (EDC) (posterior interosseous nerve [PIN])
  Extensor digiti minimi (EDM) (PIN)
  Extensor carpi ulnaris (ECU) (PIN)
Deep extensors
  Supinator (PIN)
  Abductor pollicis longus (APL) (PIN)
  Extensor pollicis brevis (EPB) (PIN)
  Extensor pollicis longus (EPL) (PIN)
  Extensor indicis proprius (EIP) (PIN)

Nerves (Fig. 11–3)

Radial
  Anterior branch—supplies the **mobile wad** (BR, ECRB, ECRL)
  Superficial—enters the distal forearm between the BR and the ECRL and is purely sensory
  Deep (posterior interosseous nerve)—splits the supinator and supplies the extensors (except for ECRB and ECRL, which are innervated by the radial nerve)
Median
  Splits the PT and runs between the FDS and the FDP in the forearm
Ulnar
  Splits the FCU and runs between the FCU and the FDP in the forearm

Vessels (see Fig. 11–3)

Radial artery
  Deep to the BR, then runs between the BR and the FCR
Ulnar artery
  Runs proximally between the FDS and the FDP; runs distally between the FCU and the FDS

Important Anatomic Relationships
(Fig. 11–4)

SURGICAL APPROACHES TO THE FOREARM

Anterior Approach (Henry)

Interval is between the BR (radial nerve) and the PT/FCR (median nerve)
Strip the supinator off the bone (proximally) or the FPL/PQ (distally)

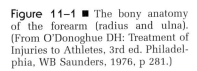
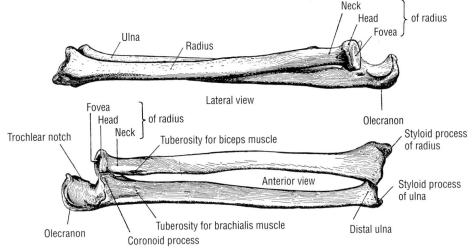

Figure 11–1 ■ The bony anatomy of the forearm (radius and ulna). (From O'Donoghue DH: Treatment of Injuries to Athletes, 3rd ed. Philadelphia, WB Saunders, 1976, p 281.)

165

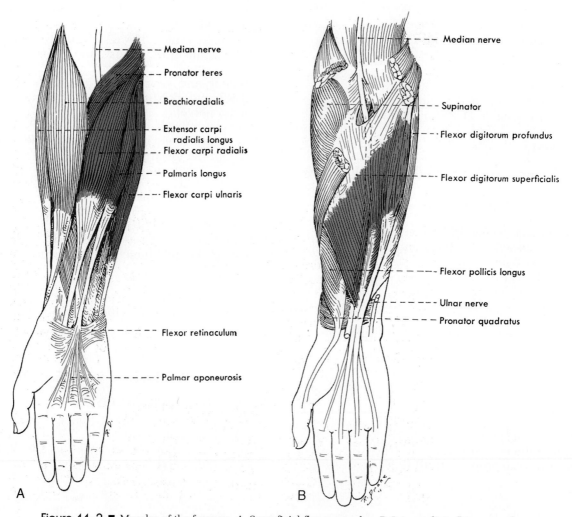

Figure 11-2 ■ Muscles of the forearm. *A*, Superficial flexor muscles. *B*, Intermediate flexor muscles.

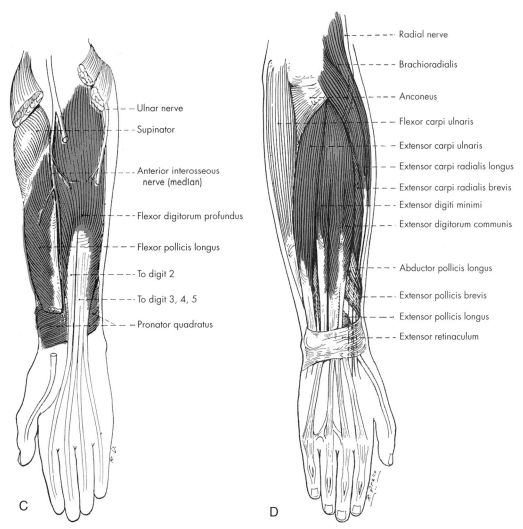

C

Ulnar nerve

Supinator

Anterior interosseous nerve (median)

Flexor digitorum profundus

Flexor pollicis longus

To digit 2

To digit 3, 4, 5

Pronator quadratus

D

Radial nerve

Brachioradialis

Anconeus

Flexor carpi ulnaris

Extensor carpi ulnaris

Extensor carpi radialis longus

Extensor carpi radialis brevis

Extensor digiti minimi

Extensor digitorum communis

Abductor pollicis longus

Extensor pollicis brevis

Extensor pollicis longus

Extensor retinaculum

Figure 11–2 ■ *Continued. C*, Deep flexor muscles. *D*, Superficial extensor muscles.
Illustration continued on following page

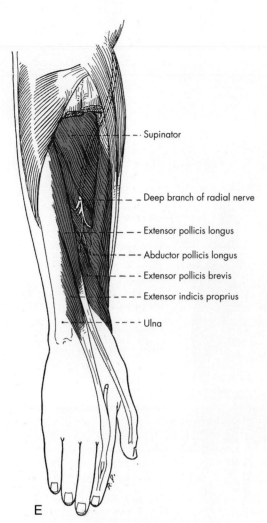

- – · Supinator

- – Deep branch of radial nerve

- – Extensor pollicis longus

- – · Abductor pollicis longus

- – · Extensor pollicis brevis

- – – Extensor indicis proprius

- – – Ulna

E

Figure 11–2 ■ *Continued. E*, Deep extensor muscles. (From Jenkins DB: Hollinshead's Functional Anatomy of the Limbs and Back, 6th ed. Philadelphia, WB Saunders, 1991, pp 126, 127, 140.)

Dorsal Approach (Thompson)

Interval is between the ECRB (radial nerve) and the EDC/EPL (PIN)

HISTORY AND PHYSICAL EXAMINATION OF THE FOREARM

History

Injury
Referred pain (from elbow)
Chronicity

Physical Examination

Observation
  Abnormal contours (muscle injuries, skin changes)
Palpation
  Radius
  Ulna (subcutaneous)
  Muscles (flexors, extensors)
  Crepitus/pseudomotion
Neurovascular examination
  Distal function (median and ulnar nerves)
  Radial and ulnar pulses
  Strength testing (forearm pronation and supination)
  (Table 11–1)

DIAGNOSTIC TESTS FOR THE FOREARM

Radiographs

Anteroposterior (AP) radiographs should be taken with the forearm supinated so that the radius and ulna do not overlap
Lateral radiographs

COMMON ADULT CONDITIONS OF THE FOREARM

Nerve Entrapments

Pronator syndrome
  Median nerve compressed in the muscle of the PT
    Nerve can also be compressed at the supracondyloid process, lacertus fibrosus (bicipital aponeurosis), arch of the flexor digitorum superficialis, and others (Fig. 11–5)
  Symptoms
    Vague, fatigue-like pain
    Exacerbated by repetitive strenuous activity

Table 11–1
MUSCLES OF THE FOREARM: THEIR ACTIONS AND INNERVATION, INCLUDING NERVE ROOT DERIVATIONS

Action	Muscles Involved	Innervation	Nerve Root Derivation
Supination of forearm	1. Supinator	Posterior interosseous (radial)	C5-6
	2. Biceps brachii	Musculocutaneous	C5-6
Pronation of forearm	1. Pronator quadratus	Anterior interosseous (median)	C8, T1
	2. Pronator teres	Median	C6-7
	3. Flexor carpi radialis	Median	C6-7

Modified from Magee DK: Orthopedic Physical Assessment, 2nd ed. Philadelphia, WB Saunders, 1992, p 185.

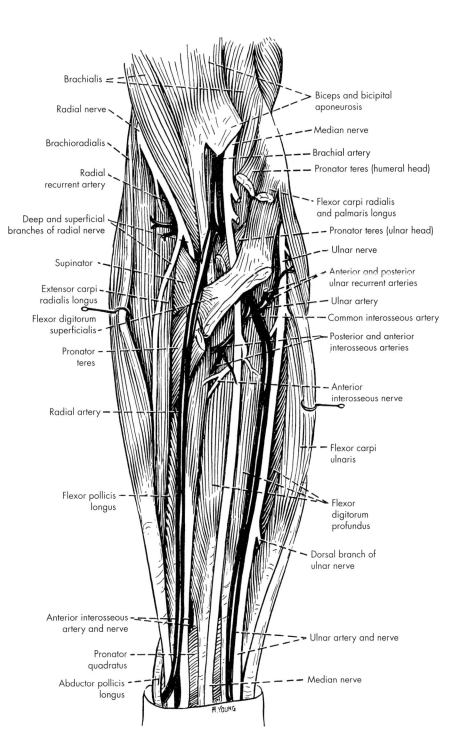

Brachialis

Radial nerve

Brachioradialis

Radial
recurrent artery

Deep and superficial
branches of radial nerve

Supinator

Extensor carpi
radialis longus

Flexor digitorum
superficialis

Pronator
teres

Radial artery

Flexor pollicis
longus

Anterior interosseous
artery and nerve

Pronator
quadratus

Abductor pollicis
longus

Biceps and bicipital
aponeurosis

Median nerve

Brachial artery

Pronator teres (humeral head)

Flexor carpi radialis
and palmaris longus

Pronator teres (ulnar head)

Ulnar nerve

Anterior and posterior
ulnar recurrent arteries

Ulnar artery

Common interosseous artery

Posterior and anterior
interosseous arteries

Anterior
interosseous nerve

Flexor carpi
ulnaris

Flexor
digitorum
profundus

Dorsal branch of
ulnar nerve

Ulnar artery and nerve

Median nerve

A. YOUNG

Figure 11–3 ■ Nerves (*white*) and arteries (*black*) of the anterior (volar) forearm. (From Jenkins DB: Hollinshead's Functional Anatomy of the Limbs and Back, 6th ed. Philadelphia, WB Saunders, 1991, p 131.)

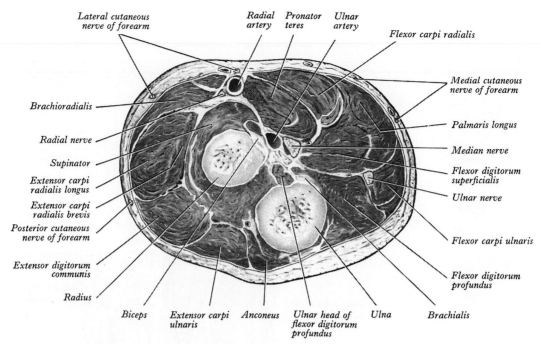

Lateral cutaneous
nerve of forearm

Radial
artery

Pronator
teres

Ulnar
artery

Flexor carpi radialis

Brachioradialis

Radial nerve

Supinator

Extensor carpi
radialis longus

Extensor carpi
radialis brevis

Posterior cutaneous
nerve of forearm

Extensor digitorum
communis

Radius

Medial cutaneous
nerve of forearm

Palmaris longus

Median nerve

Flexor digitorum
superficialis

Ulnar nerve

Flexor carpi ulnaris

Flexor digitorum
profundus

Biceps

Extensor carpi
ulnaris

Anconeus

Ulnar head of
flexor digitorum
profundus

Ulna

Brachialis

Figure 11–4 ■ Cross-sectional relationships of the forearm. (From William PL [ed]: Gray's Anatomy, 38th ed. New York, Churchill Livingstone, 1995, p 846.)

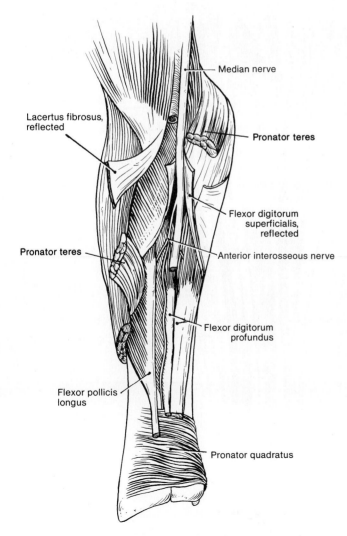

Median nerve

Lacertus fibrosus,
reflected

Pronator teres

Flexor digitorum
superficialis,
reflected

Pronator teres

Anterior interosseous nerve

Flexor digitorum
profundus

Flexor pollicis
longus

Pronator quadratus

Figure 11–5 ■ The median nerve can be compressed at several locations, including the lacertus fibrosus, flexor digitorum superficialis, and pronator teres. (From Green DP, Strickland JW: The hand. *In* DeLee JC, Drez D Jr [eds]: Orthopaedic Sports Medicine: Principles and Practice. Philadelphia, WB Saunders, 1994, p 996.)

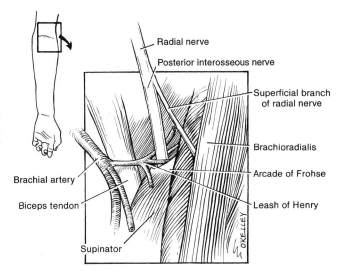

Figure 11–6 ■ The posterior interosseous nerve is most commonly compressed at the arcade of Frohse within the supinator muscle. (From Green DP, Strickland JW: The hand. *In* DeLee JC, Drez D Jr [eds]: Orthopaedic Sports Medicine: Principles and Practice. Philadelphia, WB Saunders, 1994, p 1001.)

Diagnosis
    Sensory changes to the radial 3½ digits
    Pain with prolonged resisted pronation (examiner resists the patient's attempt to pronate the forearm from a supinated position)
    Pain with pressure over the proximal portion of the PT (4 cm distal to the lateral epicondyle)
    Electromyography and nerve conduction studies are not reliable
Treatment options
    Nonoperative—activity modification
    Operative—release all structures compressing the median nerve
Posterior interosseous syndrome
    Posterior interosseous nerve (from the radial nerve) is compressed at the arcade of Frohse (within the supinator muscle proximally) (Fig. 11–6)
    Symptoms/diagnosis
        Inability to extend the metacarpophalangeal (MCP) joints of the fingers
        Pain along the course of the PIN
        Pain with resisted extension of the long finger with the elbow held in the extended position (examiner resists the patient's attempt to extend the long finger at the MCP joint)
        Pain with resisted supination (examiner resists the patient's attempt to supinate the forearm from the pronated position)

No sensory findings
Electromyography sometimes helpful
Treatment
    Surgical release (of the ECRB and the supinator)
Anterior interosseous syndrome
    Anterior interosseous nerve (from the median nerve) is compressed near the origin of the PT
    Uncommon condition that manifests as an inability to perform a precise pinch between the thumb and index finger, caused by weakness of the FDP of the index finger and the FPL of the thumb (Fig. 11–7)
Double crush syndrome
    Entrapment of a nerve at two anatomic sites along the course of the nerve
    Recognition of *both* sites of entrapment is important when planning an operative decompression

Nerve Injuries (Table 11–2; Figs. 11–8 through 11–10)

FRACTURES AND DISLOCATIONS OF THE FOREARM (Table 11–3)

Overview

Adult both-bone forearm fractures (fractures involving the radial shaft and the ulna shaft) require open reduction with internal fixation (Fig. 11–11)

Text continued on page 177

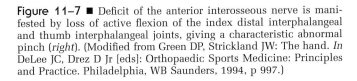
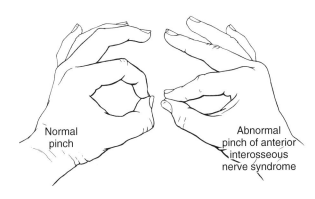

Figure 11–7 ■ Deficit of the anterior interosseous nerve is manifested by loss of active flexion of the index distal interphalangeal and thumb interphalangeal joints, giving a characteristic abnormal pinch (*right*). (Modified from Green DP, Strickland JW: The hand. *In* DeLee JC, Drez D Jr [eds]: Orthopaedic Sports Medicine: Principles and Practice. Philadelphia, WB Saunders, 1994, p 997.)

Table 11–2
NERVE INJURIES

Nerve Injured	Clinical Presentation	Specific Muscles Lost*
Radial Nerve (see Fig. 11–8)		
High	Wrist drop	EDC EPL APL ECRB ECRL BR
Low	Wrist drop	EDC EPL APL
Ulnar Nerve†		
High	Ulnar clawhand deformity (intrinsic-minus deformity) (see Fig. 11–9)	Adductor pollicis Interossei FDP (to the ring and small fingers) FCU
Low	Severe ulnar clawhand deformity	Adductor pollicis Interossei Lumbricals (to the index and long fingers)
Median Nerve		
High	Ape hand deformity (see Fig. 11–10)	PT FCR FDP (to the index and long fingers) FPL APB Lumbricals (to the index and long fingers)
Low	Thenar wasting (see Fig. 11–10)	APB Lumbricals (to the index and long fingers)

*See text for abbreviations.
†*Note*: A low ulnar nerve injury paradoxically results in a worse deformity than a high ulnar injury, because in a low ulnar nerve injury, the FDP to the ring and small fingers retains innervation and results in an even worse clawing deformity.

Table 11–3
FRACTURES OF THE ADULT FOREARM

Fracture	Eponym or Other Name	Classification	Treatment	Most Common Complications of the Injury
Radial shaft with ulna shaft (see Fig. 11–11)	Both-bone forearm		Operative treatment	Malunion, nonunion, compartment syndrome, synostosis, nerve and vessel injury
Radial shaft			ORIF	Malunion, nonunion, compartment syndrome, synostosis, nerve and vessel injury
Ulna shaft	Nightstick	Undisplaced	Long arm cast × 3 weeks, then short arm cast	
		Displaced (>10 degrees angulation or 50% displaced)	ORIF	Missed wrist or elbow injury
Radial shaft at junction of distal metaphysis/diaphysis with radioulnar dislocation; fracture is displaced by Pronator quadratus Brachioradialis Extensor/abductor pollicis longus Weight of hand (gravity)	Galeazzi/Piedmont (see Fig. 11–12)		ORIF ± pinning of distal radioulnar joint (cast in supination postoperatively)	Malunion, nonunion, distal radioulnar joint subluxation
Proximal ulna shaft with dislocation of the radial head	Monteggia (see Fig. 11–13)	Bado (I–IV)	ORIF	Injury to posterior interosseous nerve, missed radial head dislocation

ORIF, open reduction with internal fixation.

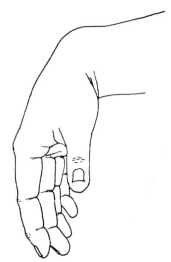

Figure 11–8 ■ Wrist drop deformity of a radial nerve injury. (From Magee DJ: Orthopedic Physical Assessment, 2nd ed. Philadelphia, WB Saunders, 1992, p 176.)

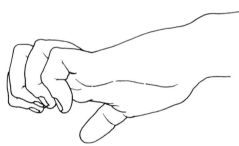

Figure 11–9 ■ Clawhand (intrinsic-minus deformity). Loss of intrinsic muscle function (usually from ulnar/median nerve injury) and overpull of the extrinsic extensors on the metacarpophalangeal (MCP) joint leads to extension at the MCP and flexion at the interphalangeal joints. (From Magee DJ: Orthopedic Physical Assessment, 2nd ed. Philadelphia, WB Saunders, 1992, p 175.)

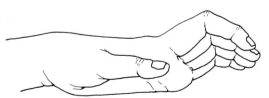

Figure 11–10 ■ Ape hand deformity (median nerve injury) associated with thenar wasting. Note the hyperextension of the metacarpophalangeal joints and the inability to flex or oppose the thumb. (From Magee DJ: Orthopedic Physical Assessment, 2nd ed. Philadelphia, WB Saunders, 1992, p 176.)

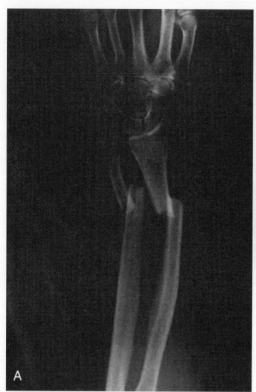

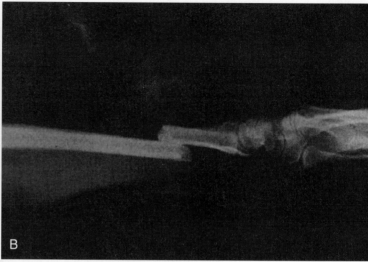

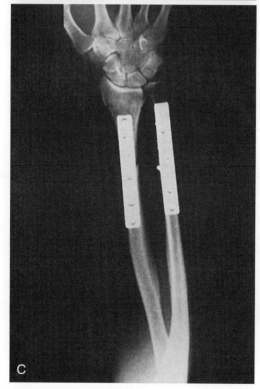

Figure 11–11 ■ Adult both-bone forearm fracture. *A*, AP view demonstrates apex radial angulation. *B*, Lateral view shows 100% dorsal displacement of the distal fragment with "bayonet apposition" of the fracture fragments. *C*, AP view after open reduction with internal fixation. (From Kellam JF, Jupiter JB: Diaphyseal fractures of the forearm. *In* Browner BD, Jupiter JB, Levine AM, et al [eds]: Skeletal Trauma. Philadelphia, WB Saunders, 1992, p 1103.)

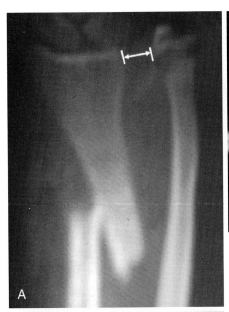

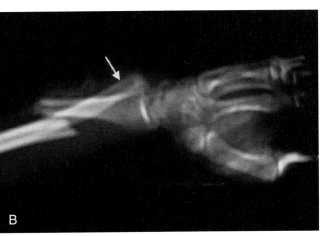

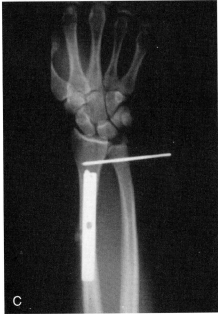

Figure 11-12 ■ Galeazzi (Piedmont) fracture. *A,* On the AP radiograph note the separation at the injured (and unstable) distal radioulnar joint (*arrow*). *B,* Lateral radiograph shows dorsal dislocation of the distal ulna (*arrow*). *C,* AP radiograph after open reduction with internal fixation of the radius and temporary K-wire stabilization of the distal radioulnar joint. (Courtesy of Fondren Orthopedic Group LLP, Texas Orthopedic Hospital, Houston, Texas.)

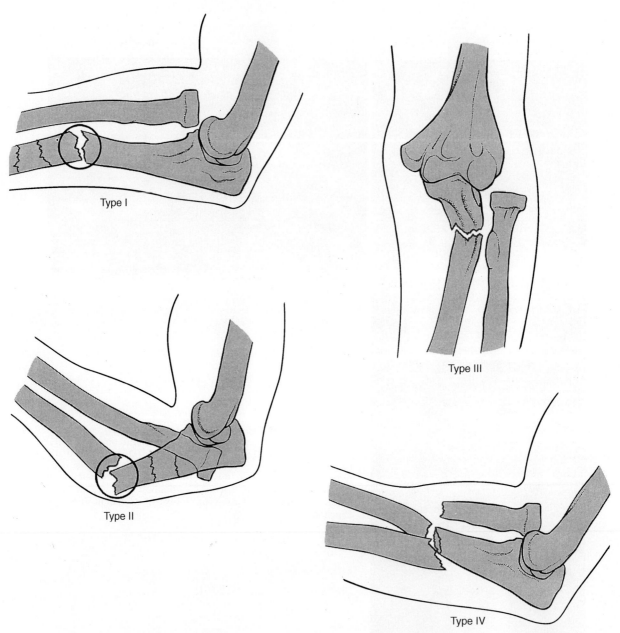

Figure 11–13 ■ Classification of Monteggia injuries. *Type I:* anterior angulation of the ulna fracture and anterior dislocation of the radial head. *Type II:* posterior angulation of the ulna fracture and posterior dislocation of the radial head. *Type III:* fracture of the proximal ulna metaphysis and lateral dislocation of the radial head. *Type IV:* anterior dislocation of the radial head and fracture of both the radius and ulna. (Modified from Kellam JF, Jupiter JB: Diaphyseal fractures of the forearm. *In* Browner BD, Jupiter JB, Levine AM, et al [eds]: Skeletal Trauma. Philadelphia, WB Saunders, 1992, p 1117.)

Isolated radial shaft fractures in the adult also require open reduction with internal fixation

An undisplaced ulna shaft fracture can be treated successfully with plaster immobilization, but it is important to remember not to immobilize in a long arm cast or splint for more than 3 weeks (because the elbow will become very, very stiff)

A displaced ulna shaft fracture requires open reduction with internal fixation

Two special types of forearm fractures, the Galeazzi (Fig. 11–12) and the Monteggia (Fig. 11–13), require open reduction with internal fixation

  A Galeazzi fracture is a distal radial shaft fracture (at the junction of the distal metaphysis and diaphysis) that is associated with a distal radioulnar dislocation and is difficult to treat nonoperatively (because of mechanical forces that tend to displace the distal radial fragment; this injury has been termed "the fracture of necessity" [because ORIF is necessary for a good result])

  A Monteggia fracture is a proximal ulna shaft fracture with an associated dislocation of the radial head; it is important not to miss a radial head dislocation; therefore, all ulna shaft fractures must include a thorough evaluation of radiographs of the elbow; the treatment of a Monteggia type injury is open reduction with internal fixation

TUMORS OF THE FOREARM

Soft Tissue

Nodular fasciitis (volar forearm)

CHAPTER 12

The Adult Wrist

WRIST ANATOMY

Bones (Fig. 12–1)

Distal radius—styloid process, lunate fossa, scaphoid fossa
Distal ulna—styloid process, head (articular surface)
Carpal bones
    Proximal row—scaphoid, lunate, triquetrum, pisiform
    Distal row—trapezium, trapezoid, capitate, hamate

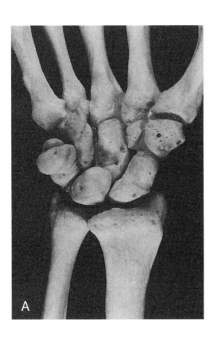

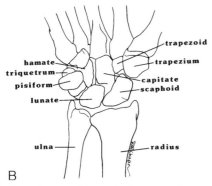

Figure 12–1 ■ Photographic and diagrammatic anatomy of the bones of the wrist. (From Weissman BNW, Sledge CB: Orthopedic Radiology. Philadelphia, WB Saunders, 1986, p 112.)

Joints

Radiocarpal
    Ellipsoid joint
    Ligaments (Fig. 12–2)
        Capsule
        Volar radiocarpal
        Dorsal radiocarpal
        Radial collateral
Ulnocarpal—includes the triangular fibrocartilage complex (TFCC) (Fig. 12–3)
Midcarpal—transverse articulation between the proximal and distal carpal rows

Muscles

Extensors (Fig. 12–4)
    Divided by the extensor retinaculum into six extensor compartments (Table 12–1)
Flexors (Fig. 12–5)
    Flexor retinaculum (transverse carpal ligament) makes up the roof of the carpal tunnel
        Carpal tunnel contents—Median nerve, flexor pollicis longus (FPL), flexor digitorum superficialis (FDS), flexor digitorum profundus (FDP)

Nerves (Fig. 12–6)

Median
    Enters the wrist through the carpal tunnel
    Innervates the **LOAF muscles** of the hand
        Lumbricals (to the long and index finger)
        Opponens pollicis
        Abductor pollicis brevis
        Flexor pollicis brevis (FPB) (superficial head)

Table 12–1
SIX EXTENSOR COMPARTMENTS

Compartment	Contents
1	APL, EPB
2	ECRL, ECRB
3	EPL
4	EDC, EIP
5	EDM
6	ECU

APL, abductor pollicis longus; EPB, extensor pollicis brevis; ECRL, extensor carpi radialis longus; ECRB, extensor carpi radialis brevis; EPL, extensor pollicis longus; EDC, extensor digitorum communis; EIP, extensor indicis proprius; EDM, extensor digiti minimi; ECU, extensor carpi ulnaris.

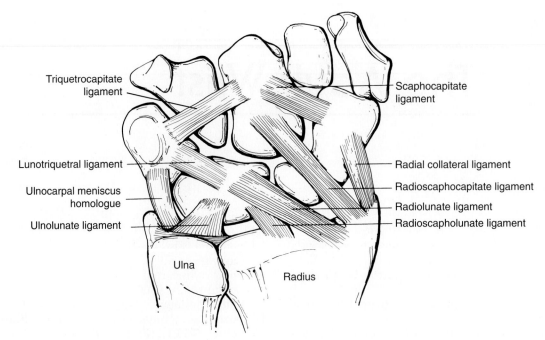

Triquetrocapitate
ligament

Scaphocapitate
ligament

Lunotriquetral ligament

Radial collateral ligament

Ulnocarpal meniscus
homologue

Radioscaphocapitate ligament

Radiolunate ligament

Ulnolunate ligament

Radioscapholunate ligament

Ulna

Radius

Figure 12–2 ■ Volar carpal ligaments. The volar carpal ligaments are more important for wrist stability than the dorsal carpal ligaments (not shown in the figure). (Modified from McCue FC, Bruce JF: The wrist. *In* DeLee JC, Drez D Jr [eds]: Orthopaedic Sports Medicine: Principles and Practice. Philadelphia, WB Saunders, 1994, p 914.)

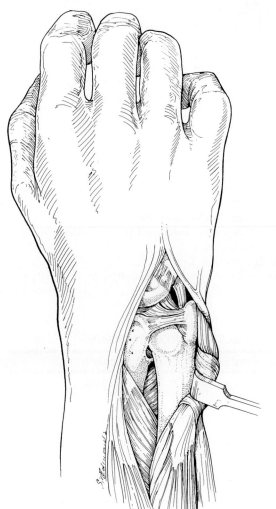

Figure 12–3 ■ Triangular fibrocartilage complex (TFCC). The TFCC is important for stabilizing the distal radioulnar joint. The structures that make up the TFCC include the articular disc (triangular fibrocartilage); meniscus homologue; ulnocarpal ligament; dorsal radioulnar ligament; volar radioulnar ligament; and tendon sheath of the extensor carpi ulnaris. (From Miller MD, Osborne JR, Warner JJP, et al [eds]: MRI-Arthroscopy Correlative Atlas. Philadelphia, WB Saunders, 1997, p 217.)

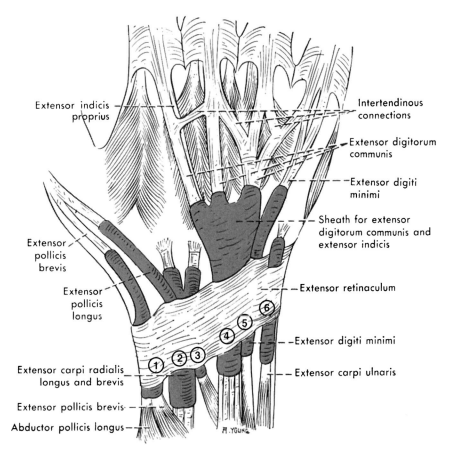

Figure 12–4 ■ Extensor compartments, labeled 1 through 6. (From Jenkins DB: Hollinshead's Functional Anatomy of the Limbs and Back, 6th ed. Philadelphia, WB Saunders, 1991, p 174.)

Extensor indicis proprius

Extensor pollicis brevis

Extensor pollicis longus

Extensor carpi radialis longus and brevis

Extensor pollicis brevis

Abductor pollicis longus

Intertendinous connections

Extensor digitorum communis

Extensor digiti minimi

Sheath for extensor digitorum communis and extensor indicis

Extensor retinaculum

Extensor digiti minimi

Extensor carpi ulnaris

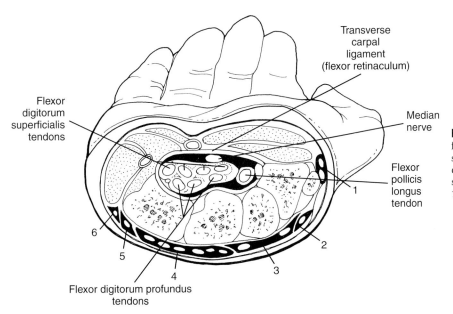

Flexor digitorum superficialis tendons

Flexor digitorum profundus tendons

Transverse carpal ligament (flexor retinaculum)

Median nerve

Flexor pollicis longus tendon

Figure 12–5 ■ Carpal tunnel. Note that the flexor digitorum profundus, flexor digitorum superficialis, flexor pollicis longus, and median nerve all reside in the carpal tunnel. The six extensor compartments have been labeled 1 through 6.

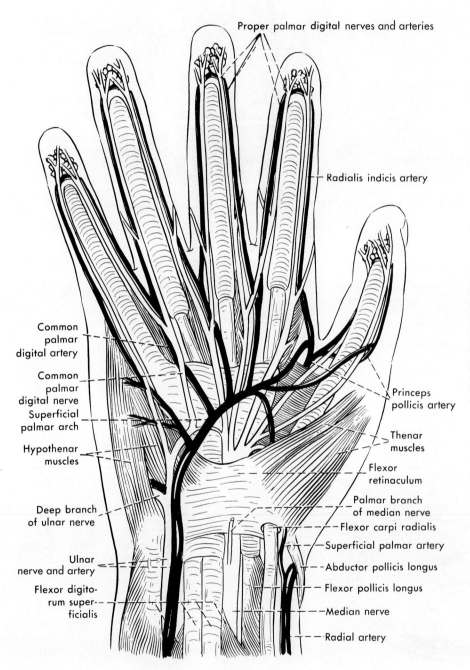

Proper palmar digital nerves and arteries

Radialis indicis artery

Common palmar digital artery

Common palmar digital nerve

Superficial palmar arch

Hypothenar muscles

Deep branch of ulnar nerve

Ulnar nerve and artery

Flexor digitorum superficialis

Princeps pollicis artery

Thenar muscles

Flexor retinaculum

Palmar branch of median nerve

Flexor carpi radialis

Superficial palmar artery

Abductor pollicis longus

Flexor pollicis longus

Median nerve

Radial artery

Figure 12–6 ■ Nerves (*white*) and arteries (*black*) of the wrist and hand. Note that the ulnar artery is the main contributor to the superficial palmar arch and that the radial artery is the main contributor to the deep palmar arch (deep to the flexor retinaculum). (From Jenkins DB: Hollinshead's Functional Anatomy of the Limbs and Back, 6th ed. Philadelphia, WB Saunders, 1991, p 169.)

Provides sensation to the radial 3½ digits

Ulnar

  Enters the wrist through Guyon's canal (the floor of Guyon's canal is the transverse carpal ligament and the roof is the volar carpal ligament)

  Innervates the hypothenar muscles, adductor pollicus, half of the FPB (the deep head), all interosseous muscles, and the lumbricales to the ring and small fingers

  Provides sensation to the ulnar 1½ digits

Vessels (see Fig. 12–6)

Radial artery

  Lies between the brachioradialis and the flexor carpi radialis (FCR) at the wrist

  Enters the anatomic "snuff box" (between the extensor pollicis longus [EPL] and the extensor pollicis brevis [EPB])

Ulnar artery

  Lies between the flexor carpi ulnaris (FCU) and the FDS at the wrist

  Enters the wrist through Guyon's canal

SURGICAL APPROACHES TO THE WRIST

Dorsal Approach to the Wrist

Between the 3rd and 4th extensor compartments

Volar Approach to the Wrist

Through the transverse carpal ligament

Volar (Russe) Approach to the Scaphoid

Between the FCR and the radial artery
Can dissect through the FCR sheath

Dorsolateral Approach to the Scaphoid

Through the anatomic snuff box (between the EPL and EPB)
Radial artery and nerve branches should be protected

HISTORY AND PHYSICAL EXAMINATION OF THE WRIST

History

Mechanism of injury
  Direction of forces involved
Aggravating motions
Onset of symptoms
  Acute (fracture, ligamentous injury)
  Chronic (arthritis, tendinitis, carpal instability)
Location of pain
  Radial side of the wrist—scaphoid fracture, deQuervain's tenosynovitis, FCR tendinitis, intersection syndrome, dorsal carpal instability patterns (DISI

= dorsal intercalated segmental instability pattern)

  Ulnar side of the wrist—extensor carpi ulnaris (ECU)/FCU tendinitis, extensor digiti minimi (EDM) tendinitis, TFCC tear, volar carpal instability patterns (VISI = volar intercalated segmental instability pattern)

  Dorsal wrist—Kienböck's disease, dorsal ganglion

  Volar wrist—carpal tunnel syndrome, volar ganglion, ulnar tunnel syndrome

Painful "click"
  TFCC injury
  Carpal instability
Age
Occupation/activities
Handedness (dominant hand)

Physical Examination

Observation
  Attitude/contour
Palpation
  Bones
    Proximal carpal row (scaphoid, lunate, triquetrum, pisiform)
    Distal carpal row (trapezium, trapezoid, capitate, hamate)
    Radius (radial styloid, Lister's tubercle)
    Ulna (ulnar styloid)
  Soft tissues
    Radial wrist—anatomic snuff box, radial artery
    Dorsal wrist—six dorsal compartments
    Ulnar wrist—FCU, Guyon's canal, ulnar artery, TFCC
    Palmar wrist—palmaris longus, carpal tunnel, FCR
Motion (Table 12–2)
  Flexion (normal, 80 degrees)
  Extension (normal, 70 degrees)
  Ulnar deviation (normal, 30 degrees)
  Radial deviation (normal, 20 degrees)
Neurovascular exam
  Pulses—radial and ulnar arteries
  Sensation (see Fig. 2–5)
  Strength testing
    Flexion (FCR, FCU)
    Extension (extensor carpi radialis longus [ECRL], extensor carpi radialis brevis [ECRB], ECU)
    Ulnar deviation (FCU, ECU)
    Radial deviation (FCR, ECRL, abductor pollicis longus [APL], EPB)
    Finger extension (extensor digitorum comminus [EDC], extensor indicis proprius [EIP], EDM)
    Finger flexion (FDP, FDS)
Special testing (condition specific)
  Instability (Fig. 12–7)
    Watson's test—palpable clunk with passive radial deviation of the wrist with the scaphoid stabilized volarly, suggests scapholunate instability
    Ballottement test—pain, crepitus, and laxity elicited by the following maneuver (tests for triquetrolunate dissociation): the lunate is stabilized

Table 12–2
MUSCLES OF THE WRIST AND HAND: THEIR ACTIONS AND INNERVATION, INCLUDING NERVE ROOT DERIVATIONS

Action	Muscles Involved	Innervation	Nerve Root Derivation
Extension of wrist	1. Extensor carpi radialis longus	Radial	C6-7
	2. Extensor carpi radialis brevis	Radial	C6-7
	3. Extensor carpi ulnaris	Posterior interosseous (radial)	C7-8
Flexion of wrist	1. Flexor carpi radialis	Median	C6-7
	2. Flexor carpi ulnaris	Ulnar	C7-8
Ulnar deviation of wrist	1. Flexor carpi ulnaris	Ulnar	C7-8
	2. Extensor carpi ulnaris	Posterior interosseous (radial)	C7-8
Radial deviation of wrist	1. Flexor carpi radialis	Median	C6-7
	2. Extensor carpi radialis longus	Radial	C6-7
	3. Abductor pollicis longus	Posterior interosseous (radial)	C7-8
	4. Extensor pollicis brevis	Posterior interosseous (radial)	C7-8
Extension of fingers	1. Extensor digitorum communis	Posterior interosseous (radial)	C7-8
	2. Extensor indicis proprius (index finger)	Posterior interosseous (radial)	C7-8
	3. Extensor digiti minimi (small finger)	Posterior interosseous (radial)	C7-8
Flexion of fingers	1. Flexor digitorum profundus	Anterior interosseous (median): lateral two digits*	C8, T1
		Ulnar: medial two digits*	C8, T1
	2. Flexor digitorum superficialis	Median	C7-8, T1
	3. Lumbricales	First and second: median; third and fourth: ulnar (deep terminal branch)	C8, T1
			C8, T1
	4. Interossei	Ulnar (deep terminal branch)	C8, T1
	5. Flexor digiti minimi (small finger)	Ulnar (deep terminal branch)	C8, T1
Abduction of fingers (with fingers extended)	1. Dorsal interossei	Ulnar (deep terminal branch)	C8, T1
	2. Abductor digiti minimi (small finger)	Ulnar (deep terminal branch)	C8, T1
Adduction of fingers (with fingers extended)	1. Palmar interossei	Ulnar (deep terminal branch)	C8, T1
Extension of thumb	1. Extensor pollicis longus	Posterior interosseous (radial)	C7-8
	2. Extensor pollicis brevis	Posterior interosseous (radial)	C7-8
	3. Abductor pollicis longus	Posterior interosseous (radial)	C7-8
Flexion of thumb	1. Flexor pollicis brevis	Superficial head: median (lateral terminal branch)	C8, T1
		Deep head: ulnar	C8, T1
	2. Flexor pollicis longus	Anterior interosseous (median)	C8, T1
	3. Opponens pollicis	Median (lateral terminal branch)	C8, T1
Abduction of thumb	1. Abductor pollicis longus	Posterior interosseous (radial)	C7-8
	2. Abductor pollicis brevis	Median (lateral terminal branch)	C8, T1
Adduction of thumb	1. Adductor pollicis	Ulnar (deep terminal branch)	C8, T1
Opposition of thumb and small finger	1. Opponens pollicis	Median (lateral terminal branch)	C8, T1
	2. Flexor pollicis brevis	Superficial head: median (lateral terminal branch)	C8, T1
	3. Abductor pollicis brevis	Median (lateral terminal branch)	C8, T1
	4. Opponens digiti minimi	Ulnar (deep terminal branch)	C8, T1

Modified from Magee DJ: Orthopedic Physical Assessment, 2nd ed. Philadelphia, WB Saunders, 1992, p 165.
*Lateral two digits = index and long fingers; medial two digits = ring and small fingers.

with the examiner's thumb and index finger of one hand; the triquetrum and pisiform are passively pistoned volar to dorsal to volar, and so on, with the other hand

Shear test—similar to the ballottement test

Carpal tunnel syndrome (Fig. 12–8)

Tinel's sign—tapping over the carpal tunnel produces paresthesias (tingling) and/or numbness in the distribution of the median nerve

Median nerve compression test—external compression of the volar wrist causes median nerve paresthesias

Phalen's test—forced wrist palmar flexion reproduces numbness/tingling in the distribution of the median nerve

DeQuervain's disease (tenosynovitis of the 1st dorsal compartment of the wrist)

Finkelstein's test (Fig. 12–9)—ulnar deviation of wrist with the thumb in the palm causes pain over the 1st dorsal compartment

Vascular disorders

Allen's test (Fig. 12–10)—evaluates the blood supply to the hand

DIAGNOSTIC TESTS FOR THE WRIST

Plain Radiographs

Posteroanterior (PA)
Lateral
Obliques (45-degree pronation PA)

Additional Radiographs

Ulnar deviation PA—scaphoid better visualized
Clenched fist PA (in both maximal ulnar and radial

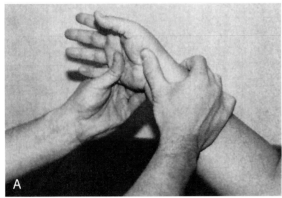

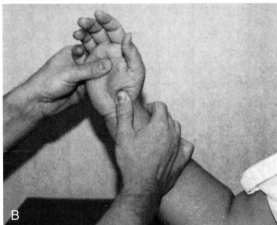

Figure 12–7 ■ *The Watson test for scapholunate instability. A, The scaphoid is stabilized with the thumb over the volar pole. B, The hand is brought from ulnar to radial deviation and a "clunk" and/or pain results. (From McCue FC, Bruce JF: The wrist. In DeLee JC, Drez D Jr [eds]: Orthopaedic Sports Medicine: Principles and Practice. Philadelphia, WB Saunders, 1994, p 919.)*

deviation)—subtle wrist instabilities may be visualized

Carpal tunnel view—visualizes carpal tunnel encroachment and hook of the hamate fractures

Cineradiography (Fluoroscopy)

Dynamic (real-time) evaluation for wrist instability

Arthrography (Fig. 12–11)

Ligamentous tears, TFCC injury, cartilaginous injuries

More accurate in younger patients

Bone Scan

Nonspecific but sensitive for wrist injuries

Tomography/Computed Tomography

Best for fracture visualization

Magnetic Resonance Imaging

TFCC injury
Ligamentous injuries

Arthroscopy (Fig. 12–12)

COMMON ADULT CONDITIONS OF THE WRIST

Entrapment Syndromes

Carpal tunnel syndrome
  Median nerve compression under the transverse carpal ligament (see Fig. 12–5)
    Symptoms/diagnosis
      Numbness/tingling in the radial 3½ digits
      Night pain
      Provocative testing (Tinel's sign, Phalen's test, compression test)
      Thenar muscle wasting (in advanced cases)
      Electromyogram/nerve conduction studies show slowed conduction velocity at the carpal tunnel and denervation of the thenar musculature (in advanced cases)
  Treatment options
    Nonoperative—splinting (volar splint with the

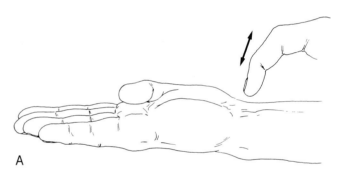

A

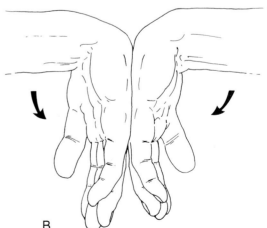

B

Figure 12–8 ■ Tests for carpal tunnel syndrome. *A, Tinel's sign is elicited by tapping over the carpal tunnel. A positive sign results in tingling and/or paresthesias into the digits in the distribution of the median nerve. B, Phalen's test. The examiner flexes the wrist and holds it in this position for 1 minute. A positive test causes tingling and/or paresthesias in the digits in the distribution of the median nerve. In the median nerve compression test (not shown), the examiner compresses the median nerve with digital pressure, causing similar symptoms. (From Magee DJ: Orthopedic Physical Assessment, 2nd ed. Philadelphia, WB Saunders, 1992, p 195.)*

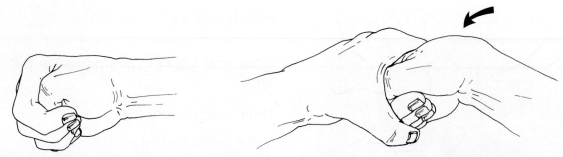

Figure 12–9 ■ Finkelstein's test. The patient makes a fist with the thumb inside the fingers. The examiner ulnarly deviates the wrist, resulting in pain over the first (dorsal) compartment in a patient with deQuervain's disease. (From Magee DJ: Orthopedic Physical Assessment, 2nd ed. Philadelphia, WB Saunders, 1992, p 192.)

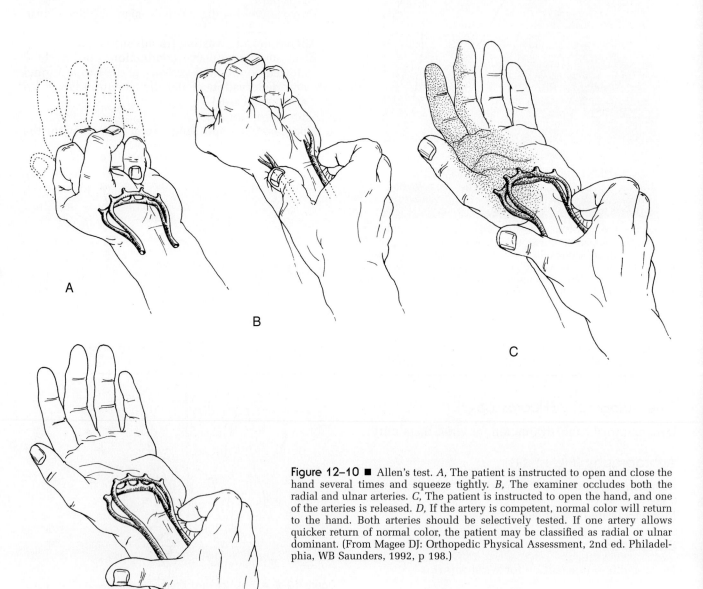

A

B

C

D

Figure 12–10 ■ Allen's test. *A*, The patient is instructed to open and close the hand several times and squeeze tightly. *B*, The examiner occludes both the radial and ulnar arteries. *C*, The patient is instructed to open the hand, and one of the arteries is released. *D*, If the artery is competent, normal color will return to the hand. Both arteries should be selectively tested. If one artery allows quicker return of normal color, the patient may be classified as radial or ulnar dominant. (From Magee DJ: Orthopedic Physical Assessment, 2nd ed. Philadelphia, WB Saunders, 1992, p 198.)

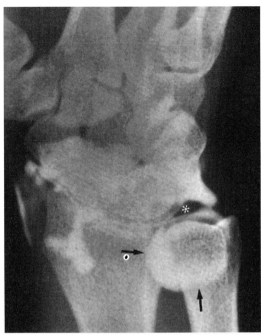

Figure 12–11 ■ Wrist arthrogram demonstrating filling of the proximal radioulnar compartment (*arrows*), suggesting a tear in the triangular fibrocartilage complex (*asterisk*). (From Weissman BNW, Sledge CB: Orthopedic Radiology. Philadelphia, WB Saunders, 1986, p 133.)

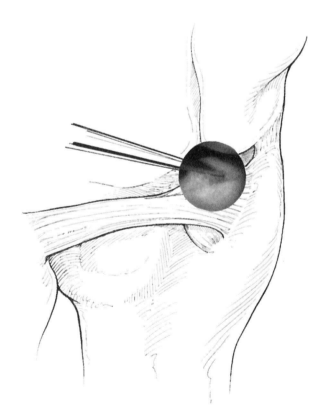

Figure 12–12 ■ Wrist arthroscopy demonstrating a tear in the triangular fibrocartilage complex. (From Miller MD, Osborne JR, Warner JJP, et al [eds]: MRI-Arthroscopy Correlative Atlas. Philadelphia, WB Saunders, 1997, p 223.)

wrist held in 10 degrees of extension), nonsteroidal anti-inflammatory drugs (NSAIDs)

Operative—surgical release of the transverse carpal ligament

Ulnar tunnel syndrome

Ulnar nerve is compressed between the transverse carpal ligament and the volar carpal ligament in Guyon's canal

Symptoms/diagnosis

Ulnar 1½ digits have symptoms (numbness, tingling)

Symptoms reproducible with compression testing over Guyon's canal

Treatment—similar to that for carpal tunnel syndrome

Wartenberg's syndrome

Isolated neuritis of the superficial radial nerve from intrinsic (anomalous muscles, fascial bands) or extrinsic (jewelry) compression

Treatment based on etiology

Post-traumatic Problems of the Wrist

Kienböck's disease

Osteonecrosis of the lunate

Related to repetitive compressive forces on the wrist

These patients tend to have negative ulnar variance (the distal ulna is proximal to distal radius; the distal ulna is relatively short compared to the distal radius)

Symptoms/diagnosis

Ulnar-sided wrist pain

Radiographs (Fig. 12–13)—negative ulnar variance of the wrist; the lunate is abnormal

Treatment

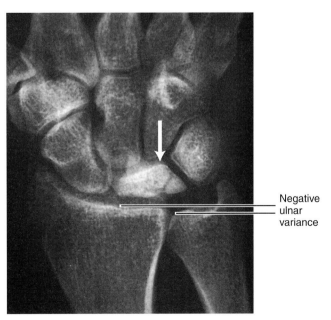

Negative ulnar variance

Figure 12–13 ■ Kienböck's disease. Note flattening and sclerosis of the lunate (*arrow*) as well as a negative ulnar variance (see radiographic lines). (Modified from Weissman BNW, Sledge CB: Orthopedic Radiology. Philadelphia, WB Saunders, 1986, p 154.)

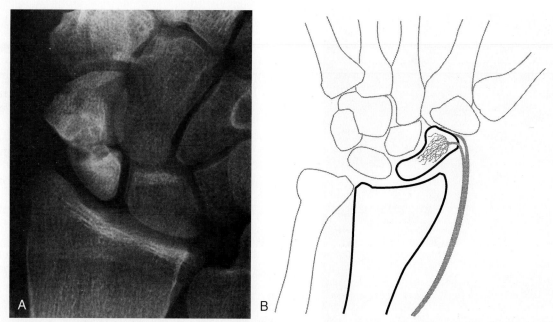

Figure 12–14 ■ *A,* Scaphoid nonunion. Note persistence of the fracture line and cystic resorption along the fracture margins. (From Weissman BNW, Sledge CB. Orthopedic Radiology. Philadelphia, WB Saunders, 1986, p 138.) *B,* Schematic representation of the unique blood supply to the scaphoid. The distal pole of the scaphoid has an abundant blood supply; the proximal pole has virtually no independent blood supply. This unique blood supply explains the high incidence of osteonecrosis and nonunions for fractures of the proximal third of the scaphoid.

Cases without fragmentation of the lunate—splinting
Cases with fragmentation of the lunate—operative treatment
TFCC injury—tear of the fibrocartilagenous complex analogous to a meniscal tear in the knee
Diagnosis—ulnar-sided wrist pain; positive arthrogram (see Fig. 12–11) or magnetic resonance imaging (MRI); well visualized on wrist arthroscopy (see Fig. 12–12)
Treatment
Acute injury—casting
Chronic—arthroscopy
Scaphoid nonunion—the scaphoid is one of the most common bones that fails to unite (heal) after a fracture; problems with fracture healing are related to the scaphoids' unique blood supply (Fig. 12–14)
Can lead to late painful arthritis (scapholunate advanced collapse [SLAC]) if left untreated
Treatment is generally operative
Carpal instability—disruption of the normal relationships of the carpal bones caused by intercarpal ligament injury can cause pain and abnormal motion
DISI pattern
Radial-sided intercarpal ligamentous injury
Increased scapholunate gap and increased dorsal tilt of the lunate seen on x-ray (Fig. 12–15)
Positive Watson's test (see Fig. 12–7)
Treatment
Early—stabilization
Late—fusion
VISI pattern
Ulnar-sided intercarpal ligamentous injury
Displays increased volar tilt of the lunate on x-ray

Treatment
Acute injury—closed reduction
Chronic—ligament reconstruction or limited intercarpal fusion

Arthritic Conditions of the Wrist

Osteoarthritis—uncommon
Rheumatoid arthritis
Can result in dorsal subluxation of the ulna

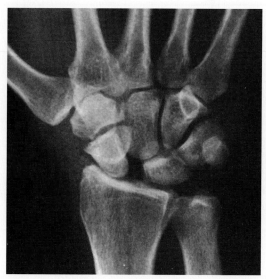

Figure 12–15 ■ Scapholunate dissociation. Note increased space between the scaphoid and lunate (Terry Thomas sign) and loss of the normal shape of the lunate. (From Weissman BNW, Sledge CB: Orthopedic Radiology. Philadelphia, WB Saunders, 1986, p 148.)

Tendon Problems (Fig. 12–16)

DeQuervain's disease (see Fig. 12–16)
  Etiology
    Stenosing tenosynovitis of the first dorsal compartment of the wrist (APL, EPB)
    Golfers, players of racket sports, clerical workers
  Symptoms/diagnosis
    Localized pain, swelling
    Positive Finkelstein's test—ulnar deviation of the wrist with the thumb in the palm reproduces painful symptoms (see Fig. 12–9)
    Pain is relieved after injection into the 1st dorsal compartment
  Treatment options
    Nonoperative—thumb spica splinting, NSAIDs, injection
    Operative—surgical decompression
FCU/FCR tendinitis
  Treatment—NSAIDs, rest, splinting, operative tenolysis
ECU problems
  Subluxation
    Represents subluxation of the ECU tendon from its groove in the 6th dorsal compartment
    Nonoperative treatment—immobilization with the wrist/forearm in pronation
    Operative treatment—reconstruction of the fibroosseous tunnel
  Tendinitis—supportive treatment
Intersection syndrome (see Fig. 12–16)
  Etiology—inflammation at the junction of the tendons of the 1st and 2nd dorsal compartments of the wrist proximal to the extensor retinaculum

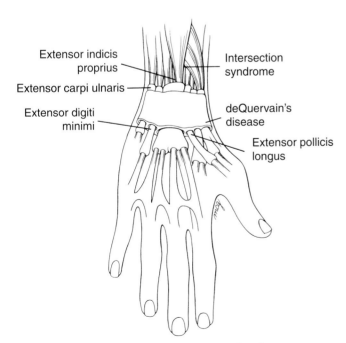

Figure 12–16 ■ Location of frequent sites of tendinitis: extensor indicis proprius; extensor carpi ulnaris; extensor digiti minimi; and extensor pollicis longus. (From Kiefhaber TR, Stern PJ: Upper extremity tendinitis and overuse syndromes in the athlete. Clin Sports Med 11[1]:43, 1992.)

Symptoms/diagnosis
  Localized pain
  Crepitus (squeakers)—can produce an audible noise on wrist flexion/extension
Treatment options
  Nonoperative—splinting, NSAIDs, local injection
  Operative—decompression (rarely required)
EPL tenosynovitis
  Pain aggravated by thumb motion
  Physical exam demonstrates pain to palpation of the EPL tendon localized around Lister's tubercle
  Treatment—NSAIDs, rest, splinting
EDM tendinitis
  Stenosing tenosynovitis of the 5th dorsal compartment
  Treatment options
    Nonoperative—ulnar gutter splinting, NSAIDs, local injection
    Operative—decompression

FRACTURES AND DISLOCATIONS OF THE WRIST

Overview (Tables 12–3 and 12–4)

Fractures of the distal radius—some of the most common injuries seen by primary care physicians and orthopaedic surgeons
  Understanding what constitutes an acceptable reduction is essential (Fig. 12–17)
  Colles' fracture (Fig. 12–18)
    Most common type of distal radius fracture
    Treatment—commonly treated with closed manipulation (to obtain reduction) and plaster immobilization
  Fractures with dorsal comminution or intra-articular fractures
    Treatment—may require operative stabilization
  Smith's fracture (Fig. 12–19)
  Dorsal and volar Barton's fractures (Fig. 12–20)
    Volar Barton's fractures often require operative intervention
  Radial styloid fracture (Fig. 12–21)
    Treatment—often requires operative intervention
Fractures of the carpal bones (see Table 12–3)
  Less common than distal radius fractures
  Most common fractures include
    Scaphoid fractures (Fig. 12–22)
      Scaphoid fractures may not become radiographically evident for up to 2 weeks after an acute injury; therefore, a patient with a traumatic injury who complains of wrist pain and demonstrates tenderness in the anatomic snuff box should alert the physician to the possibility of an underlying fracture of the scaphoid; these patients should be initially treated as if they indeed have a scaphoid fracture and should be reevaluated clinically and radiographically at 10 to 14 days after injury to rule out a scaphoid fracture and search for a fracture line that may only become apparent at 2 weeks after injury

Table 12–3
FRACTURES OF THE ADULT WRIST

Fracture	Eponym or Other Name	Classification	Treatment	Most Common Complications of the Injury
Distal radius with dorsal displacement	Colles' (see Fig. 12–18)	Frykman (I–VIII); Melone	Distract, manipulate, restore normal volar tilt of distal radius, splint in palmar flexion and ulnar deviation; operative treatment for unreducible shortening/angulation, severe comminution, or articular surface displacement	Loss of reduction, nonunion, malunion, median nerve injury, weakness, tendon adhesions, wrist instability, reflex sympathetic dystrophy, EPL rupture, post-traumatic arthritis, Volkmann's ischemic contracture
Distal radius with volar displacement	Smith's (see Fig. 12–19)	Descriptive (intra- vs. extra-articular)	Closed reduction, splint in supination; operative treatment may be necessary	Loss of reduction, nonunion, malunion, median nerve injury, weakness, tendon adhesions, wrist instability, reflex sympathetic dystrophy, EPL rupture, post-traumatic arthritis, Volkmann's ischemic contracture, missed diagnosis
Distal radius dorsal rim	Dorsal Barton's		Closed reduction and splinting; ORIF may be needed	Loss of reduction, nonunion, malunion, median nerve injury, weakness, tendon adhesions, wrist instability, reflex sympathetic dystrophy, EPL rupture, post-traumatic arthritis, Volkmann's ischemic contracture
Distal radius volar rim	Volar Barton's (see Fig. 12–20)		Closed reduction and splinting; ORIF may be needed	Loss of reduction, nonunion, malunion, median nerve injury, weakness, tendon adhesions, wrist instability, reflex sympathetic dystrophy, EPL rupture, post-traumatic arthritis, Volkmann's ischemic contracture
Radial styloid (see Fig. 12–21)	Chauffeur's		Closed reduction and splinting in ulnar deviation; operative stabilization may be necessary	Loss of reduction, nonunion, malunion, median nerve injury, weakness, tendon adhesions, wrist instability, reflex sympathetic dystrophy, EPL rupture, post-traumatic arthritis, Volkmann's ischemic contracture, missed perilunate injury
Scaphoid (see Fig. 12–22)		Anatomic location (tubercle, distal pole, waist, proximal pole) and degree of displacement		Missed diagnosis, nonunion, wrist instability, nerve injury, post-traumatic arthritis, reflex sympathetic dystrophy
		Nondisplaced (<2 mm)	Thumb spica cast (long arm cast for 3 weeks followed by short arm cast until bony union)	
		Displaced (≥2 mm)	ORIF	
Triquetrum dorsal chip			Short arm cast for 6 weeks	Missed diagnosis
Hook of hamate (see Fig. 12–23)			Splint for comfort; excise small fragment for chronic pain	Missed diagnosis

EPL, extensor pollicis longus; ORIF, open reduction with internal fixation.

Table 12–4
DISLOCATIONS OF THE ADULT WRIST

Dislocation	Classification	Treatment	Most Common Complications of the Injury
Distal radioulnar joint	Dorsal ulnar displacement	Full supination reduces displacement, long arm cast for 3 weeks, followed by short arm cast for 3 weeks	Osteochondral fracture, TFCC injury, ulnar nerve compression, wrist instability
	Volar ulnar displacement	Full pronation reduces displacement, long arm cast for 3 weeks, followed by short arm cast for 3 weeks	Osteochondral fracture, TFCC injury, wrist instability
Perilunate dislocation (carpus dislocates around lunate, lunate remains in articulation with distal radius) (see Fig. 12–24)	Mayfield	ORIF	Wrist instability, median nerve injury, late rupture of flexor tendons
Rotary lunate disassociation (≥3 mm gap between scaphoid and lunate as compared to opposite wrist on PA x-ray [Terry Thomas sign]) (see Fig. 12–15)		Closed reduction and immobilization; ORIF often needed	Post-traumatic arthritis
Carpal instability		Closed reduction and immobilization; ORIF often needed	Post-traumatic arthritis

TFCC, triangular fibrocartilage complex; ORIF, open reduction with internal fixation.

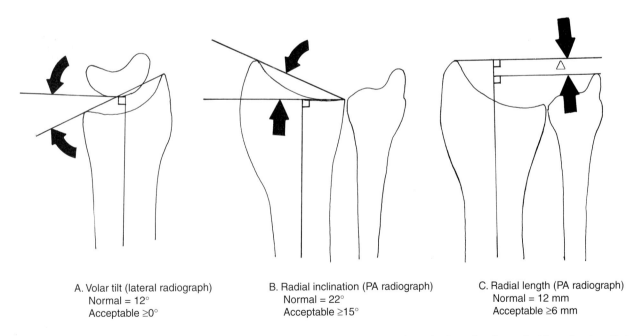

A. Volar tilt (lateral radiograph)
Normal = 12°
Acceptable ≥0°

B. Radial inclination (PA radiograph)
Normal = 22°
Acceptable ≥15°

C. Radial length (PA radiograph)
Normal = 12 mm
Acceptable ≥6 mm

Figure 12–17 ■ Postreduction radiographic measurements. *A,* Volar tilt—measured on the lateral radiograph. Normal volar tilt is 12 degrees; minimal acceptable is 0 degrees (neutral). *B,* Radial inclination—the angle formed from the line connecting the radial styloid with the ulnar margin of the radius on the PA radiographic view. Normal radial inclination is 22 degrees; acceptable is at least 15 degrees. *C,* Radial length—the distance between the tip of the radial styloid and the tip of the ulnar styloid. Normal radial length is 12 mm; acceptable is at least 6 mm. Note that for comminuted intra-articular fractures and for fractures in younger patients the acceptable values will vary.

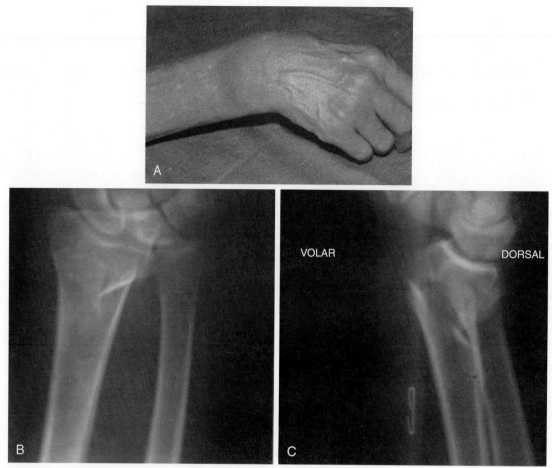

Figure 12–18 ■ Colles' fracture. *A,* Clinical view of patient with a "silver fork" deformity. *B,* PA radiograph demonstrating the distal radius fracture. *C,* Lateral radiograph shows dorsal displacement, apex volar angulation, and loss of the normal volar tilt (of the articular surface of the distal radius). (Modified from Jonas G, Masear VR: Fractures and ligament injuries of the wrist. *In* Masear VR [ed]: Primary Care Orthopaedics. Philadelphia, WB Saunders, 1996, p 171.)

Triquetrum (dorsal chip) fractures
Fractures of the hook of the hamate (Fig. 12–23)
Dislocations of the wrist (see Table 12–4)
  High-energy injuries, less common than fractures
  Dislocations at the distal radioulnar joint
  Perilunate dislocations where the carpus dislocates around the lunate and the lunate remains in its articulation with the distal radius (Fig. 12–24)
  Frank wrist dislocations where the carpus dislocates from the distal radius
  Rotary lunate disassociations

TUMORS OF THE WRIST

Bone

Giant cell tumor (distal radius)

Soft Tissue

Ganglia

DIFFERENTIAL DIAGNOSIS OF COMMON WRIST COMPLAINTS

Pain

Radial-sided
  Scaphoid fracture/nonunion
  DeQuervain's tenosynovitis
  FCR tendinitis
  Intersection syndrome
  Wartenberg's syndrome
  DISI
Ulnar-sided
  ECU/FCU tendinitis
  TFCC injury
  EDM tendinitis
  VISI
Dorsal
  Kienböck's disease
  Dorsal ganglion
Volar
  Carpal tunnel syndrome
  Volar ganglion
  Ulnar tunnel syndrome

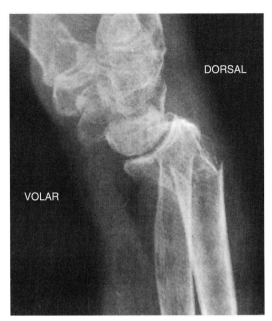

Figure 12–19 ■ Smith's fracture with volar displacement, apex dorsal angulation, and excessive volar tilt of the articular surface of the distal radius (lateral radiograph). (Modified from Weissman BNW, Sledge CB: Orthopedic Radiology. Philadelphia, WB Saunders, 1986, p 130.)

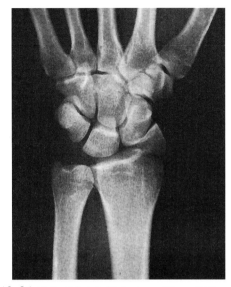

Figure 12–21 ■ Radial styloid fracture. (From O'Donoghue DH: Treatment of Injuries to Athletes. Philadelphia, WB Saunders, 1976, p 312.)

Diffuse
  Fractures
  Tumors
  Infections
  Referred pain
  Rheumatologic conditions
  Arthritis

Instability

DISI
VISI
Tendon problems

Weakness

Carpal tunnel syndrome
Ulnar tunnel syndrome
Fractures
Tumors
Tendinitis
Traumatic nerve injuries

Tingling/Loss of Sensation

Carpal tunnel syndrome
Ulnar tunnel syndrome
Wartenberg's syndrome
Other nerve entrapment syndromes
Traumatic nerve injuries

Deformity

Fractures
Dislocations
Rheumatologic conditions
Tumors/cysts
Tendon ruptures

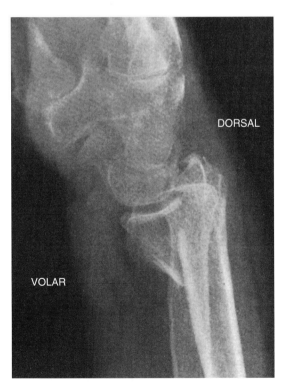

Figure 12–20 ■ Volar Barton's fracture with volar displacement of a large intra-articular fragment (volar rim) (lateral radiograph). (Modified from Weissman BNW, Sledge CB: Orthopedic Radiology. Philadelphia, WB Saunders, 1986, p 130.)

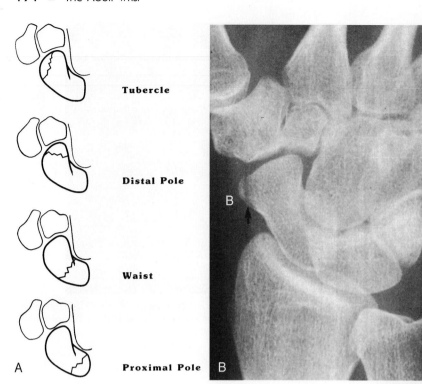

Tubercle

Distal Pole

Waist

Proximal Pole

Figure 12–22 ■ *A,* Classification of scaphoid fractures is based on the anatomic location (as shown) and displacement. *B,* AP radiograph of a minimally displaced scaphoid fracture *(arrow).* (From Weissman BNW, Sledge CB: Orthopedic Radiology. Philadelphia, WB Saunders, 1986, pp 134, 136.)

Figure 12–23 ■ Fractures of the hook of the hamate *(arrow)* are best visualized on the carpal tunnel view. (From Mirabello SC, Loeb PE, Andrews JR: The wrist: Evaluation and treatment. Clin Sports Med 11[1]:11, 1992.)

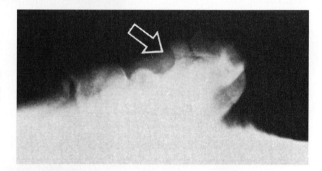

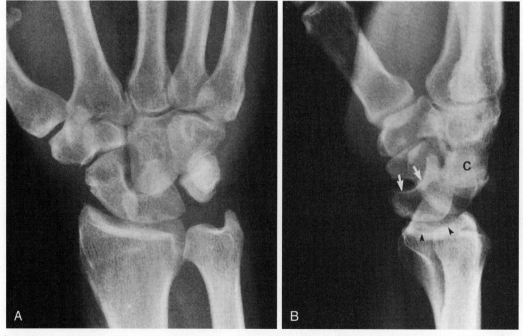

Figure 12–24 ■ Dorsal perilunate dislocation. *A,* PA view shows apparent loss of the capitate-lunate cartilage space and loss of the normal scapholunate interval. *B,* Lateral view demonstrates dorsal displacement of the capitate (C) in relation to the lunate. The distal articular surface of the lunate *(arrows)* is displaced from the articular surface of the capitate. The radiolunate joint *(arrowheads)* is intact. (From Weissman BNW, Sledge CB: Orthopedic Radiology. Philadelphia, WB Saunders, 1986, p 142.)

Snapping/Popping

Tendinitis (such as intersection syndrome)
TFCC injuries
Carpal instability

Loss of Motion

Fractures
Dislocations
Arthritis
Rheumatologic conditions
Tumors
Infections
Tendon ruptures
Tendinitis
Nerve injuries
Carpal instability

PEARLS AND PITFALLS

Always get three radiographic views of the wrist (PA, lateral, and oblique)

Scaphoid fractures are commonly missed and are not always radiographically evident initially; the patient with a history of trauma and pain in the anatomic snuff box should be presumed to have a scaphoid fracture until proven otherwise; follow-up radiographs at 10 to 14 days after injury are mandatory and may reveal the presence of a fracture line in the scaphoid

The **scapholunate interval** should always be noted on all wrist radiographs; scapholunate ligament injuries with widening of the scapholunate gap **(more than 3 mm)** will be missed unless specifically evaluated

Not all distal radial fractures are alike; before instituting treatment for a distal radius fracture, it is important to recognize exactly what type of fracture one is dealing with

It is important to understand what constitutes a final acceptable position of a distal radius fracture (reduction) (see Fig. 12–17) before attempting a reduction

CHAPTER 13

The Adult Hand

HAND ANATOMY

Bones (Fig. 13–1)

Metacarpals
Proximal phalanges
Middle phalanges (not present in the thumb)
Distal phalanges

Joints (Fig. 13–2)

Carpometacarpal (CMC)—gliding joints
Thumb CMC—mobile saddle joint
Metacarpophalangeal (MCP)—ellipsoid joints
  Volar plate (Fig. 13–3)—a thick fibrocartilagenous portion of the volar capsule that connects the metacarpal neck to the base of the proximal phalanx

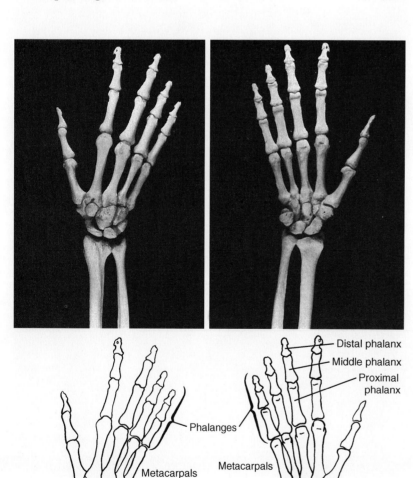

Figure 13–1 ■ Anatomy of the bones of the hand. (From Weissman BNW, Sledge CB: Orthopedic Radiology. Philadelphia, WB Saunders, 1986, p 72.)

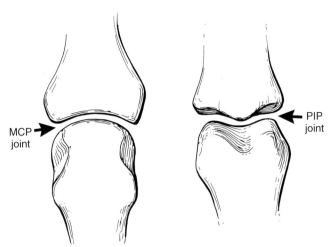

Figure 13–2 ■ Metacarpophalangeal (MCP) joints are unicondylar, and proximal interphalangeal (PIP) joints are bicondylar, giving the PIP joints more stability. (From Green DP, Strickland JW: The hand. *In* DeLee JC, Drez D Jr [eds]: Orthopaedic Sports Medicine: Principles and Practice. Philadelphia, WB Saunders, 1994, p 959.)

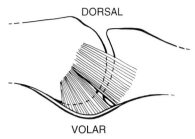

Figure 13–4 ■ Collateral ligaments have a cord-like dorsal component and a fan-shaped volar component. (Redrawn from Eaton RG: Joint Injuries of the Hand. Springfield, Charles C Thomas, 1971. From Green DP, Strickland JW: The hand. *In* DeLee JC, Drez D Jr [eds]: Orthopaedic Sports Medicine: Principles and Practice. Philadelphia, WB Saunders, 1994, p 960.)

Deep transverse metacarpal ligament (see Fig. 13–3)—connects the volar plates of the four finger metacarpals
Collateral ligaments (Figs. 13–3 to 13–5)
  Attach to the volar plates

Resist varus and valgus stresses on the MCP joint
Are tight (under tension) with the MCP joint in flexion and are lax with the MCP joint in extension ("cam effect"); this is because of the eccentric shape of the metacarpal head and the fact that the distance from the center of rotation of the metacarpal head to the phalanx in extension is less than the distance in flexion (see Fig. 13–5); the MCP joint must therefore be immobilized in flexion (when treating traumatic hand and wrist injuries) to keep the collateral liga-

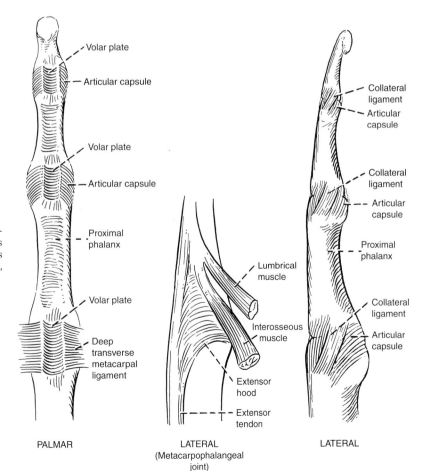

Figure 13–3 ■ Structures about the metacarpophalangeal and interphalangeal joints. (From Jenkins DB: Hollinshead's Functional Anatomy of the Limbs and Back, 6th ed. Philadelphia, WB Saunders, 1991, p 160.)

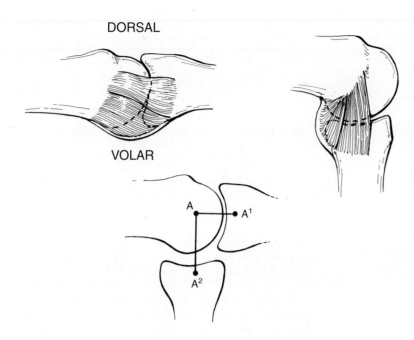

DORSAL

VOLAR

A   A¹

A²

Figure 13–5 ■ The shape of the metacarpal head is eccentric. This creates a cam effect that makes the collateral ligaments more taut in flexion than in extension. (the distance from A to A¹ is less than the distance from A to A²). (From Green DP, Strickland JW: The hand. *In* DeLee JC, Drez D Jr [eds]: Orthopaedic Sports Medicine: Principles and Practice. Philadelphia, WB Saunders, 1994, p 959.)

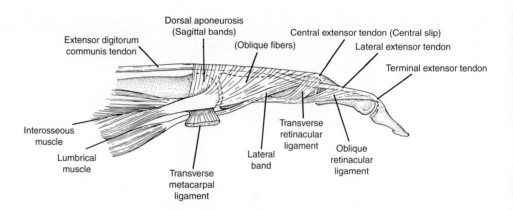

Dorsal aponeurosis (Sagittal bands)

(Oblique fibers)

Central extensor tendon (Central slip)

Lateral extensor tendon

Terminal extensor tendon

Extensor digitorum communis tendon

Transverse retinacular ligament

Oblique retinacular ligament

Lateral band

Lateral band

Transverse metacarpal ligament

Lumbrical muscle

Interosseous muscle

Figure 13–6 ■ Dorsal extensor apparatus. (Adapted from Bora FW: The Pediatric Upper Extremity. Philadelphia, WB Saunders, 1986, p 93.)

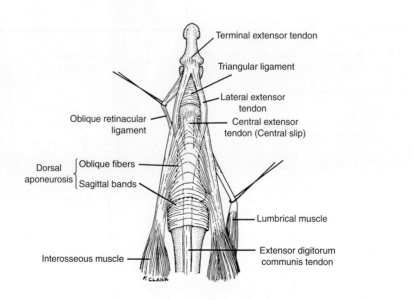

Terminal extensor tendon

Triangular ligament

Lateral extensor tendon

Central extensor tendon (Central slip)

Oblique retinacular ligament

Dorsal aponeurosis { Oblique fibers

Sagittal bands

Lumbrical muscle

Extensor digitorum communis tendon

Interosseous muscle

P. CLARK

Table 13-1
STRUCTURES OF THE EXTENSOR APPARATUS

Structure	Location	Function
Sagittal bands	MCP joint	MCP joint extension
Transverse fibers	Volar plate	MCP joint flexion
Lateral band	PIP joint	PIP joint extension
Lateral extensor tendon	Spans from the proximal phalanx to the distal phalanx	DIP joint extension
Oblique retinacular ligament	DIP joint	DIP joint extension

MCP, metacarpophalangeal; PIP, proximal interphalangeal; DIP, interphalangeal.

ments from contracting (immobilization of the MCP joint in extension leads to collateral ligament shortening and stiff [limited flexion] MCP joints)
Interphalangeal (IP)—hinge joints
　Volar plate (see Fig. 13–3)
　Collateral ligaments (see Fig. 13–3)
　　No "cam effect" and therefore can be immobilized in extension

Extensor Apparatus (Fig. 13–6)

Because the extrinsic tendons of the fingers (extensor digitorum communis) terminate proximal to the PIP joint, and because only one extrinsic extensor tendon exists per finger (as compared to two extrinsic finger flexors, flexor digitorum superficialis [FDS] and flexor digitorum profundus [FDP]), a highly complex arrangement of anatomic structures is necessary to allow for finger extension
Structures of the extensor apparatus (see Fig. 13–6) (Table 13–1)

Flexor Tendon Anatomy (Fig. 13–7)

The flexor tendons are tethered to the volar aspect of the phalanges by a series of fibrocartilaginous pulleys that prevent bowstringing (Fig. 13–8) of the flexor tendons

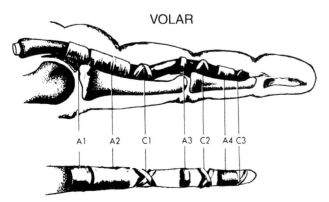

VOLAR

Figure 13-7 ■ Flexor tendon pulley system—there are four annular (A1, A2, A3, A4) and three cruciate (C1, C2, C3) pulleys. Note that A2 and A4 are the most important pulleys to preserve. (From Tubiana R: The Hand. Philadelphia, WB Saunders, 1985, vol. 3, p 173.)

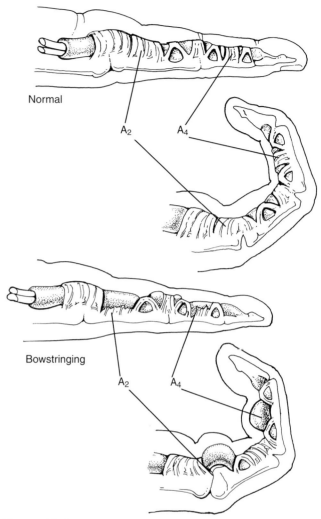

Figure 13-8 ■ Bowstringing of the flexor tendons may result from disruption of the A2 and A4 pulleys.

There are four annular (more important) and three cruciate pulleys
The odd-numbered annular pulleys overlie joints
　A1 (first annular pulley) overlies the MCP joint
　A3 (third annular pulley) overlies the PIP joint
The even-numbered annular pulleys and the cruciate pulleys overlie the phalanges
　A2 (second annular pulley) overlies the proximal phalanx
　A4 (fourth annular pulley) overlies the middle phalanx
　C1 (first cruciate pulley) is distal to A2 on the proximal phalanx
　C2 and C3 (second and third cruciate pulleys) are proximal (C2) and distal (C3) to the A4 pulley on the middle phalanx

Muscles

Extrinsic muscles (Fig. 13–9)
　Muscles are in the forearm and tendons are in the hand (and move the hand)
　　Flexor pollicis longus (FPL)

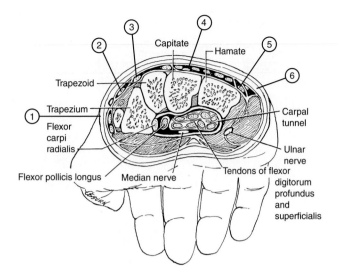

Figure 13–9 ■ Extrinsic muscles of the hand shown in cross-section. Extensor compartments 1 through 6 are numbered in circles. The contents of extensor compartment 1 (APB, EPB), 3 (EPL), 4 (EDC, EIP), and 5 (EDM) are extrinsic muscles of the hand because their muscles are in the forearm and their tendons are in the hand and move the hand. The contents of extensor compartments 2 (ECRL, ECRB) and 6 (ECU) are not considered extrinsic muscles of the hand because they move the wrist, not the hand. Extrinsic flexors of the hand include the FPL, FDP, and FDS (shown in the figure). Note that FCR is shown in the figure but is not an extrinsic muscle of the hand (although its muscle is in the forearm and its tendon is in the hand [insertion is bases of second and third metacarpals], it moves the wrist, not the hand). (From O'Donoghue DH: Treatment of Injuries to Athletes. Philadelphia, WB Saunders, 1976, p 293.)

Flexor digitorum profundus (FDP)
Flexor digitorum superficialis (FDS)
Abductor pollicis longus (APL)
Extensor pollicis brevis (EPB)
Extensor pollicis longus (EPL)
Extensor digitorum communis (EDC)
Extensor indicis proprius (EIP)

Extensor digiti minimi (EDM)
Intrinsic muscles (Fig. 13–10)
  Muscles and tendons are in the hand
    Abductor pollicis brevis (APB)
    Opponens pollicis (OP)
    Flexor pollicis brevis (FPB)
    Adductor pollicis

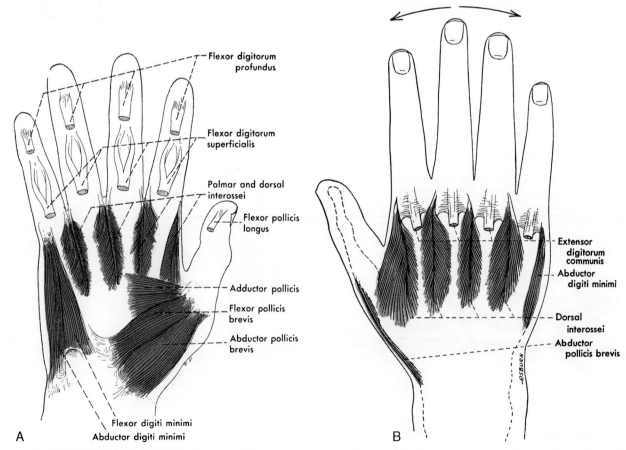

Figure 13–10 ■ Intrinsic muscles of the hand. *A*, Volar (palmar) view. *B*, Dorsal view. Intrinsic muscles of the hand not shown in the figure include opponens pollicis, opponens digiti minimi, the lumbricales, and palmaris brevis. Structures shown but that are not intrinsic muscles of the hand include FDP, FDS, FPL, and EDC. (From Jenkins DB: Hollinshead's Functional Anatomy of the Limbs and Back, 6th ed. Philadelphia, WB Saunders, 1991, pp 180, 182.)

Flexor digiti minimi (FDM)
Abductor digiti minimi (ADM)
Opponens digiti minimi (ODM)
Palmaris brevis
Interossei (seven of them—four dorsal, three palmar)
Lumbricales (four of them)

Nerves (Fig. 13–11)

Digital nerves—located volar to the digital arteries in the fingers; provide sensation to the volar aspect of the fingers; are the terminal branches of the median and ulnar nerves

Vessels (see Fig. 13–11)

Superficial palmar (arterial) arch
    Volar to the deep palmar arch
    Ulnar artery is the main contributor
Deep palmar (arterial) arch
    Radial artery is the main contributor
    Located proximal to the superficial palmar arch
Digital arteries

Arise from the superficial palmar arch
In the palm they are volar to the digital nerves
In the fingers they are dorsal to the digital nerves

Topographic Anatomy of the Hand
(Fig. 13–12)

SURGICAL APPROACHES TO THE HAND

Volar Approach to the Flexor Tendons

Zigzag incisions can be made at 90 degrees to each other and intersect at the IP flexion creases
Important to preserve the pulleys, especially the A2 and A4 pulleys

Midlateral Approach

With the finger flexed, connect the dorsal portions of the IP creases
Digital nerves and arteries will be volar to this incision
Incise the flexor tendon sheath longitudinally

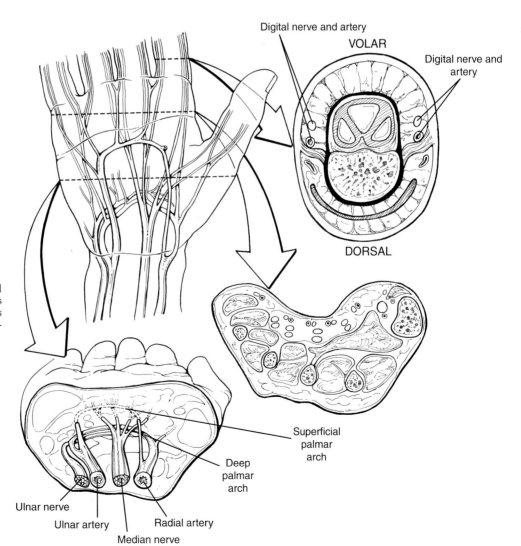

Figure 13–11 ■ The digital nerves are the terminal branches of the median and ulnar nerves and are volar to the digital arteries in the fingers.

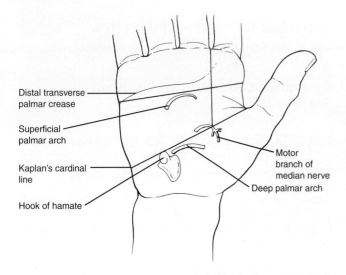

Figure 13–12 ■ Topographic anatomy of the hand. Kaplan's cardinal line, which runs from the first web space and parallel to the proximal transverse palmar crease, helps to locate the motor branch of the median nerve (at the junction of a line drawn from the radial border of the middle finger and Kaplan's cardinal line) and the hook of the hamate. The deep palmar (arterial) arch lies below Kaplan's cardinal line, and the superficial palmar (arterial) arch lies below the distal transverse palmar crease.

Labels on figure:
- Distal transverse palmar crease
- Superficial palmar arch
- Kaplan's cardinal line
- Hook of hamate
- Motor branch of median nerve
- Deep palmar arch

HISTORY AND PHYSICAL EXAMINATION OF THE HAND

History

Age
Occupation
Activities
Handedness
Injury
  Chronicity
  Mechanism
  Position of the hand and fingers at the time of injury (for example, if the fingers are flexed at the time of a volar laceration, the level of the skin laceration will be different from the level of a flexor tendon laceration)
Prior treatment(s)
Functional impairment
Exacerbating activities

Physical Examination

Observation
  Attitude—slight flexion at the MCP and IP joints is the normal resting position (cascade) (Fig. 13–13)
  Skin—thickness, irregularities
  Muscles—atrophy, abnormalities
  Knuckles—the knuckle of the middle finger (MCP joint) is normally the most prominent (make a fist to see)
  Web spaces
  Nails—spooning (fungal infections), clubbing (cardiorespiratory disorders)
Palpation
  Skin
    Normally thicker on the palmar surface
    Warm areas (infection)
    Dry areas (nerve injury)
    Scars
  Bones
    Metacarpals
    Phalanges
  Soft tissues
    Thenar eminence
    Hypothenar eminence
    Palm (aponeurosis, flexor tendons)
    Extensor tendons
    Digits
Motion (Fig. 13–14)
  MCP joint flexion (normal, 90 degrees)
  MCP joint extension (normal, 30–45 degrees)
  PIP joint flexion (normal, 90 degrees)
  PIP joint extension (normal, 0 degrees)
  Distal interphalangeal (DIP) joint flexion (normal, 90 degrees)
  DIP joint extension (normal, 0 to 10 degrees)
  Finger abduction (normal, 20 degrees)

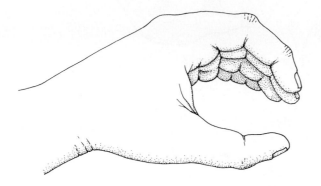

Figure 13–13 ■ Normal position of function (attitude) of the hand. (From Magee DJ: Orthopedic Physical Assessment, 2nd ed. Philadelphia, WB Saunders, 1992.)

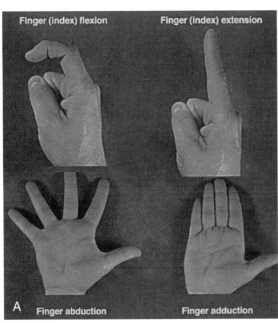
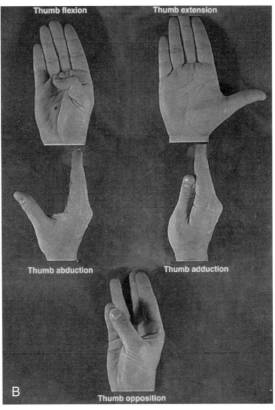

Figure 13–14 ■ Motions of the hand. *A,* Motions of the fingers include finger flexion and extension (flexion and extension of the metacarpophalangeal joints, proximal interphalangeal joints, and distal interphalangeal joints) and finger abduction and adduction. *B,* Motions of the thumb include thumb flexion (a medial movement of the thumb in the plane of the palm) and extension, thumb abduction (a forward movement of the thumb away from the palm) and adduction (a forward movement of the thumb toward the palm), and thumb opposition (a movement such that the palmar aspect of the tip of the thumb touches the palmar aspect of the tip of another finger of the same hand; when the contact between the thumb and another finger is not along the palmar aspects, the motion is known as apposition [not shown in the figure]).

Finger adduction
Thumb flexion
Thumb extension (normal, 50 degrees)
Thumb abduction (normal, 70 degrees)
Thumb adduction
Thumb opposition
Neurovascular exam
  Sensation (Fig. 13–15; see Fig. 2–5)
    Two-point discrimination (Fig. 13–16)—normal is less than 6 mm
  Strength testing (Table 13–2)
    Extrinsic muscles
      FPL—thumb flexion at the IP joint
      FDP—DIP flexion with the IP joint stabilized
      FDS—PIP flexion with the adjacent fingers stabilized in extension (blocks the shared FDP muscles)
      APL—thumb abduction and extension
      EPB—extends the thumb MCP joint
      EPL—thumb elevation off a flat surface, extends the thumb IP joint
      EDC—finger extension at the MCP joint
      EIP/EDM—extension of the index and small fingers, respectively, with the other fingers flexed into a fist
    Intrinsic muscles

    Thenar muscles
      APB—thumb abduction
      OP—thumb abduction, flexion, and medial rotation (for opposition)
      FPB—thumb flexion at the MCP joint
      Adductor pollicis—patient forcefully holds a piece of paper between the adducted thumb and index finger while the examiner attempts to remove this piece of paper; if the thumb IP joint flexes (in order to successfully hold the piece of paper), this indicates that the adductor pollicis is weak (positive Froment's sign)
    Hypothenar muscles
      FDM—small finger MCP joint flexion
      ADM—small finger abduction
      ODM—small finger abduction, flexion, and lateral rotation
      Palmaris brevis—skin retraction of the ulnar palm
    Interosseous muscles
      Dorsal interossei (four of them)—finger abduction
      Palmar interossei (three of them)—finger adduction
    Lumbrical muscles (4 of them)—flex the MCP joints and extend the IP joints

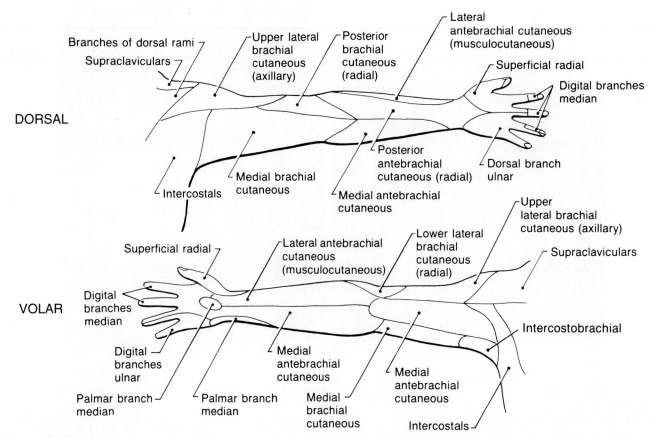

Figure 13–15 ■ Cutaneous sensation of the upper extremity. Note that the hand has cutaneous sensation provided by the following nerves: posterior antebrachial cutaneous, medial antebrachial cutaneous, lateral antebrachial cutaneous, palmar branch of the median nerve, superficial radial nerve, dorsal branches of the ulnar nerve, and digital branches of the median and ulnar nerves. (Redrawn from Hollinshead WH: Anatomy for Surgeons, 3rd ed. Philadelphia, Harper & Row, 1982. From Jobe CM: Gross anatomy of the shoulder. *In* Rockwood CA Jr, Matsen FA III [eds]: The Shoulder. Philadelphia, WB Saunders, 1990, p 90.)

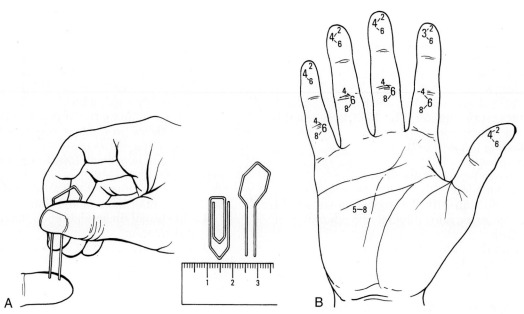

Figure 13–16 ■ Two-point discrimination. *A*, Technique of testing. *B*, Normal values (in millimeters) for discrimination (larger figures indicate average values; smaller figures indicate the minimum and maximum normal values). (From Tubiana R: The Hand. Philadelphia, WB Saunders, 1981, pp 645, 646.)

Table 13–2
MUSCLES ABOUT THE WRIST AND HAND: THEIR ACTIONS AND INNERVATION, INCLUDING NERVE ROOT DERIVATIONS

Action	Muscles Involved	Innervation	Nerve Root Derivation
Extension of wrist	1. Extensor carpi radialis longus	Radial	C6-7
	2. Extensor carpi radialis brevis	Radial	C6-7
	3. Extensor carpi ulnaris	Posterior interosseous (radial)	C7-8
Flexion of wrist	1. Flexor carpi radialis	Median	C6-7
	2. Flexor carpi ulnaris	Ulnar	C7-8
Ulnar deviation of wrist	1. Flexor carpi ulnaris	Ulnar	C7-8
	2. Extensor carpi ulnaris	Posterior interosseous (radial)	C7-8
Radial deviation of wrist	1. Flexor carpi radialis	Median	C6-7
	2. Extensor carpi radialis longus	Radial	C6-7
	3. Abductor pollicis longus	Posterior interosseous (radial)	C7–8
	4. Extensor pollicis brevis	Posterior interosseous (radial)	C7-8
Extension of fingers	1. Extensor digitorum communis	Posterior interosseous (radial)	C7-8
	2. Extensor indicis proprius (index finger)	Posterior interosseous (radial)	C7-8
	3. Extensor digiti minimi (small finger)	Posterior interosseous (radial)	C7-8
Flexion of fingers	1. Flexor digitorum profundus	Anterior interosseous (median): lateral two digits*	C8, T1
		Ulnar: medial two digits*	C8, T1
	2. Flexor digitorum superficialis	Median	C7-8, T1
	3. Lumbricales	First and second: median; third and fourth: ulnar (deep terminal branch)	C8, T1 — C8, T1
	4. Interossei	Ulnar (deep terminal branch)	C8, T1
	5. Flexor digiti minimi (small finger)	Ulnar (deep terminal branch)	C8, T1
Abduction of fingers (with fingers extended)	1. Dorsal interossei	Ulnar (deep terminal branch)	C8, T1
	2. Abductor digiti minimi (small finger)	Ulnar (deep terminal branch)	C8, T1
Adduction of fingers (with fingers extended)	1. Palmar interossei	Ulnar (deep terminal branch)	C8, T1
Extension of thumb	1. Extensor pollicis longus	Posterior interosseous (radial)	C7-8
	2. Extensor pollicis brevis	Posterior interosseous (radial)	C7-8
	3. Abductor pollicis longus	Posterior interosseous (radial)	C7-8
Flexion of thumb	1. Flexor pollicis brevis	Superficial head: median (lateral terminal branch)	C8, T1
		Deep head: ulnar	C8, T1
	2. Flexor pollicis longus	Anterior interosseous (median)	C8, T1
	3. Opponens pollicis	Median (lateral terminal branch)	C8, T1
Abduction of thumb	1. Abductor pollicis longus	Posterior interosseous (radial)	C7-8
	2. Abductor pollicis brevis	Median (lateral terminal branch)	C8, T1
Adduction of thumb	1. Adductor pollicis	Ulnar (deep terminal branch)	C8, T1
Opposition of thumb and small finger	1. Opponens pollicis	Median (lateral terminal branch)	C8, T1
	2. Flexor pollicis brevis	Superficial head: median (lateral terminal branch)	C8, T1
	3. Abductor pollicis brevis	Median (lateral terminal branch)	C8, T1
	4. Opponens digiti minimi	Ulnar (deep terminal branch)	C8, T1

Modified from Magee DJ: Orthopedic Physical Assessment, 2nd ed. Philadelphia, WB Saunders, 1992, p 165.
*Lateral two digits = index and long fingers; medial two digits = ring and small fingers.

Arterial testing
　Pulses (radial and ulnar)
　Allen's test—the patient makes a fist and opens and closes it several times (to exsanguinate the finger to be tested); with the hand still in a fist, the examiner compresses the radial and ulnar digital arteries; the patient then straightens the finger and the examiner selectively releases the digital radial or ulnar artery to check for patency with restoration of normal color to the finger (Fig. 13–17)
Special testing
　Extrinsic muscle tightness (Fig. 13–18)—the PIP joint can passively flex with the MCP held in extension but is unable to do so with the MCP joint held in flexion because the extensor digitorum communis (EDC) is scarred to the bone or retinaculum at the wrist or the dorsal metacarpal;

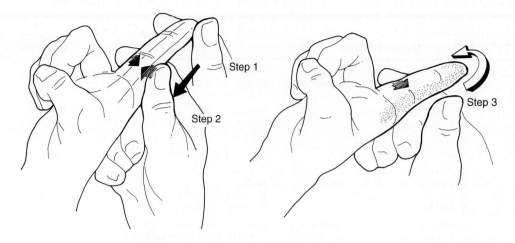

Figure 13–17 ■ Digital Allen's test. Note similarity to Allen's test at the wrist (see Fig. 12–10).

Figure 13–18 ■ Test for extrinsic tightness. Note that the proximal interphalangeal (PIP) joint cannot be flexed with the metacarpophalangeal (MCP) joint held in flexion when there is extrinsic muscle tightness.

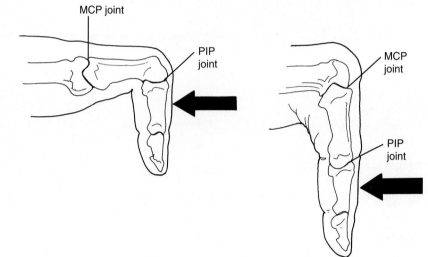

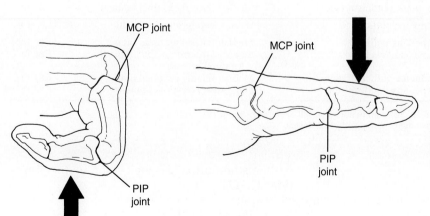

Figure 13–19 ■ Test for intrinsic tightness. Note that the proximal interphalangeal (PIP) joint cannot be flexed with the metacarpophalangeal (MCP) joint held in extension when there is intrinsic muscle tightness.

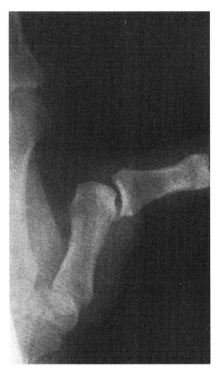

Figure 13–20 ■ Thumb ulnar collateral ligament stress test demonstrates significant lateral deviation (and angulation) at the thumb metacarpophalangeal joint (as seen on this stress radiograph). (From O'Donoghue DH: Treatment of Injuries to Athletes. Philadelphia, WB Saunders, 1976, p 347.)

the EDC tendon lacks the necessary excursion to allow simultaneous flexion of both the MCP and the PIP joints

Intrinsic muscle tightness (intrinsic plus deformity) (Fig. 13–19)—the PIP joint can passively flex with the MCP joint held in flexion but is unable to do so with the MCP joint held in extension because the intrinsic muscles are foreshortened and lack the necessary excursion to allow for simultaneous MCP joint extension and PIP joint flexion

Thumb ulnar collateral ligament stress test (for gamekeeper's or skier's thumb) (Fig. 13–20)—valgus stress testing demonstrates increased opening of the thumb MCP joint; greater than 45 degrees of opening without a firm end point suggests a complete tear

Grind test (for thumb CMC arthritis)—axial compression with rotation (of the thumb) causes pain at the CMC joint

DIAGNOSTIC TESTS FOR THE HAND

Plain Radiographs

Posteroanterior (PA)
Lateral
Obliques
Digits—views of the digit are helpful for finger injuries
Special obliques

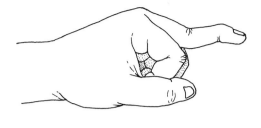

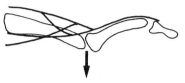

Figure 13–21 ■ Swan-neck deformity from dorsal subluxation of the lateral bands. (From Magee DJ: Orthopedic Physical Assessment, 2nd ed. Philadelphia, WB Saunders, 1992, p 175.)

10 degrees of supination (to view the fourth and fifth metacarpals)
10 degrees of pronation (to view the second and third metacarpals)

COMMON ADULT CONDITIONS OF THE HAND

Tendon Injuries

Mallet injuries

Traumatic avulsion of the terminal portion of the extensor apparatus (terminal extensor tendon [see Fig. 13–6]) caused by sudden flexion of the DIP joint while the finger is in the extended position

Can be a soft tissue or bony avulsion

Physical examination shows inability of the patient to extend the DIP joint

If left untreated, can lead to a swan-neck deformity (hyperextension of the PIP joint with flexion of the DIP joint) caused by dorsal subluxation of the lateral bands (Fig. 13–21)

Treatment

Extension splinting of the DIP joint (full time for 6 weeks, followed by night-time splinting for 6 more weeks) (Fig. 13–22)

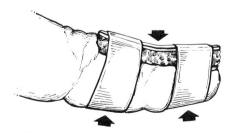

Figure 13–22 ■ Extension splinting of the distal interphalangeal joint for mallet injuries. The dorsal padded aluminum splint employs the three-point fixation principle (*arrows*). (From Green DP, Strickland JW: The hand. *In* DeLee JC, Drez D Jr [eds]: Orthopaedic Sports Medicine: Principles and Practice. Philadelphia, WB Saunders, 1994, p 951.)

Central slip injury (Fig. 13–23)

Commonly results from a volar dislocation of the PIP joint

Physical examination reveals tenderness over the central slip (dorsal finger just distal to the PIP joint), loss of active extension of the DIP joint with the PIP joint stabilized on a flat surface (Elson's test)

If left untreated, can lead to a boutonnière deformity (hyperextension of the DIP joint with flexion of the PIP joint) caused by volar subluxation of the lateral bands because of disruption of the central slip and extensor apparatus (see Figs. 13–6 and 13–23)

Treatment

Reduce the volar PIP joint dislocation followed by testing for active PIP joint extension; if PIP joint extension is near normal (within 30 degrees of full extension), then splint the PIP joint in extension; if PIP joint extension is absent or poor, the patient needs an operative repair

FDP avulsion (jersey finger)

Traumatic avulsion of the FDP is a common sports injury caused by grabbing an opponent (finger gets caught in opponent's jersey or other part of the uniform)

The ring finger is most commonly affected

Physical examination shows inability of the patient to actively flex the DIP joint with the PIP joint held in extension (by holding the PIP joint in extension, the effect of the FDS is eliminated, thus isolating the action of the FDP) (Fig. 13–24)

Treatment

Early—operative reattachment (to the tendon insertion site)

Late—two-stage operative reconstruction

FDS rupture

Physical examination demonstrates inability to flex the PIP joint with the MCP joints of the uninvolved fingers held by the examiner in maximal forced extension; by hyperextending the MCP joints of the uninvolved fingers, the ability of the FDP to flex both the PIP and the DIP joints is eliminated; therefore, any active flexion at the PIP

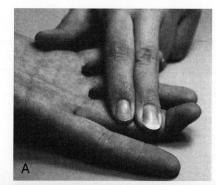

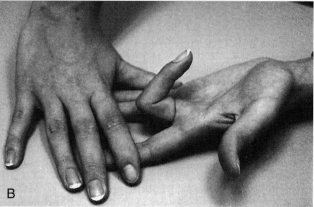

Figure 13–24 ■ Testing finger flexors. *A*, The flexor digitorum profundus (FDP) can be tested by holding the proximal interphalangeal (PIP) joint in extension and testing for distal interphalangeal joint flexion. In this example the FDP is intact. *B*, The flexor digitorum superficialis (FDS) can be tested by holding the adjacent digits in extension and testing for PIP joint flexion of the affected digit. In this example the FDS is intact. (From Rettig AC: Closed tendon injuries of the hand and wrist in the athlete. Clin Sports Med 11:93, 1992.)

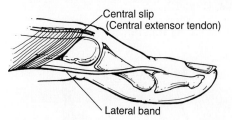

Figure 13–23 ■ Central slip injuries, if left untreated, can result in volar displacement of the lateral bands and a boutonnière deformity. Volar dislocations of the proximal interphalangeal (PIP) joint, although uncommon, can result in central slip injuries. Splinting the PIP joint (not the distal interphalangeal [DIP] joint) in extension and encouraging passive DIP flexion is the correct treatment for acute central slip injuries as long as the patient has active PIP joint extension to within 30 degrees of full extension. (From Green DP, Strickland JW: The hand. *In* DeLee JC, Drez D Jr [eds]: Orthopaedic Sports Medicine: Principles and Practice. Philadelphia, WB Saunders, 1994, p 956.)

Central slip
(Central extensor tendon)

Lateral band

joint during this maneuver is from the FDS (and with an FDS rupture there can be no flexion at the PIP joint during this maneuver) (see Fig. 13–24)

Ligamentous Injuries

PIP joint ligamentous injuries

Collateral ligament injury

Caused by varus or valgus stress on the joint usually in the extended position

Physical examination reveals local tenderness over the collateral ligament with joint opening to varus/valgus stress testing

Treat with buddy taping (Fig. 13–25)

Volar plate injury

Usually results from a hyperextension injury with dorsal dislocation at the PIP joint (often reduced by the patient or an observer [team trainer] at the time of injury)

It is important to check the reduction (of the dislocation) for congruency of the joint with a lateral radiograph

If the reduction is congruent, buddy tape; if the reduction is incongruent, apply an extension block splint

MCP joint ligamentous injuries

Collateral ligament injury

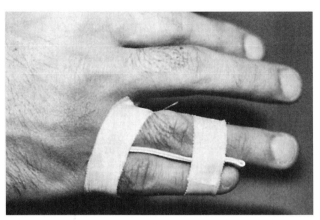

Figure 13–25 ■ Buddy taping for proximal interphalangeal joint injury. Note that absorbent padding is placed between the fingers to prevent skin maceration. (From Loeb PE, Mirabello SC, Andrews JR: The hand: Field evaluation and treatment. Clin Sports Med 11:30, 1992.)

Similar to PIP joint injuries
Treat with splinting of the MCP joint in flexion for 3 weeks; associated displaced avulsion fractures may require open reduction with internal fixation (ORIF)
Volar plate injury
Usually results from a hyperextension injury with dorsal dislocation at the MCP joint
It is important to differentiate a simple MCP joint dislocation (volar plate not trapped within the MCP joint) from a complex MCP joint dislocation (volar plate trapped within the MCP joint) (Fig. 13–26)
Simple dislocations are treated with closed reduction via longitudinal traction and splinting in flexion
Complex dislocations (see Fig. 13–26) are treated with open reduction and are recognized by
Puckering of the palmar skin
Parallelism of the metacarpal and proximal phalanx (this is abnormal) seen on a lateral radiograph
Entrapment of a sesamoid within a widened joint space (seen on radiograph)
Thumb MCP joint ulnar collateral ligament injury
Caused by sudden valgus stress to the thumb MCP joint
Also known as gamekeeper's thumb because British gamekeepers would kill rabbits by breaking the rabbits' necks using their hands (first web space), which stressed the thumb MCP joint ulnar collateral ligament
Also known as skier's thumb because of this common mechanism of injury (valgus stress from a ski pole)
Physical examination reveals local tenderness over the thumb MCP joint ulnar collateral ligament with opening of the ulnar side of the joint to valgus stress testing (see Fig. 13–20)
Treatment—partial ligament injuries display opening of less than 45 degrees and are treated with thumb spica splinting or casting for 3 to 6 weeks based on symptoms; complete ligamentous injuries display more than 45 degrees of joint opening to valgus stress and require an operative repair
A Stener lesion represents interposition of the adductor pollicis aponeurosis between the two torn ends of the ulnar collateral ligament
Thumb MCP joint radial collateral ligament injury
Uncommon injury
Treatment is casting until symptoms resolve
Lacerations of the finger
Important to assess the status of the **digital nerves**
Two-point discrimination testing (see Fig. 13–16)
Important to assess the status of the **digital arteries**
Digital Allen's test (see Fig. 13–17)
With a volar laceration, normal sensation on physical examination typically rules out an injury to the digital arteries (because the digital nerves are volar to the digital arteries in the finger and would presumably be lacerated prior to the digital arteries with a volar laceration)
Important to assess the status of the **flexor tendons**
Motor examination is the key to making the diagnosis of a lacerated flexor tendon
Flexor tendon lacerations require operative repair; it is crucial not to allow shortening of the FDP tendon during repair; excessive shortening of the FDP tendon can result in loss of full flexion of not only the involved finger but also adjacent fingers because of the **quadriga effect** (the four FDP tendons have a common muscle belly, and therefore DIP flexion of any finger normally results in flexion of the other three fingers; a limitation of DIP flexion in any finger results in a limitation of DIP flexion in the other three fingers; this is in contrast to the FDS, which maintains independent muscle function to each finger)
Important to assess the status of the **extensor tendons**
Motor examination is the key to making the diagnosis of a lacerated extensor tendon
Extensor tendon lacerations may be sutured in the emergency department (injuries involving less than 50% of the tendon do not require repair)

Late Effects of Traumatic Injuries

Intrinsic-plus deformity (see Fig. 13–19)
Caused by foreshortening of the intrinsic muscles
Treatment is operative soft tissue release
Intrinsic-minus deformity (see Fig. 11–9)
Caused by an injury to the ulnar nerve (with or without a median nerve injury) that causes a claw-hand deformity (hyperextension of the MCP joint and flexion at the PIP joint) resulting from loss of the intrinsic muscles that are normally responsible for flexion at the MCP joint and extension at the PIP joint and the unapposed action of the extrinsic muscles (FDS, FDP, and EDC)
Treatment typically includes tendon transfers (from

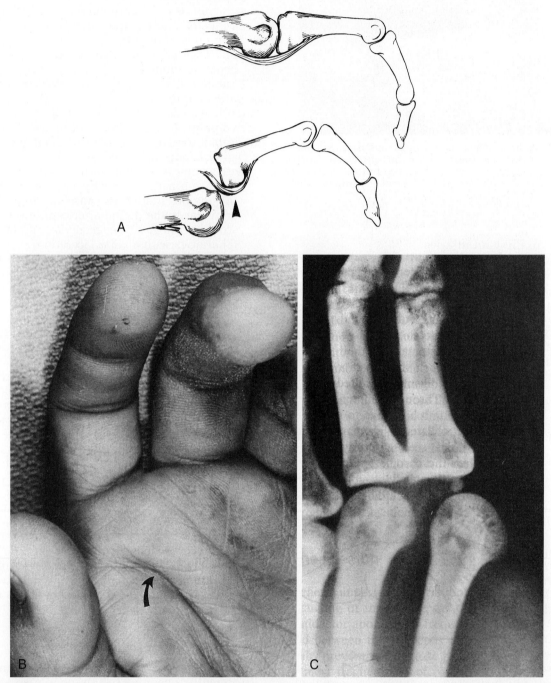

Figure 13–26 ■ Complex dorsal dislocation of the metacarpophalangeal (MCP) joint. *A,* Diagram demonstrating how the volar plate can become displaced dorsally, blocking reduction of the MCP joint dorsal dislocation. *B,* Clinical photograph demonstrating puckering (*arrow*) of the palmar skin. *C,* Radiograph showing entrapment of a sesamoid within the (widened) MCP joint. (From Green DP, Strickland JW: The hand. *In* DeLee JC, Drez D Jr [eds]: Orthopaedic Sports Medicine: Principles and Practice. Philadelphia, WB Saunders, 1994, pp 974, 975.)

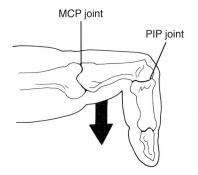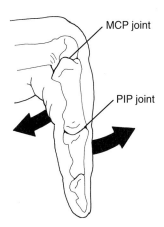

Figure 13–27 ■ Lumbrical-plus deformity. With the metacarpophalangeal (MCP) joint in extension and the proximal interphalangeal (PIP) joint in flexion, active flexion of the MCP joint will cause paradoxical extension of the PIP joint.

MCP joint

PIP joint

MCP joint

PIP joint

tendons that are still functional [such as the FDS]) that reroute a tendon to correct the deformity

Lumbrical-plus deformity

Caused by lumbrical tightness

This can occur as a late effect of an FDP laceration distal to the lumbrical origin on the FDP

Physical examination reveals paradoxical extension of the PIP joint when the MCP joint is actively flexed (with the PIP joint beginning in the flexed position) (Fig. 13–27)

Treatment is operative soft tissue release/repair

Boutonnière deformity (see Fig. 13–23)

Can occur as a late effect of a central slip injury

Treatment is operative reconstruction

Swan-neck deformity (see Fig. 13–21)

Can occur as a late effect of a mallet injury or an FDS rupture

Treatment is operative reconstruction

Arthritic Conditions

Rheumatoid arthritis (Fig. 13–28; see Fig. 3–3)

Can be associated with debilitating hand problems that include

Tenosynovitis

Trigger finger

Carpal tunnel syndrome

Tendon ruptures

EPL

Vaughn-Jackson syndrome—rupture of the EDC tendon of the ring and small fingers

Mannerfelt's syndrome—rupture of the FPL tendon

Joint destruction

Ulnar deviation (subluxation) of the MCP joints (ulnar drift) caused by ulnar subluxation of the extensor tendons

Intrinsic-plus deformity

Boutonnière deformity

Swan-neck deformity

Thumb deformities

Rheumatoid nodules

Treatment

Complex operative reconstructions based on the specific problems

Osteoarthritis

Common in the thumb CMC joint

DIP involvement with **Heberden's nodes** is also common (Fig. 13–29)

Treatment

Nonsteroidal anti-inflammatory drugs (NSAIDs)

Joint injections

Figure 13–28 ■ Rheumatoid arthritis of the hand. AP radiograph demonstrates ulnar deviation of the metacarpophalangeal joints, a thumb deformity, and joint destruction. (From Weissman BNW, Sledge CB: Orthopedic Radiology. Philadelphia, WB Saunders, 1986, p 105.)

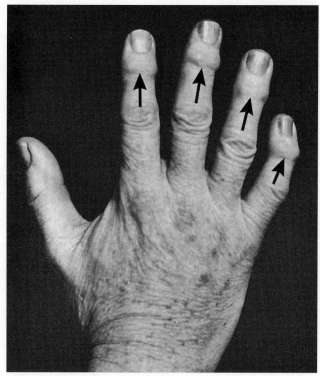

Figure 13–29 ■ Clinical photograph demonstrating Heberden's nodes (*arrows*), which are common in osteoarthritis. Note distal interphalangeal joint enlargement. (From Gartland JJ: Fundamentals of Orthopaedics, 4th ed. Philadelphia, WB Saunders, 1986, p 125.)

Arthrodesis (IP joints)
Arthroplasty (thumb CMC joint)

Infections

Paronychia (Fig. 13–30)
   Infection of the paronychial fold(s) on the side of the fingernail
   Commonly results from a hangnail with introduction of *Staphylococcus aureus* into the paronychial tissue
   Treatment is débridement, nail trimming, warm soaks, and oral antibiotics
Eponychia (see Fig. 13–30)
   Infection of the eponychial fold at the base of the nail
   Treatment is similar to that for paronychia
Felon (Fig. 13–31)
   Subcutaneous abscess of the distal pulp of a finger or the thumb
   May follow a penetrating injury or spread from a paronychia/eponychia
   Treatment is débridement
Herpetic whitlow
   Viral infection of the hand caused by herpes simplex
   Common in medical and dental personnel and small children
   The patient presents with pain and clear, fluid-filled vesicles of the distal finger

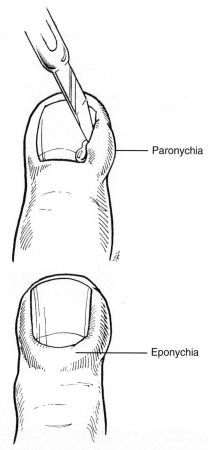

Figure 13–30 ■ Paronychia (the figure shows operative débridement) and eponychia. (From Bora FW: The Pediatric Upper Extremity. Philadelphia, WB Saunders, 1986, pp 362, 363.)

Treatment is with acyclovir
Débridement of the vesicles is contraindicated
Suppurative flexor tenosynovitis (Fig. 13–32)
   Infection of the flexor tendon sheath of the hand (a surgical emergency)
   The four classic signs (Kanavel's signs) to make the diagnosis
      Tenderness along the flexor tendon sheath
      Sausage-appearing digits

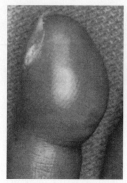

Figure 13–31 ■ Felon. (From Bogumill GP: The hand. *In* Wiesel SW, Delahay JN, Connell MC [eds]: Essentials of Orthopaedic Surgery. Philadelphia, WB Saunders, 1993, p 229.)

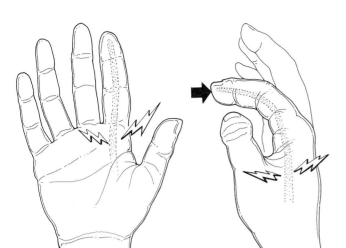

Figure 13–32 ■ Kanavel's signs of suppurative flexor tenosynovitis: tenderness along the flexor tendon sheath, sausage-appearing digits, flexed position of the finger, and pain on passive extension of the finger.

The finger is held in a flexed position
Pain on passive extension of the finger
Treatment—emergent operative débridement
Deep infections of the hand
Include
Web space (collar button) abscess
Palmar space infection
Thenar space infection
Hypothenar space infection
Ulnar and radial bursal infections
Parona's space infection (distal forearm)
The patient presents with
Pain
Swelling
Tenderness to palpation
Erythema
Localized warmth
Systemic symptoms in some cases (fever, chills, etc.)
Treatment is emergent operative débridement
Bite injuries (see Chapter 3)
Can lead to significant infections
Human bites are worse than most animal bites because they commonly involve virulent anaerobic organisms; one should have a high index of suspicion for an open MCP joint injury in the patient presenting with a laceration over the dorsal aspect of the MCP joint (fight bite)
For animal bites, it is important to isolate the animal and obtain a history for immunization (rabies)
Treatment is débridement and administration of the appropriate antibiotic (based on the suspected organisms present in the oral flora of the animal; see Chapter 3)
Marine injuries
Commonly involve anaerobic organisms and atypical mycobacteria
Organisms are typically difficult to culture
Treatment is débridement and antibiotics
Paint/grease gun injuries

Accidental injection of foreign matter by paint and grease guns can cause significant morbidity because of the high injection pressures and toxicity of the paint or grease
Initial presentation may be deceptively benign
Rapid, relentless progression to limb-threatening fulminant infection
Emergent operative débridement with a wide surgical exploration is mandatory
Nail gun and fish hook injuries
In addition to irrigation and débridement, these objects must be removed by advancing them in the same direction that they entered (they must by pushed out, not pulled out) because of the configuration of their barbs

Other Conditions

Dupuytren's contracture (Fig. 13–33)
Cords and nodules (proliferative fibrodysplasia) in the subcutaneous palmar fascia
Common in alcoholics, diabetics, and smokers
The patient presents with palmar nodules and flexion contractures that may limit hand function
Surgical release of contractures may be indicated depending on the extent of the functional disability
Trigger finger
Stenosing tenosynovitis (nonsuppurative) of the flexor tendon, resulting in abnormal gliding of the flexor tendon within the tendon sheath with catching or locking as the affected tendon is caught at the proximal edge of the A1 pulley
The patient presents with a demonstrable catching during flexion/extension of the finger; the triggering is palpable to the examiner immediately proximal to the MCP joint (at the proximal edge of the A1 pulley)
Treatment is operative release of the A1 pulley if conservative management (splinting) fails
Neuromas
Represent a nodule that develops on the stump of the proximal end of a severed nerve

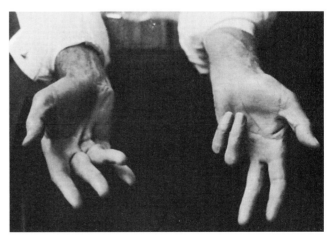

Figure 13–33 ■ Dupuytren's contracture. (From Polley HF, Hunder GG: Rheumatologic Interviewing and Physical Examination of the Joints. Philadelphia, WB Saunders, 1978, p 98.)

Table 13–3
TRAUMATIC AMPUTATIONS

Replant	Do Not Replant
All thumb injuries	Mangled digits
Injuries involving multiple digits	Severe degloving injuries
Injuries in children	Elderly patients with arteriosclerosis
Amputations proximal to the MCP joint or distal to the FDS insertion	Injuries more than 8 hours old
	Single-digit amputations between the MCP joint and the insertion of the FDS
	Psychiatric patients (self-mutilators)
	Patients with other life-threatening injuries that take priority

MCP, metacarpophalangeal; FDS, flexor digitorum superficialis.

Can cause pain (burning) and discomfort
Arise as a result of
    Nerve injuries
    Nerve repairs
    Traumatic or surgical amputations
Treatment options
    Local injection (can also aid in making the diagnosis)

    Operative decompression or resection
Vaso-occlusive disorders
    Etiologies
      Emboli
      Vasospasm
      Connective tissue disorders (such as scleroderma, Raynaud's syndrome)
    Clinical presentation includes hand pain, paresthesias, and cold intolerance
    Treatment is based on the etiology
Traumatic amputations (Table 13–3)
    Normal function should not be expected regardless of the type of treatment

FRACTURES AND DISLOCATIONS OF THE HAND

Overview (Tables 13–4 and 13–5)

Fractures and dislocations of the hand can be challenging problems and often require operative intervention
Treatment must be based on the exact anatomic na-

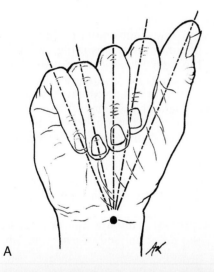

A

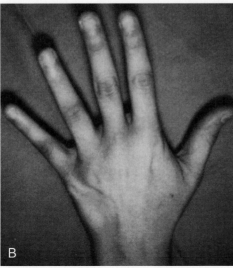

B

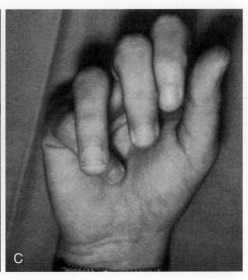

C

Figure 13–34 ■ Assessment for rotational deformity of the fingers. *A*, Normally, the four flexed fingers converge at the scaphoid tubercle and the nails are aligned. *B*, Rotational malalignment cannot be appreciated with the fingers extended. *C*, Same patient as *B* with the fingers flexed. Note malrotation of the ring finger. (*A* from Tubiana R: The Hand. Philadelphia, WB Saunders, 1981, p 22. *B* and *C* from Culver JE, Anderson TE: Fractures of the hand and wrist in the athlete. Clin Sports Med 11:103, 1992.)

Table 13–4
FRACTURES OF THE ADULT HAND

Fracture	Eponym or Other Name	Classification	Treatment	Most Common Complications of the Injury
Distal phalanx Extensor digitorum communis terminal tendon avulsion	Mallet finger	Descriptive Extensor tendon tear (Fig. 13–35) Bony avulsion (see Fig. 13–35)	Splint DIP joint × 4 weeks Volar splint × 6–10 weeks ORIF	Nail bed injury Residual deformity
Flexor digitorum profundus avulsion	Jersey finger	Leddy; Smith	Operative repair	Deformity (lumbrical-plus)
Proximal and middle phalanges		Extra-articular, good fracture stability	Buddy tape	Decreased ROM, contractures, malunion, nonunion, tendon adhesions
		Extra-articular, poor fracture stability	Operative reduction and fixation	
		Intra-articular, nondisplaced	Buddy tape, early ROM, observe closely for fracture displacement	
		Intra-articular, displaced	Operative reduction and fixation	
Intra-articular fracture of the base of the middle phalanx		Descriptive	Splint PIP joint in extension × 6 weeks; ORIF if large fragment (external fixation if comminuted)	
Metacarpal head		Descriptive	ORIF for large displaced fragment, otherwise early ROM	Malunion (rotation), prominent metacarpal head in palm, loss of reduction, nonunion
Metacarpal neck (Fig. 13–36)	Boxer's fracture	4th and 5th	Closed reduction and splinting	
		2nd and 3rd	Operative reduction and fixation	
Metacarpal shaft (Fig. 13–37)		Transverse	Closed reduction and splint or operative reduction and fixation if irreducible by closed methods	
		Oblique/Spiral Comminuted and nondisplaced Comminuted and displaced	ORIF if shortened or rotated Splint Operative reduction and fixation	
First (thumb) metacarpal base (intra-articular volar lip)	Bennett's fracture (Fig. 13–38)		Operative reduction and fixation	Fracture displacement by abductor pollicis longus
First (thumb) metacarpal base ("Y" or "T" configuration or comminuted)	Rolando's fracture (see Fig. 13–38)	Intra-articular	Operative reduction and fixation	Post-traumatic osteoarthritis
		Extra-articular	Closed reduction and thumb spica cast	
Fifth metacarpal base	Baby Bennett's fracture		Operative reduction and fixation	Fracture displacement by extensor carpi ulnaris

DIP, distal interphalangeal; ORIF, open reduction with internal fixation; ROM, range of motion; PIP, proximal interphalangeal.

ture of the injury, and recognition of specific injury patterns is crucial

Treatment should be aimed at obtaining early joint motion to avoid stiffness and contractures

Intra-articular fractures require anatomic reduction to obtain the best possible clinical result

Careful clinical evaluation for a rotational deformity of the fingers caused by a malaligned fracture is essential (Fig. 13–34)

50% of all hand fractures involve the distal phalanx

Residual angulation of metacarpal fractures is better tolerated in the ring and small finger metacarpals (as compared to the long and index metacarpals) because of their relative increased mobility, which is able to compensate for the deformity

TUMORS OF THE HAND

Bone

Enchondroma
Chondrosarcoma

Table 13–5
DISLOCATIONS OF THE ADULT HAND

Dislocation	Eponym or Other Name	Classification	Treatment	Most Common Complications of the Injury
Distal interphalangeal joint		Dorsal	Closed reduction, immobilize × 2 weeks	
		Collateral ligament sprain	Buddy tape × 3–6 weeks	
		Collateral ligament tear	Operative repair	
Proximal interphalangeal joint (Fig. 13–39)		Dorsal (volar plate disruption)	Closed reduction and buddy tape; extension block splint for loss of reduction	Stiffness, contractures
		Dorsal with fracture of the middle phalanx (fracture-dislocation)	Operative reduction and fixation	Stiffness, contractures
		Volar	Closed reduction and extension splint × 4–6 weeks	Missed diagnosis (late recognition), central slip injury
		Rotatory	Operative treatment	
Metacarpophalangeal joint		Collateral ligament injury	Splint in 50 degrees MCP joint flexion × 3 weeks (operative treatment if displaced >2 mm)	Missed diagnosis (failure to recognize), stiffness, contractures, neurovascular injury
		Simple, dorsal	Closed reduction and immobilize × 1 week	
		Complex, dorsal (volar plate interposed at dislocation site) (see Fig. 13–26)	Open reduction	
		Volar	Open reduction	
Carpometacarpal joint			Open reduction	
Thumb metacarpophalangeal joint with ulnar collateral ligament injury	Gamekeeper's thumb (see Fig. 13–20)	Sprain (<45 degree joint opening on stress test)	Thumb spica cast	Unrecognized Stener's lesion (interposition of adductor aponeurosis between the two ends of the torn UCL); chronic pain, instability
		Rupture (≥45 degree joint opening on stress test)	Operative repair	
Thumb metacarpophalangeal joint with radial collateral ligament injury			Splint	
Thumb metacarpophalangeal joint without ligament injury		Simple, dorsal	Reduce, immobolize × 3 weeks	
		Complex, dorsal (volar plate or flexor pollicis longus interposed)	Open reduction	
Thumb carpometacarpal joint			Operative reduction (hyperpronation), immobilize × 6–10 weeks	

MCP, metacarpophalangeal; UCL, ulnar collateral ligament.

Soft Tissue

Glomus tumor
Epidermoid (inclusion) cyst
Ganglion cyst
Superficial fibromatoses
Giant cell tumor of tendon sheath
Kaposi's sarcoma
Epithelioid sarcoma

Mucous cyst
Volar retinacular cyst
Foreign body granuloma
Calcinosis
Squamous cell carcinoma
False aneurysm
True aneurysm
Arteriovenous fistula
Neurofibroma

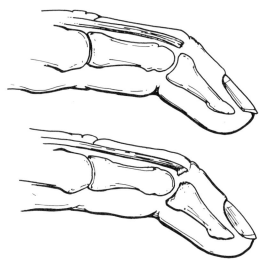

Figure 13–35 ■ Mallet finger. Soft tissue (terminal extensor tendon tear) mallet (*top*) and bony mallet (*bottom*). (From Green DP, Strickland JW: The hand. *In* DeLee JC, Drez D Jr [eds]: Orthopaedic Sports Medicine: Principles and Practice. Philadelphia, WB Saunders, 1994, p 951.)

Neuroma
Neurilemmoma
Lipoma

DIFFERENTIAL DIAGNOSIS OF COMMON HAND COMPLAINTS

Pain

Tendon injuries
Ligamentous injuries
Fractures
Dislocations
Nerve injuries/disorders
Arthritis
Rheumatologic conditions
Infections
Tumors
Vaso-occlusive disorders

Instability

Ligamentous injuries
Fractures
Dislocations
Rheumatologic conditions

Weakness

Tendon injuries
Nerve injuries/disorders

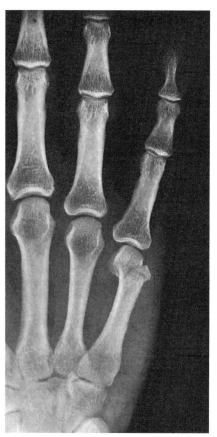

Figure 13–36 ■ Boxer's fracture of the fifth metacarpal neck. (From Gartland JJ: Fundamentals of Orthopaedics, 4th ed. Philadelphia, WB Saunders, 1994, p 267.)

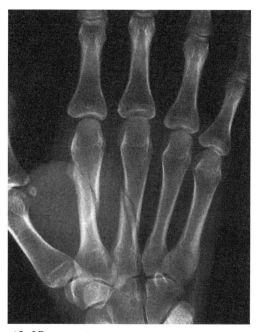

Figure 13–37 ■ Spiral metacarpal shaft fractures of the index and middle fingers. (From Culver JE, Anderson TE: Fractures of the hand and wrist in the athlete. Clin Sports Med 11:116, 1992.)

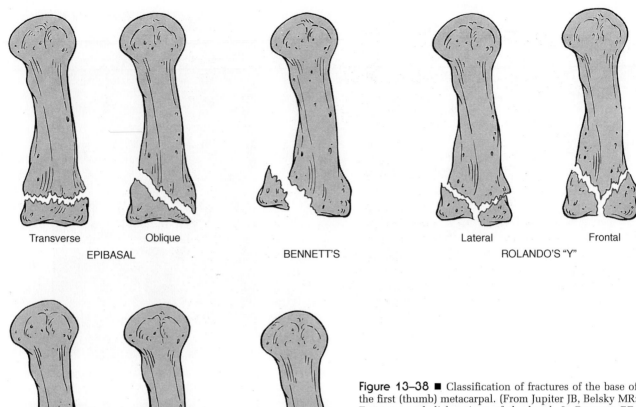

Transverse   Oblique
EPIBASAL

BENNETT'S

Lateral   Frontal
ROLANDO'S "Y"

Lateral   Frontal
ROLANDO'S "T"

ROLANDO'S
COMMINUTED

Figure 13–38 ■ Classification of fractures of the base of the first (thumb) metacarpal. (From Jupiter JB, Belsky MR: Fractures and dislocations of the hand. *In* Browner BD, Jupiter JB, Levine AM, et al [eds]: Skeletal Trauma. Philadelphia, WB Saunders, 1992, p 967.)

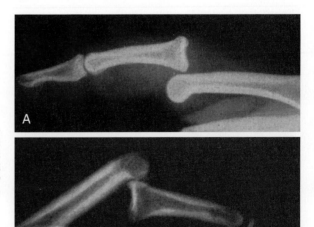

Figure 13–39 ■ Proximal interphalangeal (PIP) joint dislocation. *A,* Dorsal dislocation (most common) can usually be treated by closed reduction and buddy taping. Loss of reduction in extension may require extension block splinting. *B,* Volar dislocation (unusual) requires extension splinting of the PIP joint only. (From Green DP, Strickland JW: The Hand. *In* DeLee JC, Drez D Jr [eds]: Orthopaedic Sports Medicine: Principles and Practice. Philadelphia, WB Saunders, 1994, pp 964, 965.)

Tingling/Loss of Sensation

Traumatic nerve injuries
Nerve entrapments
Cervical radiculopathy
Neuromas
Tumors
Vaso-occlusive disorders

Deformity

Fractures
Dislocations
Ligamentous injuries
Nerve injuries/disorders (atrophy, clawing)
Late effects of trauma (intrinsic-plus deformity, lumbrical-plus deformity, boutonnière deformity, swanneck deformity)
Rheumatologic conditions
Infections
Tumors
Dupuytren's contracture

Catching/Locking

Trigger finger

Loss of Motion

Tendon injuries
Ligamentous injuries
Fractures
Dislocations
Late effects of trauma

Arthritis
Rheumatologic conditions
Infections
Tumors
Dupuytren's contracture
Trigger finger

PEARLS AND PITFALLS

Thorough knowledge of hand anatomy and techniques of physical examination must be mastered; there are no shortcuts to understanding the hand

When evaluating a patient with a hand injury, all of the patient's jewelry must be removed

The hand should always be immobilized with the wrist extended (20 degrees); the MCP joints flexed (to 70 degrees); and the PIP and DIP joints in extension

Prolonged immobilization of the PIP joint can lead to permanent residual stiffness

If you are not sure, refer to a specialist

Rotational malalignment is a common problem with hand fractures and must not be overlooked (see Fig. 13–34)

The digital nerves are very superficial in the fingers and thumb and are easily injured

A high index of suspicion is needed to diagnose an early hand infection before it becomes limb-threatening

When evaluating a hand laceration, it is more important to test for the function of the structures at risk than to attempt to visualize damaged structures in the depth of the wound

CHAPTER 14

The Adult Cervical Spine

CERVICAL SPINE ANATOMY

Bones (Fig. 14–1)

Cervical vertebrae
  Seven of them (C1-7)
  Foramina in each transverse process
  Atlas (C1) has no body or spinous process
  Axis (C2) has the odontoid (dens) and both superior and inferior articular facets

Joints

The atlantoaxial joint (C1-2) is unique (Fig. 14–2)
Facet (apophyseal) joints (Fig. 14–3)
  Oriented 45 degrees in the sagittal plane and neutrally in the coronal plane
  Superior facet (of the lower vertebra) is anterior and inferior to the inferior articular process of the vertebra above (see Fig. 14–3)

Intervertebral discs lie between the vertebrae (Fig. 14–4)
Supporting ligaments
  Entire length
    Anterior longitudinal ligament
    Posterior longitudinal ligament
    Ligamentum nuchae
  Each level
    Ligamentum flavum
    Interspinous ligaments

Muscles (Fig. 14–5) (see Fig. 15–4)

Anterior
  Platysma (innervated by cranial nerve VII)
  Stylohyoid and digastrics (innervated by cranial nerve XII)
  "Strap" muscles (innervated by the ansa cervicalis)
  Sternohyoid
  Omohyoid
  Thyrohyoid
  Sternothyroid

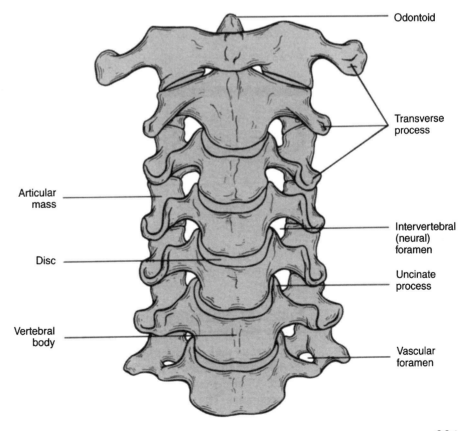

Figure **14–1** ■ Anterior view of the bony anatomy of the cervical spine. (From Bucholz RW: Lower cervical spine injuries. *In* Browner BD, Jupiter JB, Levine AM, et al [eds]: Skeletal Trauma. Philadelphia, WB Saunders, 1992, p 700.)

Odontoid

Transverse process

Articular mass

Intervertebral (neural) foramen

Disc

Uncinate process

Vertebral body

Vascular foramen

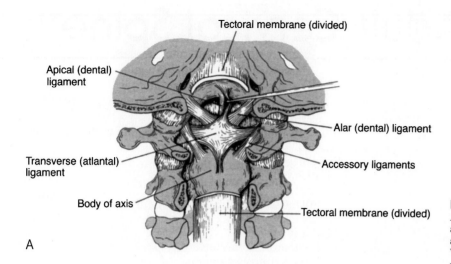

Tectoral membrane (divided)

Apical (dental) ligament

Alar (dental) ligament

Transverse (atlantal) ligament

Accessory ligaments

Body of axis

Tectoral membrane (divided)

A

Figure 14–2 ■ Atlantoaxial joint and cranium. *A,* Posterior coronal view: Note alar, transverse, and apical ligaments. *B,* Superior view of the atlantoaxial articulation. (From Jarrett PJ, Whitesides TE Jr: Injuries of the cervicocranium. *In* Browner BD, Jupiter JB, Levine AM, et al [eds]: Skeletal Trauma. Philadelphia, WB Saunders, 1992, pp 666, 667.)

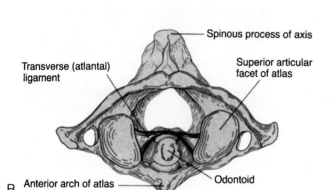

Spinous process of axis

Transverse (atlantal) ligament

Superior articular facet of atlas

Anterior arch of atlas

Odontoid

B

Figure 14–3 ■ Superior and lateral view of a typical C5 vertebra showing the orientation of the superior (1) and inferior (7) articular processes of the facet joints in the cervical spine. (Modified from Bucholz RW: Lower cervical spine injuries. *In* Browner BD, Jupiter JB, Levine AM, et al [eds]: Skeletal Trauma. Philadelphia, WB Saunders, 1992, p 700.)

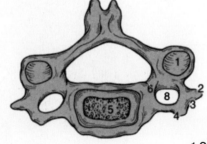

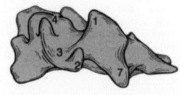

1 Superior articular process
2 Posterior tubercle
3 Costotransverse bar   } of transverse process
4 Anterior tubercle
5 Body
6 Pedicle
7 Inferior articular process
8 Vascular foramen

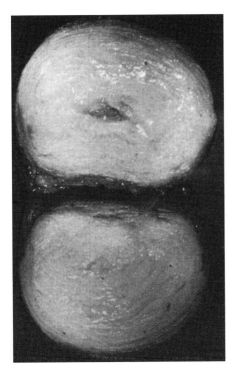

Figure 14–4 ■ Cross-section of an intervertebral disc. Note circumferential fibers of the annulus fibrosus (type I collagen) and the gelatinous central disc of the nucleus pulposus (type II collagen). (From Gartland JJ: Fundamentals of Orthopaedics, 4th ed. Philadelphia, WB Saunders, 1986, p 328.)

Lateral—sternocleidomastoid (innervated by cranial nerve XI and the ansa cervicalis)
Posterior—obliquus capitis, rectus capitis

Nerves

Spinal cord (Fig. 14–6)
Nerve roots (Fig. 14–7)

Nerve Root Level	Muscles Innervated
C3	Diaphragm (breathing)
C4	Diaphragm
C5	Diaphragm
	Elbow flexors
	Deltoid
C6	Elbow flexors
	Wrist extensors
C7	Elbow extensors
	Wrist flexors
C8	Finger flexors (extrinsics)
T1	Hand intrinsics

Cervical sympathetic chain
  The cervical sympathetic chain is made up of various ganglia (superior cervical ganglion, middle cervical ganglion, vertebral ganglion, and stellate ganglion) that are located in the neck region

Vessels

Vertebral arteries (Fig. 14–8)
  Branch from the subclavian arteries
  Run anterior to C7 and then through the vascular foramen (in the transverse processes of C6 through C1); the vertebral arteries enter the skull through the foramen magnum and unite to become the basilar artery
  Supply the spinal cord and vertebrae in the cervical spine and the cerebellum and circle of Willis in the cranium
Carotid arteries (Fig. 14–9)
  Common carotid artery
  Internal carotid artery
  External carotid artery
Jugular veins (see Fig. 14–9)
  Internal jugular vein
  External jugular vein
  Anterior jugular vein

Important Anatomic Relationships (Figs. 14–10 to 14–12)

SURGICAL APPROACHES TO THE CERVICAL SPINE

Anterior Approach

Interval is between the carotid sheath and the trachea
Contents of the carotid sheath—vagus nerve, common carotid artery, internal jugular vein
Longus colli muscle protects the recurrent laryngeal nerve (a branch of the vagus nerve)

Posterior Approach

Midline approach through the trapezius, splenius capitis/semispinalis, and longissimus capitis
Vertebral artery must be protected during the approach

HISTORY AND PHYSICAL EXAMINATION OF THE CERVICAL SPINE

History

Age
  Young patients—develop instability
  Older patients—develop osteoarthritis
Characterization of symptoms
  Localized pain—trauma, tumor, infection
  Radicular pain (pain that radiates peripherally along the distribution of an affected nerve root)—herniated nucleus pulposus (HNP [of disc]), cervical spinal stenosis
  Mechanical pain—instability, disc disease
Mechanism of injury/onset of symptoms

Physical Examination

Observation
  Attitude and posture of the head
  Scars, skin problems
  Abnormal contours to the neck
Palpation
  Bones

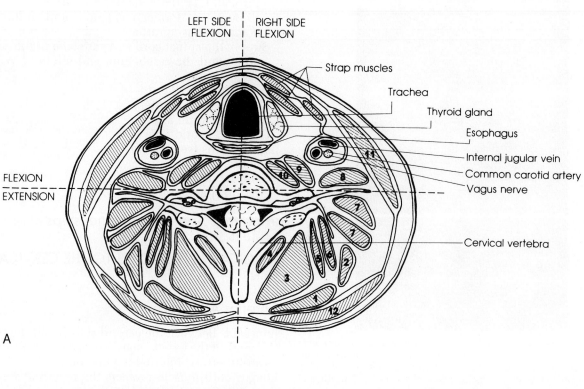

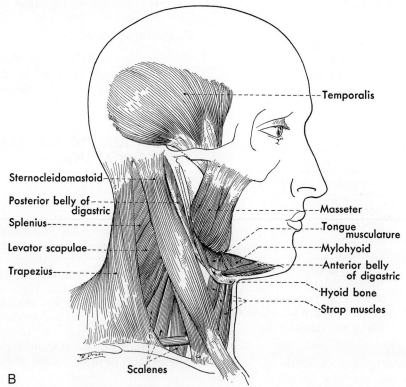

Figure 14–5 ■ Muscles of the neck. *A,* Cross-section of the lower cervical spine demonstrating (1) splenius capitis; (2) splenius cervicis; (3) semispinalis; (4) multifidus and rotatores; (5) longissimus capitis; (6) longissimus cervicis; (7) levator scapulae; (8) scalenus posterior; (9) scalenus medius; (10) scalenus anterior; (11) sternocleidomastoid; and (12) trapezius. *B,* Dissection of the muscles of the neck. (*A* from Magee DJ: Orthopedic Physical Assessment, 2nd ed. Philadelphia, WB Saunders, 1992, p 46. *B* from Jenkins DB: Hollinshead's Functional Anatomy of the Limbs and Back, 6th ed. Philadelphia, WB Saunders, 1991, p 343.)

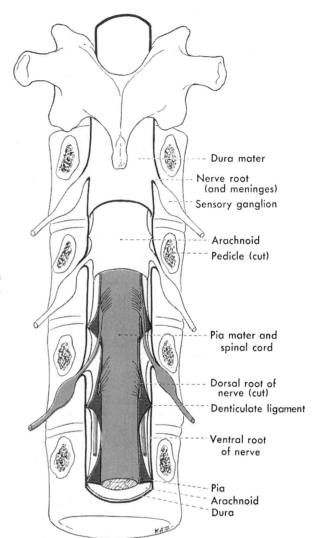

Figure 14–6 ■ The spinal cord runs from the base of the skull to L1 and is covered by dura mater, arachnoid, and pia mater. (From Jenkins DB: Hollinshead's Functional Anatomy of the Limbs and Back, 6th ed. Philadelphia, WB Saunders, 1991, p 204.)

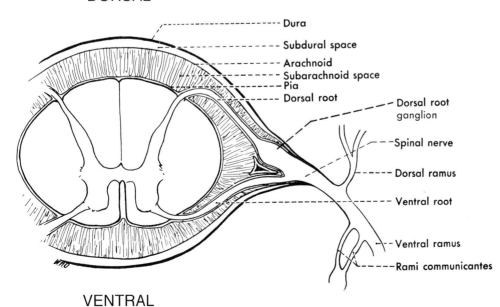

Figure 14–7 ■ Spinal nerve root nomenclature. (From Jenkins DB: Hollinshead's Functional Anatomy of the Limbs and Back, 6th ed. Philadelphia, WB Saunders, 1991, p 205.)

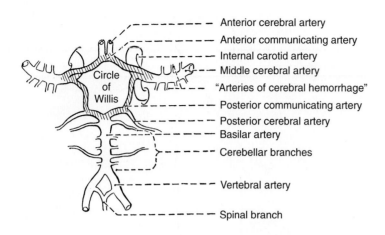

Circle
of
Willis

Anterior cerebral artery

Anterior communicating artery

Internal carotid artery

Middle cerebral artery

"Arteries of cerebral hemorrhage"

Posterior communicating artery

Posterior cerebral artery

Basilar artery

Cerebellar branches

Vertebral artery

Spinal branch

Figure 14–8 ■ Vertebral arteries, which are branches of the subclavian arteries at the base of the neck, run through the vascular foramina of cervical vertebrae 2 to 7 and combine to form the basilar artery (which contributes to the circle of Willis). (From Jenkins DB: Hollinshead's Functional Anatomy of the Limbs and Back, 6th ed. Philadelphia, WB Saunders, 1991, p 337.)

Anterior
  Angle of the mandible—at the level of C2-3
  Hyoid bone—at the level of C3
  Thyroid cartilage (Adam's apple)—at the level of C4-5
  Cricoid cartilage—at the level of C6
Posterior
  Occiput
  Spinous processes of cervical vertebrae—C7 is the most prominent
  Facet joints
Soft tissues
  Anterior
    Sternocleidomastoid muscle
    Thyroid gland
    Carotid pulse
  Posterior
    Trapezius muscle
    Nuchal ligament
Motion (Fig. 14–13)
  Flexion (normal—chin to chest)
  Extension (normal—look directly at the ceiling)
  Rotation (normal—chin almost in line with the shoulder)
  Lateral bending (normal—45 degrees to each side)
Neurovascular exam
  Sensation (see Figure 2–5)
  Reflexes
    Biceps (C5)
    Brachioradial (C6)
    Triceps (C7)
  Strength testing
    Deltoid, biceps (C5)
    Wrist extensors (C6)
    Triceps, wrist flexors, finger extensors (C7)
    Interossei, finger flexors (C8)
Special testing (condition specific)
  Encroachment on the nerve roots (Fig. 14–14)
    Compression test—axial pressure on the top of the head increases symptoms and radicular pain
    Distraction test—traction on the head relieves radicular symptoms
    Spurling's test—lateral flexion and rotation with compression causes nerve root encroachment and pain on the side of the nerve root encroachment

Encroachment on the spinal cord
  Valsalva's test—Valsalva's maneuver (patient attempts expiratory effort while closing his glottis [bears down as if having a bowel movement]) increases intrathecal pressure and causes radicular pain
Encroachment on the anterior cervical structures
  Swallowing test—difficulty or pain on swallowing may be a sign of anterior cervical pathology

DIAGNOSTIC TESTS FOR THE CERVICAL SPINE

Plain Radiographs

Anteroposterior (AP)—check for overall alignment
Lateral (Fig. 14–15)—must see the bottom of C7 and the top of T1
  Vertebral alignment—posterior borders of the vertebral bodies should form an unbroken line; translation of any vertebra greater than 3.5 mm is abnormal (see Fig. 14–15)
  Increased angulation between adjacent vertebral bodies—angulation of more than 11 degrees is abnormal
  Segmental disc or facet joint widening
  Avulsion fractures
  Anterior soft tissue space (see Fig. 14–15)
    At the level of C3—more than 3 mm of **soft tissue shadow** is abnormal
    At the level of C4—more than 8 to 10 mm of **soft tissue shadow** is abnormal
AP open-mouth (odontoid) view of the atlantoaxial articulation (Fig. 14–16)
Oblique views—evaluate the pedicles and intervertebral (neural) foramen

Special Radiographs

Lateral flexion/extension views—evaluate for subluxation of adjacent cervical vertebrae
Pillar views—rotate the head one direction, off-center the x-ray cassette 2 cm from the midline toward the opposite direction, angle the x-ray beam 30 degrees caudad; used to evaluate the articular masses

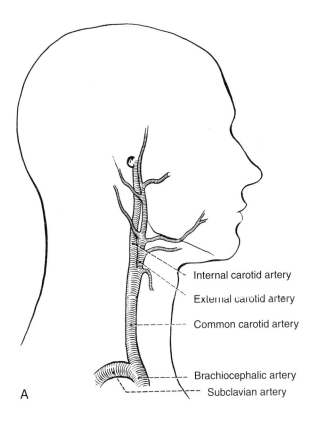

A

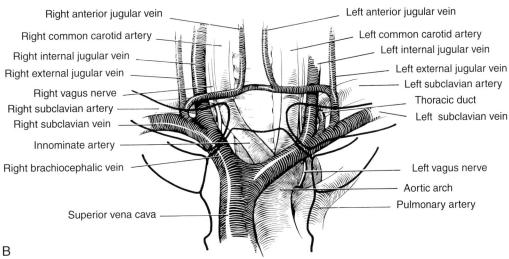

Right anterior jugular vein

Right common carotid artery

Right internal jugular vein

Right external jugular vein

Right vagus nerve

Right subclavian artery

Right subclavian vein

Innominate artery

Right brachiocephalic vein

Superior vena cava

Left anterior jugular vein

Left common carotid artery

Left internal jugular vein

Left external jugular vein

Left subclavian artery

Thoracic duct

Left subclavian vein

Left vagus nerve

Aortic arch

Pulmonary artery

Internal carotid artery

External carotid artery

Common carotid artery

Brachiocephalic artery

Subclavian artery

B

Figure 14–9 ■ *A,* Carotid arteries. *B,* Diagram of the origin of the carotid arteries and jugular veins. There are actually three paired jugular veins. The anterior jugular veins are midline; the external jugular veins are subcutaneous; and the internal jugular veins accompany the carotid arteries. (*A* from Jenkins DB: Hollinshead's Functional Anatomy of the Limbs and Back, 6th ed. Philadelphia, WB Saunders, 1991, p 350. *B* from Rockwood CA Jr, Green DP [eds]: Fractures, 2nd ed. Philadelphia, JB Lippincott, 1984.)

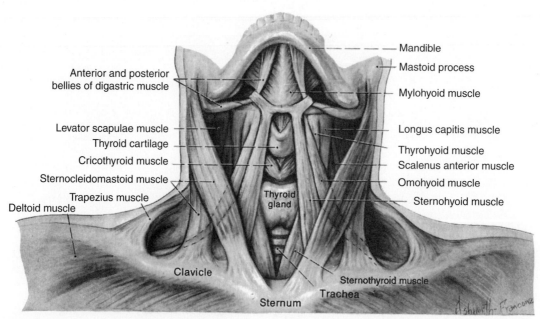

Figure 14–10 ■ The anterior triangle of the neck is bounded by the sternocleidomastoid, the sternohyoid, and the lower border of the mandible. (From Jacob SW, Francone C, Lossow WJ: Structure and Function in Man, 5th ed. Philadelphia, WB Saunders, 1982, p 192.)

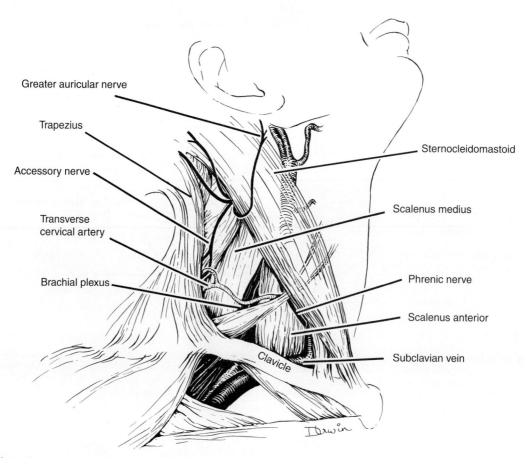

Figure 14–11 ■ The posterior triangle is bounded by the trapezius, the sternocleidomastoid, and the middle third of the clavicle. (From Bateman JE: The Shoulder and Neck. Philadelphia, WB Saunders, 1972, p 63.)

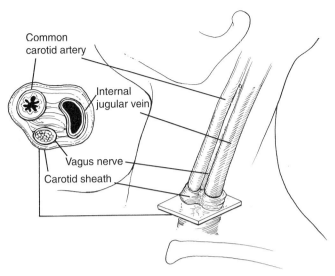

Figure 14-12 ■ Contents of the carotid sheath include the common carotid artery, the internal jugular vein, and the vagus nerve.

Swimmer's view (Fig. 14–17)—lateral view with the arm abducted 180 degrees; used to evaluate the lower cervical spine when the lateral view is inadequate (fails to visualize C7 and T1)

Computed Tomography (Fig. 14–18)

Helpful in evaluating fractures

Magnetic Resonance Imaging (Fig. 14–19)

Helpful in the evaluation of disc disease and ligamentous injuries

Electromyography/Nerve Conduction Studies/Somatosensory Evoked Potentials

Sensitive but nonspecific for nerve root impingement

COMMON ADULT CONDITIONS OF THE CERVICAL SPINE

Cervical Strains/Sprains

Trapezial strain
  Very common
  Patient presents with pain localized to the posterior cervical region
  Pain is reproducible with palpation of the trapezius muscles
  Treatment is supportive
    Nonsteroidal anti-inflammatory drugs (NSAIDs)
    Physical therapy
Whiplash
  Represents a hyperextension/hyperflexion injury of the neck commonly associated with a motor vehicle accident
  Does not imply any specific injury or syndrome
  Treatment is similar to that for a trapezial strain

Cervical Spondylosis

Chronic disc degeneration and facet joint arthropathy (degenerative arthritis)
Represents nerve root compression from a herniated nucleus pulposus or a bone spur (osteophyte)
Symptoms
  Neck pain
  Radicular pain—pain radiating from the neck peripherally to the upper extremity (Fig. 14–20)
  Myelopathy—impingement upon the spinal cord leads to
    Upper motor neuron findings
    Lower-extremity weakness
    Wide-based gait
    Urinary urgency/frequency
Diagnosis is made based on history, physical examination, and plain radiographs (including obliques [Fig. 14–21]) and may be confirmed via MRI (see Fig. 14–19)
Treatment options
  NSAIDs
  Exercises
  Soft cervical collar
  Cervical traction
  Operative anterior decompression

Cervical Stenosis

Narrowing of the space available for the spinal cord (SAC)
Can be congenital or acquired (traumatic or degenerative)
The patient presents with symptoms of radiculopathy to the upper extremities and/or myelopathy to the lower extremities
Radiographs distinguish this condition from cervical spondylosis
  The absolute AP canal diameter is less than 10 mm in cases of cervical stenosis
  Pavlov ratio—The ratio of the AP canal diameter to the AP diameter of the vertebral body is less than 0.80 in cases of cervical stenosis (Fig. 14–22)
Treatment
  Supportive
  Operative decompression for severe myelopathy or radiculopathy

Rheumatoid Spondylitis

Cervical spine involvement is common in rheumatoid arthritis and can lead to a variety of conditions
  Atlantoaxial subluxation (abnormal motion of C1 on C2)
    Displays more than 3.5 mm of atlantodens interval differences on the flexion and extension lateral radiographs
    Treatment—supportive unless flexion/extension lateral radiographs show atlantoaxial subluxation of more than 10 mm, in which case a fusion is required

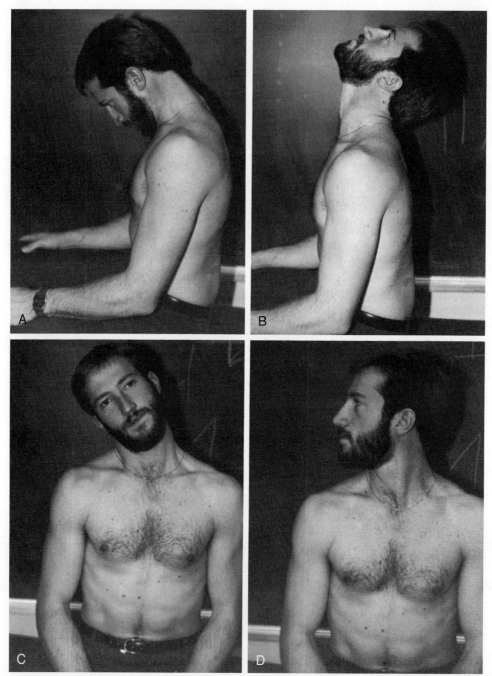

Figure 14–13 ■ Normal motion of the cervical spine. *A,* Flexion; *B,* Extension; *C,* Lateral bending; *D,* Rotation. (From Magee DJ: Orthopedic Physical Assessment, 2nd ed. Philadelphia, WB Saunders, 1992, p 41.)

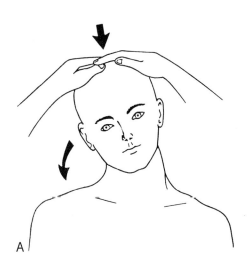

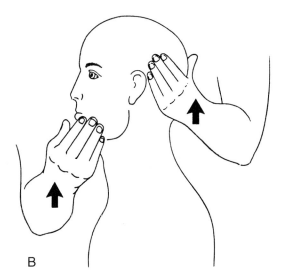

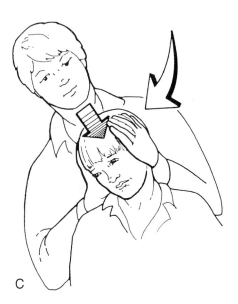

Figure 14–14 ■ Nerve root encroachment tests. *A,* Compression test can cause radicular symptoms on the affected side. *B,* Distraction can relieve these symptoms. *C,* Spurling's test. Lateral flexion and rotation with compression may cause nerve root encroachment and pain on the ipsilateral side in patients with cervical root impingement. (*A* and *B* from Magee DJ: Orthopedic Physical Assessment, 2nd ed. Philadelphia, WB Saunders, 1992, p 50. *C* from Miller MD, Cooper DE, Warner JJP: Review of Sports Medicine and Arthroscopy. Philadelphia, WB Saunders, 1995, p 129.)

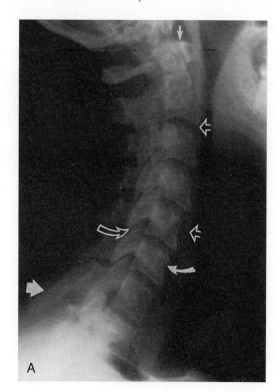

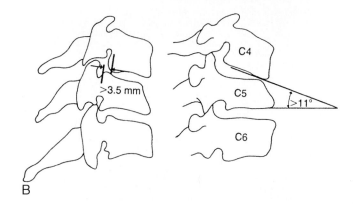

Figure 14–15 ■ *A,* Lateral radiograph demonstrating vertebral body (*solid curved arrow*), facet joint (*open curved arrow*), spinous process (*solid large straight arrow*), C1-2 (atlantodens) interval (*solid small straight arrow*), and retropharyngeal soft tissue shadow (*open straight arrows*). *B,* Anterior displacement of >3.5 mm or angulation >11 degrees on flexion/extension lateral radiographs is associated with cervical spine instability. (*A* from Kirkpatricks JS, Ghavam C: Injuries to the spinal column. *In* Masear VR [ed]: Primary Care Orthopaedics. Philadelphia, WB Saunders, 1996, p 54. *B* from Miller MD, Cooper DE, Warner JJP: Review of Sports Medicine and Arthroscopy. Philadelphia, WB Saunders, 1995, p 204.)

Figure 14–16 ■ AP open-mouth (odontoid) view illustrating the lateral mass of C1 (*open curved arrow*), the odontoid (*solid large arrow*), and the lateral mass/odontoid space (*solid small arrows*). (From Kirkpatricks JS, Ghavam C: Injuries to the spinal column. *In* Masear VR [ed]: Primary Care Orthopaedics. Philadelphia, WB Saunders, 1996, p 55.)

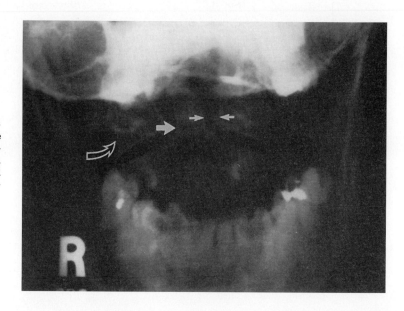

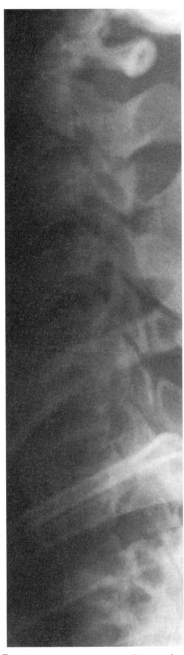

Figure 14–17 ■ Swimmer's view; used to evaluate the cervicothoracic junction. (From Harris JH: Spinal imaging. *In* Browner BD, Jupiter JB, Levine AM, et al [eds]: Skeletal Trauma. Philadelphia, WB Saunders, 1992, p 618.)

Basilar invagination or basilar impression (cranial settling)

Etiology is bone erosions, loss, or softening

Progressive migration of C1 and C2 (odontoid) proximally into the foramen magnum (Fig. 14–23) can lead to neurologic compromise and may require operative stabilization

Lower cervical spine subluxation

Related to rheumatologic involvement (destruction) of the facet joints

Posterior fusion may be required for subluxation of two adjacent cervical vertebrae greater than 4

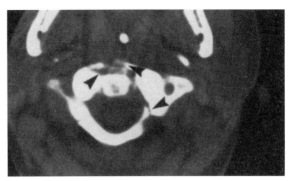

Figure 14–18 ■ CT scan of a Jefferson-type burst fracture of C1 (*arrowheads* show fracture lines). (From Harris JH: Spinal imaging. *In* Browner BD, Jupiter JB, Levine AM, et al [eds]: Skeletal Trauma. Philadelphia, WB Saunders, 1992, p 607.)

mm with intractable pain and neurologic compromise

All patients with rheumatoid arthritis should have a lateral flexion/extension radiograph of the cervical spine (to rule out subluxation) before undergoing intubation for an operative procedure

Injuries to the Cervical Spine

Result from high-energy accidents

Motor vehicle

Diving

Falls

Handguns

A high index of suspicion is needed to evaluate for

Fractures and dislocations

Spinal cord injuries

Rapid, accurate evaluation helps to protect the spinal cord from further injury and progression of any neurologic deficit

Immobilization of the cervical spine at the scene of the accident is via a spine board with a rigid cervical collar and sandbags

The best initial radiographic screen for bony injury

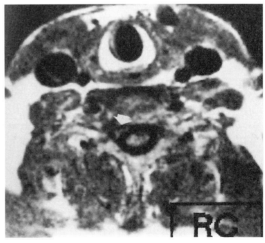

Figure 14–19 ■ Axial MRI demonstrating occlusion of the right C6-7 neural foramen (*arrow*). (From Boden S, Wiesel SW, Laws E, et al: The Aging Spine. Philadelphia, WB Saunders, 1991, p 58.)

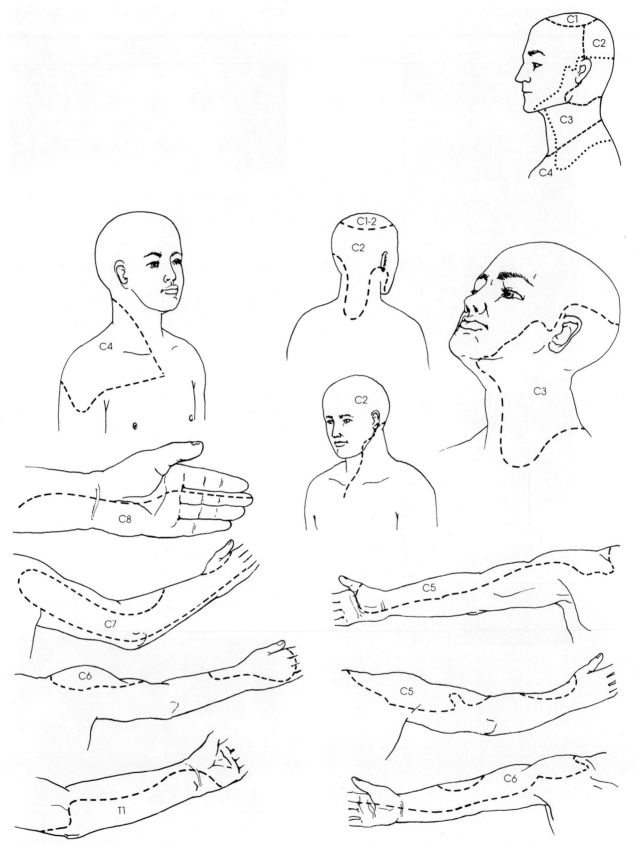

Figure 14–20 ■ Dermatomes for radicular pain of cervical origin. (From Magee DJ: Orthopedic Physical Assessment, 2nd ed. Philadelphia, WB Saunders, 1992, p 57.)

is the cross-table lateral with the patient remaining immobilized on the spine board

During the initial evaluation, head gear (such as a football helmet) **should not** be removed

A thorough neurologic exam follows the initial trauma survey

Methylprednisolone (bolus of 30 mg/kg followed by administration at 5.4 mg/kg/hr for 23 hours) should be administered to all patients with an acute spinal cord injury

Spinal shock—a period after spinal cord injury that lasts for less than 48 hours that limits the ability to predict recovery of spinal cord function; during spinal shock the bulbocavernosus reflex is absent; the return of the bulbocavernosus reflex signifies the end of spinal shock and indicates that further neurologic improvement is unlikely; the bulbocavernosus reflex will be present even in the presence of a complete spinal cord injury once the patient is out of spinal shock

Bulbocavernosus reflex—anal sphincter contraction with squeezing of the glans penis or clitoris; the presence of this reflex signifies the end of spinal shock and indicates that significant further neurologic recovery is unlikely

Prognosis is based on the extent of neurologic injury

A spinal cord injury can be classified as **complete** (no neurologic function below the level of injury) or **incomplete** (partial neurologic function below the level of injury)

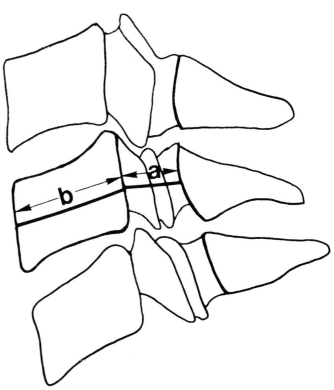

Figure 14-22 ■ Cervical stenosis can be determined by the Pavlov ratio (a/b); a is the AP diameter of the spinal canal, and b is the AP diameter of the verebral body. Ratios of <0.8 are consistent with cervical stenosis. (From Pavlov H, Proter IS: Criteria for cervical instability and stenosis. Op Tech Sports Med 1:170, 1993.)

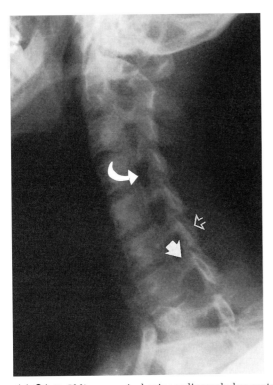

Figure 14-21 ■ Oblique cervical spine radiograph demonstrating the pedicle (*solid arrow*) and the facet joints (*open arrow*). Facet hypertrophy and disc space narrowing may reduce the size of the intervertebral (neural) foramen (*curved arrow*) and cause nerve root impingement. (From Kirkpatricks JS, Ghavam C: Injuries to the spinal column. *In* Masear VR [ed]: Primary Care Orthopaedics. Philadelphia, WB Saunders, 1996, p 55.)

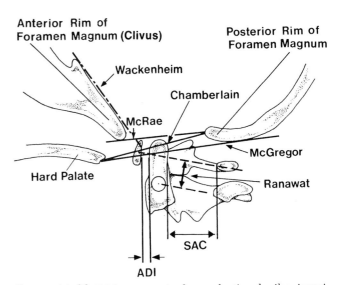

Figure 14-23 ■ Measurements for evaluating basilar invagination. Acknowledgment of migration of the tip of the odontoid (dens) superior to Chamberlain's line is the most useful tool for making the diagnosis of basilar invagination. ADI, atlantodens interval; SAC, space available for the (spinal) cord. (From Lauerman WC, Regan M: Spine. *In* Miller MD [ed]: Review of Orthopaedics, 2nd ed. Philadelphia, WB Saunders, 1996, p 273.)

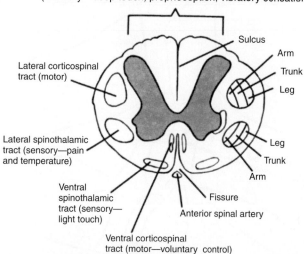

Figure 14–24 ■ An understanding of the effects of various cord syndromes is based on an appreciation of the cross-section of the spinal cord and the various tracts. (From Gomez BA: Anatomy. *In* Miller MD [ed]: Review of Orthopaedics, 2nd ed. Philadelphia, WB Saunders, 1996, p 454.)

Four incomplete cervical spinal cord injury syndromes have been described (Fig. 14–24)

Central cord syndrome

Hyperextension injury

Common especially with preexisting spondylosis

Upper extremity motor function is more affected than lower extremity motor function

Perianal sensation is preserved (sacral sparing)

Anterior cord syndrome

Posterior cord (proprioception and vibratory sensation) is spared

Motor loss is greater in the lower extremity

Worst prognosis

Brown-Séquard syndrome

Damage to half of the cord

Ipsilateral motor loss and contralateral pain loss

Best prognosis

Posterior cord syndrome

Only crude touch sensation is spared below the level of injury

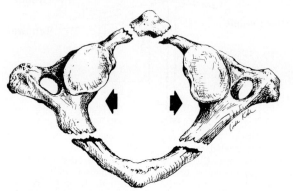

Figure 14–25 ■ Jefferson fracture. (From Urbaniak JR: Fractures of the spine. *In* Sabiston DC Jr [ed]: Davis-Christopher Textbook of Surgery. Philadelphia, WB Saunders, 1977, p 1528.)

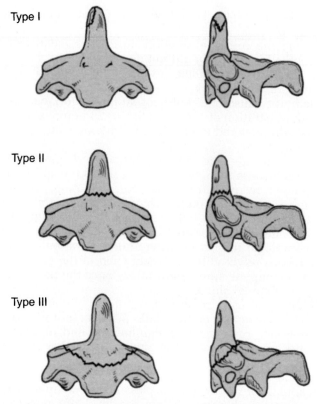

Figure 14–26 ■ Odontoid fractures. (From Fredrickson BE, Yuan HA: Nonoperative treatment of the spine: External immobilization. *In* Browner BD, Jupiter JB, Levine AM, et al [eds]: Skeletal Trauma. Philadelphia, WB Saunders, 1992, p 634.)

FRACTURES AND DISLOCATIONS OF THE CERVICAL SPINE

Overview (Table 14–1)

Careful evaluation of the lateral radiograph is essential in the early management of cervical spine injur-

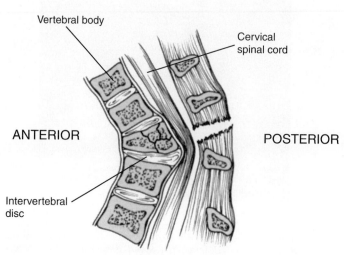

Figure 14–27 ■ Lower cervical burst fracture. (From Bucholz RW: Lower cervical spine injuries. *In* Browner BD, Jupiter JB, Levine AM, et al [eds]: Skeletal Trauma. Philadelphia, WB Saunders, 1992, p 724.)

Table 14-1
INJURIES OF THE ADULT CERVICAL SPINE

Injury	Eponym or Other Name	Classification	Treatment	Most Common Complications of the Injury
Occiput-C1 dislocation		Descriptive	Halo and operative treatment	Usually fatal
C1 fracture	Jefferson (from axial load) (Fig. 14-25)		Halo (± traction) or orthosis	Vertebral artery injury, cranial nerve VIII injury, malunion
C1-2 subluxation			Operative treatment	
C1-2 dislocation	Cock robin		Halo traction for reduction followed by operative treatment	
Odontoid process (C2) fracture (Fig. 14-26)		Anderson and D'Alonzo (Types I-III) I. Upper tip II. At junction of odontoid and body of C2 III. Through the body of C2	Orthosis Operative treatment Halo for 12 weeks	Nonunion
C2 isthmus fracture	Hangman's		Halo vest; may require operative treatment	Missed diagnosis of other cervical spine injuries, loss of reduction
Lower cervical spine compression injuries (C3-7) (Fig. 14-27)	Burst/crush	Stable fracture pattern with no neurologic deficit Unstable fracture pattern or stable pattern with neurologic deficit	Halo Operative treatment	Compression of cervical spinal canal, neurologic injury, post-traumatic cervical kyphosis
Lower cervical spinous process fractures (C3-7)	Clay shoveler's (spinous process avulsion)		Symptomatic	
Lower cervical spine facet dislocations (C3-7) (Fig. 14-28)	Jumped facets	Unilateral (<25% step-off seen radiographically between adjacent vertebrae on a lateral radiograph) Bilateral (25-50% step-off)	Traction; may require operative treatment Traction; may require operative treatment	Neurologic injury, disc herniation Neurologic injury, disc herniation
Lower cervical spine fracture/ subluxations (C3-7)			Requires operative treatment for translation of >3.5 mm or angulation >11 degrees between adjacent cervical vertebrae	

ies; this should include a survey of the bones and soft tissues

These injuries are best managed by a specialist

Proper early immobilization of the cervical spine diminishes the risk of further injury

A thorough baseline neurologic evaluation aids in the tracking of neurologic impairment

The injury pattern is related to the mechanism of injury

Pure flexion—anterior vertebral body compression fracture; a stable fracture without ligamentous or facet joint involvement

Flexion-rotation—unilateral or bilateral facet dislocation with or without a fracture through the lamina or vertebral body

Axial load—burst fracture (disruption of the entire vertebral body generally with retropulsion [in the posterior direction] of bony elements into the spinal canal)

Hyperextension—fracture of the anterior superior margin of the vertebral body that is avulsed by the anterior longitudinal ligament (teardrop fracture)

Lateral flexion—may produce fractures through the lateral masses, pedicles, vertebral foramen, or facet joints; these are usually stable injuries

TUMORS OF THE CERVICAL SPINE

Bone

Paget's disease
Aneurysmal bone cyst
Multiple myeloma
Hemangioma
Angiosarcoma
Metastatic lesions
Giant cell tumor

DIFFERENTIAL DIAGNOSIS OF COMMON CERVICAL SPINE COMPLAINTS

Neck Pain

Trapezial strain
Whiplash

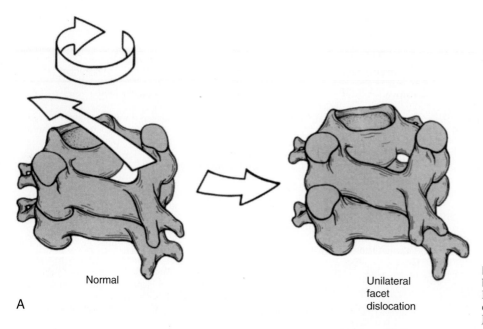

A

Normal

Unilateral
facet
dislocation

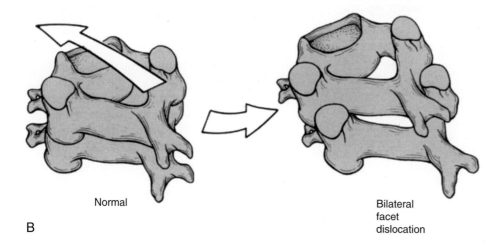

B

Normal

Bilateral
facet
dislocation

Figure 14–28 ■ *A*, Unilateral, and *B*, bilateral cervical spine facet joint dislocations. (From Bucholz RW: Lower cervical spine injuries. *In* Browner BD, Jupiter JB, Levine AM, et al [eds]: Skeletal Trauma. Philadelphia, WB Saunders, 1992, pp 702, 703.)

Cervical spondylosis
Cervical stenosis
Arthritis
Rheumatologic conditions
Fractures
Facet dislocations
Referred pain from the mediastinum

Neck Pain and Radicular Upper-Extremity Pain

Cervical spondylosis
Cervical stenosis
Fractures
Facet dislocations
Referred pain from the mediastinum

Neck Pain and Lower-Extremity Weakness

Cervical spondylosis
Cervical stenosis

Rheumatologic conditions (with myelopathy)
Fractures
Facet dislocations
Spinal cord injuries

CERVICAL SPINE ALGORITHM (Fig. 14–29)

PEARLS AND PITFALLS

C3, C4, and C5 keep the diaphragm alive
Evaluation of lateral radiographs includes an assessment of alignment, soft tissue swelling, and fractures/dislocations
There are seven cervical vertebrae and eight cervical nerve roots
Nerve roots exit above the cervical vertebra of the named level; for example, the C3 nerve root exits above the C3 vertebra

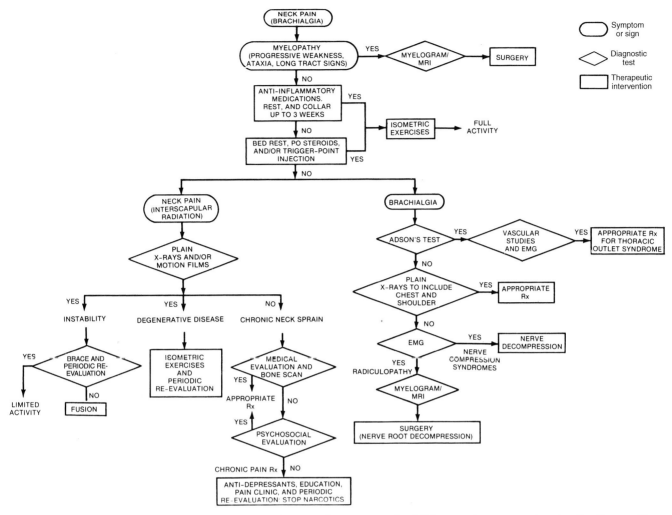

Figure 14-29 ■ Cervical spine algorithm. PO, by mouth; EMG, electromyography; MRI, magnetic resonance imaging; Rx, therapy. (From Wiesel SW, Delahay JN: Essentials of Orthopaedic Surgery, 2nd ed. Philadelphia, WB Saunders, 1997, p 199.)

Nerve root impingement by a herniated cervical disc or osteophyte will affect the exiting nerve root; for example, a C5-6 herniated disc will affect the C6 nerve root

Radiculopathy implies impingement on a nerve root; myelopathy implies impingement on the spinal cord

The classification of incomplete cervical spinal cord injury syndromes is based on the portion of the cord affected

CHAPTER 15

The Adult Thoracolumbar Spine

THORACOLUMBAR SPINE ANATOMY

Bones (Fig. 15–1)

Thoracic vertebrae—12 of them (T1-12)
Lumbar vertebrae—5 of them (L1-5)

Joints (Fig. 15–2)

Facet (apophyseal) joints
  Oriented 60 degrees in the sagittal plane and 20 degrees posterior in the coronal plane in the thoracic spine
  Oriented 90 degrees in the sagittal plane and 45 degrees anterior in the coronal plane in the lumbar spine
  The superior articular facet (of the lower vertebra) of a facet joint is anterior and lateral to the inferior facet of the vertebra above in the thoracic and lumbar spine; this is in contrast to the cervical spine, where the superior articular facet (of the lower vertebra) is anterior and inferior to the inferior articular facet of the vertebra above (see Figs. 14–3 and 15–2)
Intervertebral disc (like a jelly-filled donut) (see Fig. 14–4)
  Annulus (type I collagen)—peripheral disc
  Nucleus pulposus (type II collagen)—central disc (jelly)
Supporting ligaments (Fig. 15–3)
  Entire length of the spine
    Anterior longitudinal ligament
    Posterior longitudinal ligament
    Supraspinous ligament
  Each level of the spine
    Ligamentum flavum
    Interspinous ligaments

Muscles (Fig. 15–4)

Superficial
  Trapezius
  Latissimus dorsi
Deep
  Levator scapulae
  Rhomboids
Paraspinous muscles
  Erector spinae (sacrospinalis muscles)—spinalis, longissimus, iliocostalis
  Transversospinalis—multifidus, rotatores, semispinalis

Nerves (Fig. 15–5)

The spinal cord terminates at the conus medullaris at the L1 vertebral level; individual nerve roots continue as the cauda equina
Nerve roots exit below the pedicle of their named root; for example, the L4 nerve root exits below the pedicle of L4
Nerve roots are impinged by a herniated disc above the pedicle; for example, an L3-4 herniated disc will affect the traversing L4 nerve root

Vessels

The aorta lies on the left side of the vertebral column and gives off segmental arteries at each vertebral level
The segmental arteries cross anteriorly at the midbody level of each vertebra
There are approximately eight anterior medullary feeder arteries that are branches of the segmental arteries that enter the vertebral canal to supply the vertebrae and spinal cord; the largest of these anterior medullary feeder arteries is the **artery of Adamkiewicz**, which enters the vertebral canal through the left intervertebral foramen in the lower thoracic spine and must be protected during surgical approaches to this region

SURGICAL APPROACHES TO THE THORACOLUMBAR SPINE

Anterior Approach to the Thoracic Spine

Retroplural approach through the ribs and the thoracic cage

Posterior Approach to the Thoracolumbar Spine

Midline
Paraspinal muscles stripped

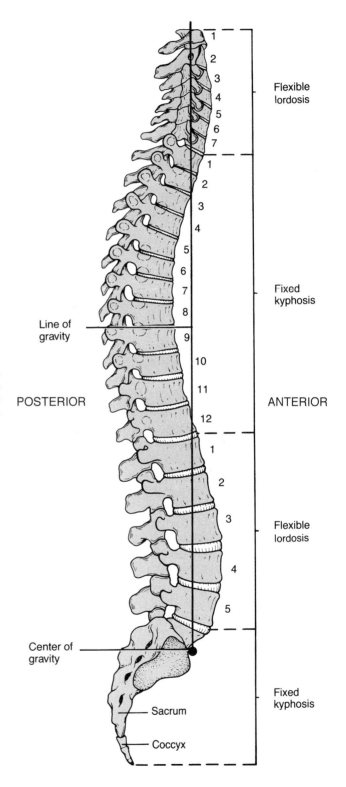

Figure 15–1 ■ Vertebral spine. Note that the thoracic spine has relative fixed kyphosis, and the lumbar spine has relative flexible lordosis. (From Levine AM: Lumbar and sacral spine trauma. *In* Browner BD, Jupiter JB, Levine AM, et al [eds]: Skeletal Trauma. Philadelphia, WB Saunders, 1992, p 806.)

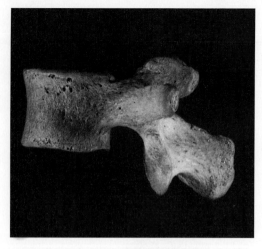

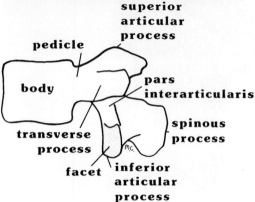

superior
articular
process

pedicle

pars
interarticularis

body

transverse
process

spinous
process

facet

inferior
articular
process

Figure 15–2 ■ Lateral view of a lumbar vertebra and a schematic drawing demonstrating the superior and inferior articular processes (and facets). (From Weissman BNW, Sledge CB: Orthopedic Radiology. Philadelphia, WB Saunders, 1986, p 280.)

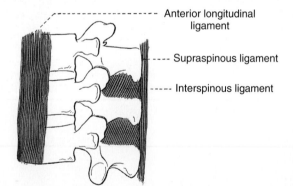

Anterior longitudinal ligament

Supraspinous ligament

Interspinous ligament

Figure 15–3 ■ Supporting ligaments of the spine. (From Jenkins DB: Hollinshead's Functional Anatomy of the Limbs and Back, 6th ed. Philadelphia, WB Saunders, 1991, p 191.)

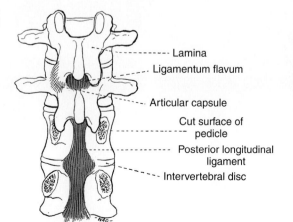

Lamina

Ligamentum flavum

Articular capsule

Cut surface of pedicle

Posterior longitudinal ligament

Intervertebral disc

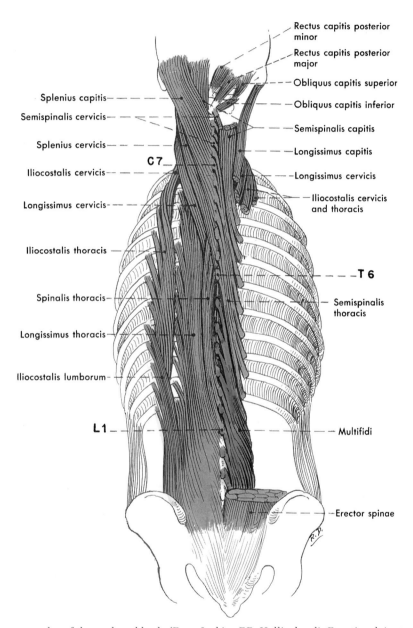

Figure 15–4 ■ Paraspinous muscles of the neck and back. (From Jenkins DB: Hollinshead's Functional Anatomy of the Limbs and Back, 6th ed. Philadelphia, WB Saunders, 1991, p 199.)

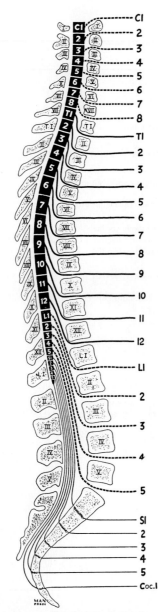

Figure 15–5 ■ Spinal cord and nerve roots in relation to the vertebrae. Note that the spinal cord terminates at the L1 vertebra. (From Haymaker W, Woodhall B: Peripheral Nerve Injuries, 2nd ed. Philadelphia, WB Saunders, 1953.)

Anterior Approach to the Lumbar Spine

Through the lower ribs
Retroperitoneal

HISTORY AND PHYSICAL EXAMINATION OF THE THORACOLUMBAR SPINE

History

Age
  Younger patients develop instability
  Older patients develop osteoarthritis
Characterization of symptoms
  Localized pain—trauma, tumor, infection
  Radicular pain—herniated nucleus pulposus (HNP), stenosis of the neural foramen
  Mechanical pain—instability, disc disease
Mechanism of injury/onset of symptoms
Bowel or bladder incontinence/symptoms—**Caution!**—beware of cauda equina syndrome
Areas of numbness—beware of "saddle" anesthesia
Leg pain
Psychosocial evaluation
Onset of symptoms

Physical Examination

Observation
  Skin—redness, skin markings, unusual hair patches
  Posture—loss of normal lumbar lordosis
Palpation
  Bones
    Spinous processes
    Coccyx
    Sacral promontory
    Iliac crests
    Posterior superior iliac spines
    Ischial tuberosities
  Soft tissues
    Paraspinal muscles
    Sciatic nerve
    Inguinal nodes
    Psoas muscle
    Rectal examination
Motion (Fig. 15–6) (Table 15–1)
  Flexion (normal, bend over to touch the toes)
  Extension (normal, 30 to 40 degrees)
  Lateral bending (normal, 30 degrees to each side)
  Rotation (symmetric)
Neurovascular examination
  Sensation (see Fig. 2–5)
  Reflexes
    L4 (knee jerk)
    S1 (ankle jerk)
    S2–4 (rectal exam; bulbocavernosus reflex)
  Strength testing
    Iliopsoas—hip flexion (T12-L3)
    Quadriceps—knee extension, hip adduction (L2-4)
    Tibialis anterior—ankle dorsiflexion and inversion (L4)
    Extensor hallicus longus—great toe extension (L5)
    Gluteus medius—hip abduction (L5)
    Peroneus longus and brevis—ankle eversion (S1)
    Bowel/bladder (S2–4)
Special testing (condition specific)
  Nerve root impingement (tension signs) (Fig. 15–7)—HNP, foraminal stenosis, others
    Straight leg raise (see Fig. 15–7)—Passive lifting of the leg reproduces radicular symptoms (pain radiating down the posterior or lateral aspect of the leg distal to the knee and often into the foot), not back pain; dorsiflexion of the foot (Lasègue maneuver) should make these symptoms worse and lead to onset of symptoms with the leg in a less elevated position

Figure 15–6 ■ Motion of the thoracic and lumbar spine. *A,* Forward flexion. *B,* Extension. *C,* Side flexion (lateral bending). *D,* Rotation. (From Magee DJ: Orthopedic Physical Assessment, 2nd ed. Philadelphia, WB Saunders, 1992, p 256.)

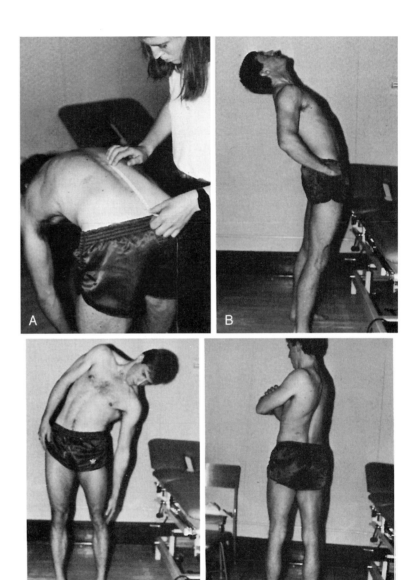

Table 15–1
MUSCLES OF THE THORACOLUMBAR SPINE: THEIR ACTIONS AND INNERVATION IN THE THORACIC AND LUMBAR SPINE

Action	Muscles Involved	Innervation
Flexion of thoracic spine	1. Rectus abdominis	T6-12
	2. External abdominal oblique (both sides acting together)	T7-12
	3. Internal abdominal oblique (both sides acting together)	T7-12, L1
Extension of thoracic spine	1. Spinalis thoracis	T1-12
	2. Iliocostalis thoracis (both sides acting together)	T1-12
	3. Longissimus thoracis (both sides acting together)	T1-12
	4. Semispinalis thoracis (both sides acting together)	T1-12
	5. Multifidus (both sides acting together)	T1-12
	6. Rotatores (both sides acting together)	T1-12
	7. Interspinalis	T1-12
Rotation and side flexion (lateral bending) of thoracic spine	1. Iliocostalis thoracis (to same side)	T1-12
	2. Longissimus thoracis (to same side)	T1-12
	3. Intertransverse (to same side)	T1-12
	4. Internal abdominal oblique (to same side)	T7-12, L1
	5. Semispinalis thoracis (to opposite side)	T1-12
	6. Multifidus (to opposite side)	T1-12
	7. Rotatores (to opposite side)	T1-12
	8. External abdominal oblique (to opposite side)	T7-12
	9. Transversus abdominis (to opposite side)	T7-12, L1
Forward flexion of lumbar spine	1. Psoas major	L1-3
	2. Rectus abdominis	T6-12
	3. External abdominal oblique	T7-12
	4. Internal abdominal oblique	T7-12, L1
	5. Transversus abdominis	T7-12, L1
Extension of lumbar spine	1. Latissimus dorsi	Thoracodorsal (C6-8)
	2. Erector spinae	L1-3
	3. Transversospinalis	L1-5
	4. Interspinales	L1-5
	5. Quadratus lumborum	T12, L1-4
Side flexion (lateral bending) of lumbar spine	1. Latissimus dorsi	Thoracodorsal (C6-8)
	2. Erector spinae	L1-3
	3. Transversospinalis	L1-5
	4. Intertransversarii	L1-5
	5. Quadratus lumborum	T12, L1-4
	6. Psoas major	L1-3
	7. External abdominal oblique	T7-12
Rotation* of lumbar spine	—	—

*Very little rotation occurs in the lumbar spine because of the shape of the facet joints. Any rotation would be due to a shearing movement. If shear does occur, the transversospinal muscles would be responsible for the movement.
From Magee DJ: Orthopedic Physical Assessment, 2nd ed. Philadelphia, WB Saunders, 1992, pp 235, 262.

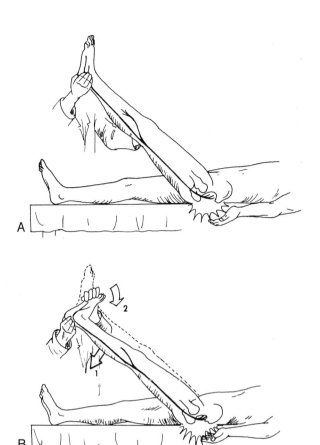

Figure 15–7 ■ Tension signs. Straight leg raising. *A,* Radicular symptoms are precipitated with straight leg raising. *B,* The symptoms resolve with lowering the leg slightly, but dorsiflexion of the foot (Lasègue maneuver) makes the symptoms recur. (From Reilly BM: Practical Strategies in Outpatient Medicine. Philadelphia, WB Saunders, 1991, p 912.)

Crossed straight leg raise—raising the contralateral leg can cause symptoms in the affected leg when there is a central disc herniation

Bowstring signs—after straight leg raising, the knee is flexed approximately 20 degrees to reduce radicular pain; digital pressure is applied to the popliteal area by the examiner; return of radicular pain during this maneuver constitutes a positive test

Femoral nerve traction test—the patient lies on the unaffected side and the examiner passively extends the hip and flexes the knee of the affected (up) side; development of radicular pain during this maneuver constitutes a positive test

Tests for malingering (Fig. 15–8)

Hoover's test (see Fig. 15–8)—the examiner cups one hand under the heel of the unaffected leg while the patient performs a straight leg raise; if the patient does not exert pressure on the examiner's hand (with the unaffected leg) as he or she attempts to raise the affected leg, the patient is probably not really trying

Burn's test (see Fig. 15–8)—if the patient is unable to touch the floor even when kneeling on a chair, then the patient is probably malingering

Waddell described several clinical indicators of emotional distress consistent with malingering (Table 15–2)

DIAGNOSTIC TESTS FOR THE THORACOLUMBAR SPINE

Plain Radiographs (Fig. 15–9)

Anteroposterior (AP)
Lateral
Oblique views

Computed Tomography
(Fig. 15–10)

Helpful in the evaluation of fractures

Magnetic Resonance Imaging
(Fig. 15–11)

Helpful in the evaluation of disc disease and ligamentous injuries

Table 15–2
NONORGANIC PHYSICAL SIGNS IN LOWER BACK PAIN

Category	Test	Comment
Tenderness	Superficial palpation	Inordinate, widespread sensitivity to light touch of the superficial soft tissues over the lumbar spine is nonanatomic and suggests amplified symptoms
	Nonanatomic testing	Tenderness is poorly localized
Simulation (to assess patient cooperation and reliability)	Axial loading	Light pressure to the skull of a standing patient should not significantly increase symptoms
	Rotation	Physician should rotate the standing patient's pelvis and shoulders in the same plane—this does not move the lumbar spine and should not increase pain
Distraction	Straight leg raising	Physician asks the seated patient to straighten the knee—patients with true sciatic tension will arch backward and complain; these results should closely match those of the traditional, recumbent straight leg raising test
Regional		Diffuse motor weakness or bizarre sensory deficits suggest functional regional disturbances if they involve multiple muscle groups and cannot be explained by neuroanatomy principles
Overreaction		Excessive and inappropriate grimacing, groaning, or collapse during a simple request is disproportionate

Adapted from Waddell G, McCulloch JA, Kummel E, et al: Nonorganic physical signs in low-back pain. Spine 5:117–125, 1980.

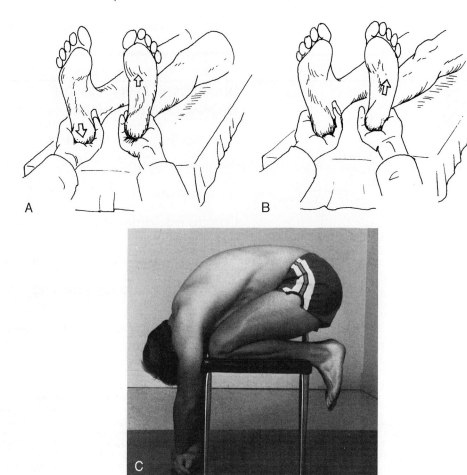

Figure 15–8 ■ Hoover's test. *A*, Normally, when a patient who is lying supine raises one leg off the exam table it will be accompanied by downward pressure by the opposite leg. *B*, If there is no downward pressure on the opposite leg, the patient is probably feigning at least part of his weakness. *C*, Burn's test. If the patient is unable to touch the floor even in this position, he is probably malingering. (*A* and *B* from Reilly BM: Practical Strategies in Outpatient Medicine. Philadelphia, WB Saunders, 1991, p 946. *C* from Magee DJ: Orthopedic Physical Assessment, 2nd ed. Philadelphia, WB Saunders, 1992, p 277.)

Myelography

Useful technique that outlines the spinal cord and nerve roots

Electrodiagnostic Studies

Can help confirm clinical impressions but are not specific

Psychological Evaluation

Personality tests such as the Minnesota Multiphasic Personality Inventory (MMPI) can be helpful in identifying poor surgical candidates
Pain drawings (Fig. 15–12)—help differentiate organic from nonorganic symptoms

COMMON ADULT CONDITIONS OF THE THORACOLUMBAR SPINE

Musculoskeletal Lower Back Pain

Nonradiating back pain
No clear etiology

Pain may be referred in a nondermatomal pattern
Physical examination notable only for localized tenderness and limitation of motion (from pain)
Treatment is physical therapy

Herniated Nucleus Pulposus of the Lumbar Spine

Displacement of the central area of the disc (nucleus) resulting in impingement on a nerve root
Classification based on the degree of disc displacement (Fig. 15–13)
Most commonly involves the L4-5 disc (L5 nerve root)
History
  Radicular leg pain
  May also have lower back pain
Physical findings
  Motor weakness
    L4 nerve root—tibialis anterior weakness
    L5 nerve root—extensor hallucis longus weakness
  Asymmetric reflexes
    Knee jerk (L4)
    Ankle jerk (S1)

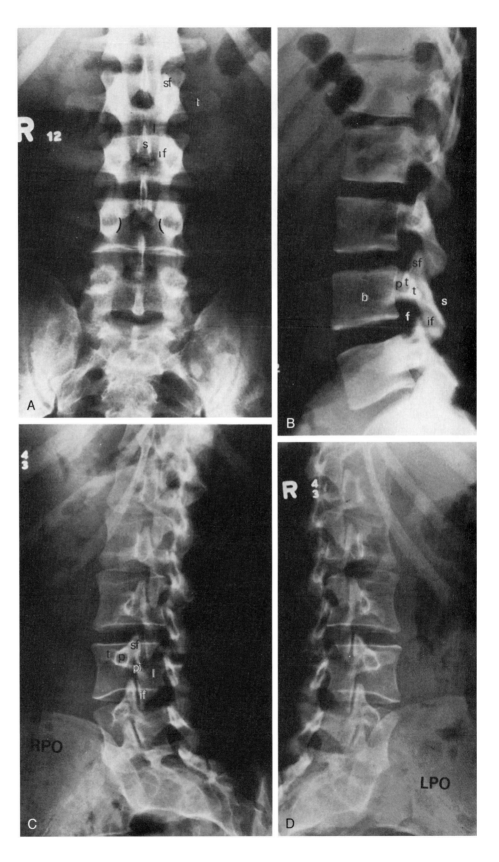

Figure 15–9 ■ Plain radiographs of the lumbar spine. *A,* AP view. *B,* Lateral view. *C* and *D,* Oblique views. b, body of vertebra; f, intervertebral (neural) foramen; if, inferior facet; l, lamina; p, pedicle; pi, pars interarticularis; s, spinous process; sf, superior facet; t, transverse process;) (denotes the interpedicular distance; RPO, right posterior oblique view; LPO, left posterior oblique view. (From Weissman BNW, Sledge CB: Orthopedic Radiology. Philadelphia, WB Saunders, 1986, p 287.)

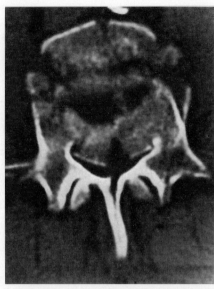

Figure 15–10 ■ CT scan of a lumbar burst fracture with significant retropulsion of bony fragments into the spinal canal. (From Levine AM: Lumbar and sacral spine trauma. *In* Browner BD, Jupiter JB, Levine AM, et al [eds]: Skeletal Trauma. Philadelphia, WB Saunders, 1992, p 812.)

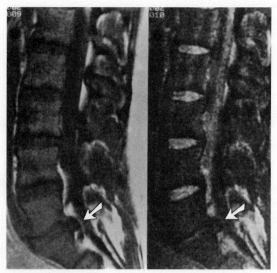

Figure 15–11 ■ Sagittal T1 (*left*) and sagittal T2 (*right*) MR images of a patient with a large L5-S1 herniated nucleus pulposus (*arrows*). (From Boden S, Wiesel SW, Laws E, et al: The Aging Spine. Philadelphia, WB Saunders, 1991, p 147.)

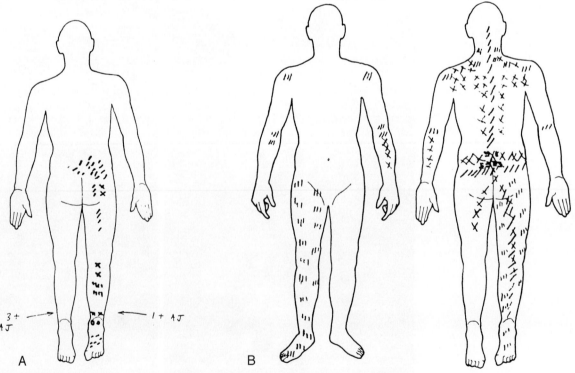

Figure 15–12 ■ Pain drawings. *A,* Patient with a confirmed L5-S1 right-sided herniated nucleus pulposus. Note the precise anatomic distribution of the symbols (areas of pain). *B,* Patient without true findings of any objective disc pathology. Note the nonanatomic distribution of pain and the use of various symbols. A pain drawing such as this does not rule out organic pathology, but it should alert the examiner to search for nonorganic and psychological issues. (From American Academy of Orthopaedic Surgeons: Orthopaedic Knowledge Update 2: Home Study Syllabus. Park Ridge, IL, AAOS, 1987, p 320.)

Sensory findings (see Fig. 2–5)
Positive tension signs (see Fig. 15–7)
Diagnostic tests
Magnetic resonance imaging (MRI) (see Fig. 15–11)
Myelography
Electromyography/nerve conduction studies
Treatment (most patients' symptoms resolve with time)
Symptomatic
Physical therapy
Nonsteroidal anti-inflammatory drugs (NSAIDs)
Aerobic conditioning
Lumbar epidural steroids
Surgical discectomy (for cases that fail to improve with 6 to 12 months of nonoperative therapy)
Prerequisites for surgery
Failure of nonoperative management
Predominately leg symptoms
Neurologic findings
Positive tension signs
Positive imaging studies (MRI, computed tomography [CT], myelography)
No psychosocial overlay

Cauda Equina Syndrome

A massive central herniation of a lumbar disc (see Fig. 15–13) that presents with
Progressive motor weakness and numbness
Saddle anesthesia (buttock anesthesia)
Loss of bowel and bladder control
This represents a surgical emergency

Herniated Nucleus Pulposus of the Thoracic Spine

Far less common than lumbar HNPs
Most commonly involves the lower thoracic discs
The patient presents with thoracic back pain with or without circumferential radiating pain around the thorax

Pain exacerbated by sneezing or coughing
MRI makes the diagnosis
Treatment similar to lumbar HNP

Spinal Stenosis

Narrowing of the spinal canal (central stenosis) or neural (intervertebral) foramen (lateral recess stenosis)
Central stenosis (Fig. 15–14)
Congenital or acquired (most common) narrowing of the spinal canal from facet joint hypertrophy or hypertrophy of the supporting soft tissues
Symptoms
Insidious pain and paresthesias
Neurogenic claudication—takes longer for relief of symptoms upon sitting than does vascular claudication (Table 15–3)
Diagnosis
Symptoms of neurogenic claudication
CT/MRI shows narrowing of the central canal
Treatment options
Nonoperative—rest, exercises, lumbar epidural steroids
Operative indications (decompression with or without fusion)—positive findings on physical exam and diagnostic studies with persistent impairment of quality of life
Lateral recess stenosis (Fig. 15–15)
Narrowing of the neural (intervertebral) foramen most commonly as a result of bone spurs (osteophytes)
Can cause nerve root compression
Clinical presentation is similar to that for HNP, but the patient is usually older
Operative decompression may be necessary
Far-out syndrome
Extraforaminal lateral root compression
Involves L5 root impingement between the sacral ala and the L5 transverse process

Table 15–3
COMPARISON OF NEUROGENIC AND VASCULAR CLAUDICATION

	Neurogenic Claudication	Vascular Claudication
Classic Symptoms	Pain and weakness in the muscles of the thighs and calves (usually bilateral)	Cramping muscle pain without paresthesias
Effect of Specific Activities on Symptoms		
Walking on level ground	Symptoms more proximal (thigh)	Symptoms more distal (primarily calf)
Walking uphill	Symptoms develop later	Symptoms develop sooner
Standing	Symptoms relieved only if the patient assumes a flexed position	Symptoms relieved
Resting	Symptoms relieved with sitting or bending (flexed position)	Symptoms relieved
Bicycling	Symptoms typically do not develop	Symptoms develop
Lying flat	Symptoms exacerbated unless the patient assumes a flexed position while lying flat	Symptoms relieved

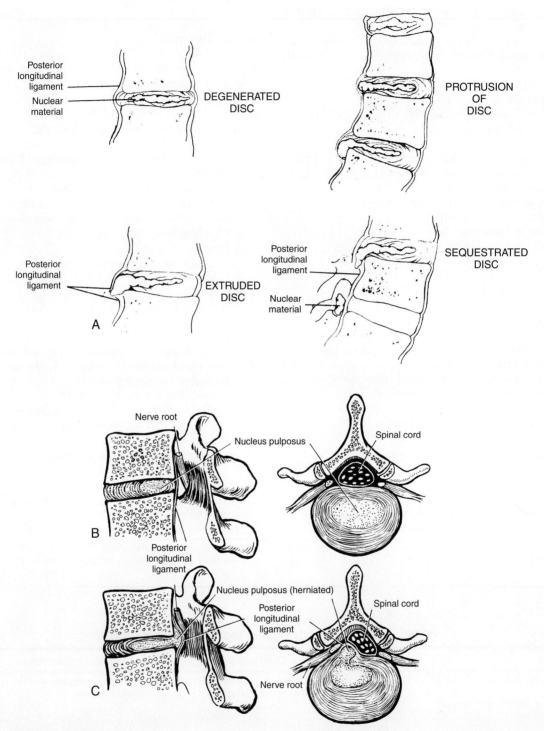

Figure 15–13 ■ *A,* Nomenclature of disc pathology. *B,* Normal position of the nucleus pulposus. *C,* Course taken by a herniated disc. (*A* from Wiltse LL: Lumbosacral spine reconstruction. *In* Orthopaedic Knowledge Update. I. Chicago, AAOS, p 247, 1984. *B* and *C* from Gartland JJ: Fundamentals of Orthopaedics, 4th ed. Philadelphia, WB Saunders, 1986, p 332.)

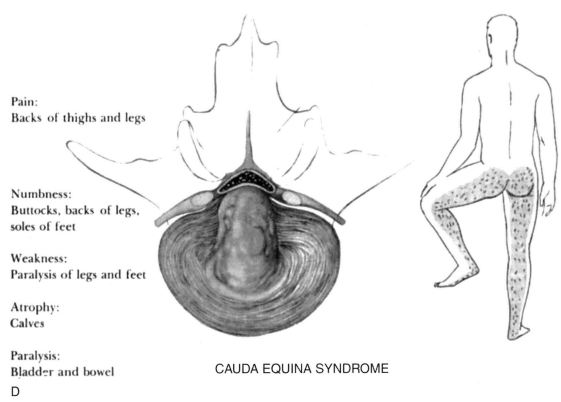

Pain:
Backs of thighs and legs

Numbness:
Buttocks, backs of legs,
soles of feet

Weakness:
Paralysis of legs and feet

Atrophy:
Calves

Paralysis:
Bladder and bowel

D

CAUDA EQUINA SYNDROME

Figure 15–13 *Continued* ■ *D,* Massive central herniation of a lumbar disc can cause a cauda equina syndrome. (*D* from DePalma AF, Rothman RH: The Intervertebral Disc. Philadelphia, WB Saunders, 1970, p 194.)

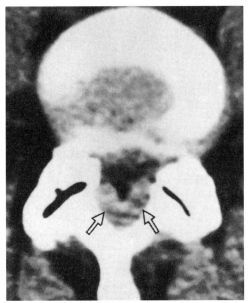

Figure 15–14 ■ CT scan of a patient with central spinal stenosis. Note thickening of the ligamentum flavum (*arrows*). (From Kricun ME: Imaging Modalities in Spinal Disorders. Philadelphia, WB Saunders, 1988.)

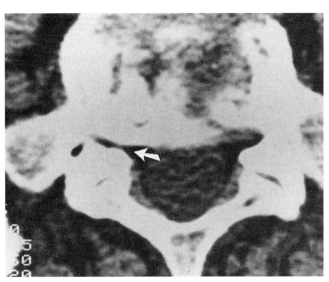

Figure 15–15 ■ Lateral recess stenosis. CT scan shows marked narrowing of the right lateral recess (neural foramen) (*arrow*). (From Weissman BNW, Sledge CB: Orthopedic Radiology. Philadelphia, WB Saunders, 1986, p 320.)

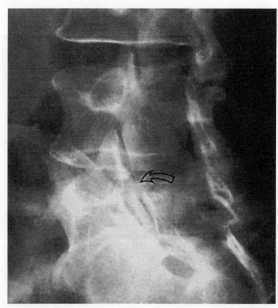

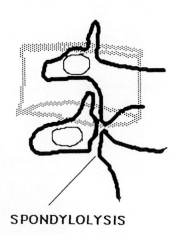

SPONDYLOLYSIS

Figure 15–16 ■ Spondylolysis. Oblique radiograph (*left*) and drawing (*right*); both show a "collar" (break) in the neck of the "Scottie dog," which is diagnostic of spondylosis. (From Helms CA: Fundamentals of Skeletal Radiology. Philadelphia, WB Saunders, 1989, p 101.)

Spondylolysis (Fig. 15–16)

Represents a defect in the pars interarticularis (see Fig. 15–16)

Common cause of back pain in adolescents

Hyperextension stress activities are a common history (gymnasts, football linemen)

Symptoms/diagnosis

  Activity-related back pain

  Radiographs (especially obliques) are helpful in visualizing the pars defect (see Fig. 15–16)

  Bone scan—an excellent screening test

  CT scan—may be helpful in identifying the pars defect

Treatment

  Activity restriction

  Stretching exercises

  Bracing

Spondylolisthesis (Fig. 15–17)

Forward slippage of one vertebra on another

Presents as lower back pain

Classification (Table 15–4)

Severity of slip

  Grade I: 0 to 25%

  Grade II: 25% to 50%

  Grade III: 50% to 75%

  Grade IV: 75% to 100%

  Grade V: >100% (spondyloptosis)

Treatment

  Grades I and II

    Symptomatic

    Avoid football and gymnastics

    Fusion in situ for intractable pain that fails nonoperative management

  Grades III, IV, and V

    Bilateral posterolateral fusion with or without decompression

Facet Syndrome

Inflammation/degeneration of the facet joints

Lower back pain becomes worse with extension; patients may also have some referred pain to the buttock and posterior thigh

Facet joint injections may be helpful in making the diagnosis and also in the treatment

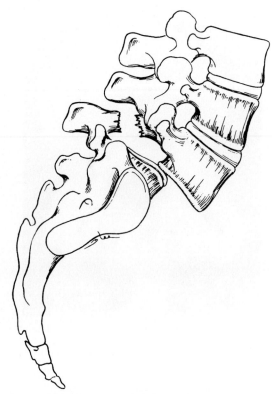

Figure 15–17 ■ Isthmic spondylolisthesis, which is the most common type. In this example, the slip is grade IV.

Table 15–4
TYPES OF SPONDYLOLISTHESIS

Type	Age Group	Pathology
Congenital	Children	Congenital dysplasia of the superior facet of S1
Isthmic (see Fig. 15–17) (most common type)	Children and adults	Elongation/fracture of the pars interarticularis (L5-S1)
Degenerative	Older adults	Facet arthrosis that leads to (facet) joint subluxation (L4-5)
Traumatic	Children and younger adults	Acute fracture (other than a fracture of the pars interarticularis)
Pathologic	Any age	Incompetence of the bony elements
Postsurgical	Adults	Caused by excessive operative resection of the neural arches, the facet joints, or both

Syndesmophytes (Fig. 15–18)

Vertical bony connections of adjacent vertebrae
Common in two disease processes
  Diffuse idiopathic skeletal hyperostosis (DISH)
    Nonmarginal syndesmophytes at three successive levels
    Most commonly occurs on the right side of the thoracic spine
    Patients are at an increased risk of forming heterotopic ossification
  Ankylosing spondylitis
    HLA-B27 positive
    Marginal syndesmophytes
    Sacroiliac involvement
    Epidural bleeding common after spinal injury (high morbidity and mortality)

Adult Scoliosis

Lateral spinal curvature greater than 50 degrees in a patient older than 20 years
Etiology is usually idiopathic
Main presenting complaints are back pain at the convexity of the curve and a cosmetic deformity
Treatment options
  Nonoperative—NSAIDs, weight reduction, physical therapy, soft spinal braces for activities

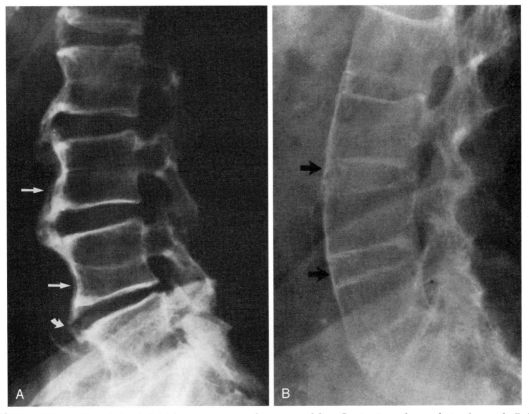

Figure 15–18 ■ *A,* Diffuse idiopathic skeletal hyperostosis is characterized by "flowing" syndesmophytes (*arrows*). *B,* In ankylosing spondylitis, syndesmophytes (*arrows*) connect the vertebral bodies. (From Weissman BNW, Sledge CB: Orthopedic Radiology. Philadelphia, WB Saunders, 1986, pp 302, 321.)

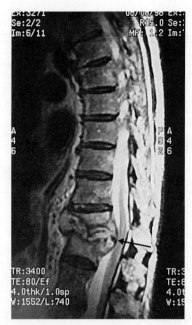

Figure 15–19 ■ MRI of a disc space infection. Note disc space infection (*arrow*) with destruction of adjacent vertebral bodies and compression of the spinal cord. (Courtesy of Jeffrey A. Kozak, MD, Fondren Orthopedic Group LLP, Texas Orthopedic Hospital, Houston, Texas.)

Operative—instrumentation and fusion (anterior and posterior surgical approaches for large curves [>70 degrees]); these procedures have a relatively high complication rate

Adult Kyphosis

Forward bending (apex posterior angulation) of the thoracic spine greater than 50 degrees

Etiology may be old Scheuermann's disease, post-traumatic condition, metabolic bone disease, ankylosing spondylitis, or idiopathic

Posterior fusion is required for refractory pain (combined with anterior decompression for curves not correcting to less than 55 degrees on a hyperextension lateral radiograph)

See Chapter 5 for Scheuermann's kyphosis

Spinal Infections

Disc space infection
　More common in children but does occur in adults (spreads from adjacent osteomyelitis)
　MRI is diagnostic (Fig. 15–19)
　Treatment—rest, immobilization, antibiotics
Vertebral osteomyelitis
　Risk factors—intravenous (IV) drug abuse, immunologic compromise
　Symptoms—spinal pain, tenderness, spasm
　Clinical findings/diagnostic tests
　　Fever
　　Elevated white blood cell (WBC) count
　　Elevated erythrocyte sedimentation rate (ESR)
　　Positive technetium bone scan
　　CT-guided needle biopsy allows identification of the organism (*Staphylococcus aureus* is the most common)
　　MRI is diagnostic (95% accurate)
　Treatment—IV antibiotics, operative débridement sometimes needed
Tuberculosis of the spine (Pott's disease)
　May present with a psoas abscess (pain on passive extension of the hip [stretches the psoas muscle])
　Clinical findings similar to vertebral osteomyelitis
　MRI of the pelvis shows the abscess and is diagnostic
　Treatment is antibiotics and operative débridement (anterior approach)

FRACTURES AND DISLOCATIONS OF THE THORACOLUMBAR SPINE

Overview (Table 15–5)

Classification of fractures of the thoracolumbar spine is based on involvement of the three columns described by Denis (Fig. 15–20)
　Anterior column—anterior longitudinal ligament, anterior aspect of the vertebral body, and anterior aspect of the annulus fibrosus
　Middle column—posterior longitudinal ligament, posterior aspect of the vertebral body, and posterior annulus fibrosus

Table 15–5
INJURIES OF THE ADULT THORACIC AND LUMBAR SPINE

Injury	Eponym or Other Name	Classification	Treatment	Most Common Complications of the Injury
Compression fracture (see Fig. 15–21)		Descriptive (based on percent decrease in anterior body height)	Bed rest, orthosis	Progressive kyphosis
Burst fracture (see Fig. 15–22)	Blowout fracture	Based on the amount of bone retropulsion into the spinal canal	Operative decompression and stabilization	Missed diagnosis (confused as a compression fracture), dural tears, neurologic injury
Flexion-distraction injuries (see Fig. 15–23)	Chance injury	Bony chance injury	Hyperextension casting	Spinal instability
		Soft tissue chance injury	Operative stabilization	Spinal instability
Fracture-dislocations			Operative stabilization with early mobilization	Severe neurologic compromise, dural tears, intra-abdominal injuries

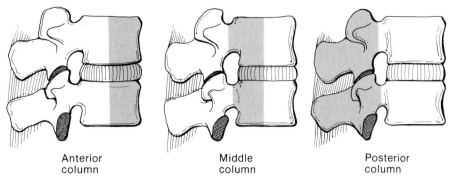

Figure 15–20 ■ Three-column spine classification of Denis. (From Eismont FJ, Kitchel SH: The thoracolumbar spine. *In* DeLee JC, Drez D Jr [eds]: Orthopaedic Sports Medicine: Principles and Practice. Philadelphia, WB Saunders, 1994, p 1048.)

Posterior column—pedicles, facet joints and capsules, ligamentum flavum, osseous neural arch, and interspinous and supraspinous ligaments

Columns can fail individually, or in combination, in the following manners

Compression

Distraction

Rotation

Shear

Resulting thoracolumbar spine injuries are of four main types

Compression fracture (Fig. 15–21)—failure of the anterior column; the middle column remains intact

Burst fracture (Fig. 15–22)—failure of the anterior and middle columns with retropulsion of bony fragments into the spinal canal

Flexion-distraction injuries (chance injuries) (Fig. 15–23)

Involve all three columns

Bony chance injuries are stable because the posterior ligaments remain intact

Soft tissue chance injuries are unstable because of disruption of the posterior ligaments

Fracture-dislocations—failure of all three columns with resultant instability

Types of fracture-dislocations

Flexion-rotation

Shear

Flexion-distraction—results in bilateral facet dislocation

TUMORS OF THE THORACOLUMBAR SPINE

Bone

Paget's disease

Aneurysmal bone cyst

Multiple myeloma

Hemangioma

Angiosarcoma

Metastatic lesions

Giant cell tumor

DIFFERENTIAL DIAGNOSIS OF COMMON THORACOLUMBAR SPINE COMPLAINTS

Back Pain

Musculoskeletal lower back pain

Spondylolysis

Facet syndrome

Adult scoliosis

Adult kyphosis

Spondylolisthesis

Infections

Tumors

Fractures

Dislocations

Arthritis

Rheumatologic conditions

Referred pain from the viscera

Back Pain and Radicular Lower Extremity Pain or Weakness

HNP

Spinal stenosis (central or lateral recess)

Fractures

Dislocations

Cauda equina syndrome

LOWER BACK PAIN ALGORITHM
(Fig. 15–24)

PEARLS AND PITFALLS

There are five lumbar vertebrae and five lumbar nerve roots

Nerve roots exit below the lumbar pedicle of the same named level; for example, the L4 nerve root exits below the pedicle of L4

Nerve root impingement by a herniated lumbar disc will affect the traversing nerve root; for example, an L4-5 herniated disc will affect the L5 nerve root

Beware of inappropriate signs and symptoms in the examination of a patient with lower back pain; secondary gain, litigation, work-related injuries, and psychological disturbances can make the evaluation difficult

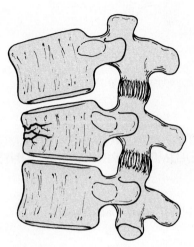

Figure 15–21 ■ Vertebral compression fracture. (From Eismont FJ, Garfin SR, Abitbol JJ: Thoracic and upper lumbar spine injuries. *In* Browner BD, Jupiter JB, Levine AM, et al [eds]: Skeletal Trauma. Philadelphia, WB Saunders, 1992, p 746.)

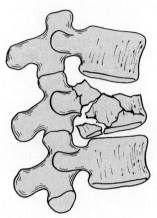

Figure 15–22 ■ Vertebral burst fracture. (From Eismont FJ, Garfin SR, Abitbol JJ: Thoracic and upper lumbar spine injuries. *In* Browner BD, Jupiter JB, Levine AM, et al [eds]: Skeletal Trauma. Philadelphia, WB Saunders, 1992, p 753.)

Figure 15–23 ■ Flexion-distraction (chance) injuries. *A,* One-level injury with the injury through bone. *B,* One-level injury with the injury through the soft tissues. (From Eismont FJ, Garfin SR, Abitbol JJ: Thoracic and upper lumbar spine injuries. *In* Browner BD, Jupiter JB, Levine AM, et al [eds]: Skeletal Trauma. Philadelphia, WB Saunders, 1992, p 754.)

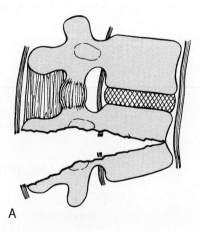

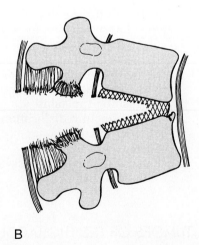

A

B

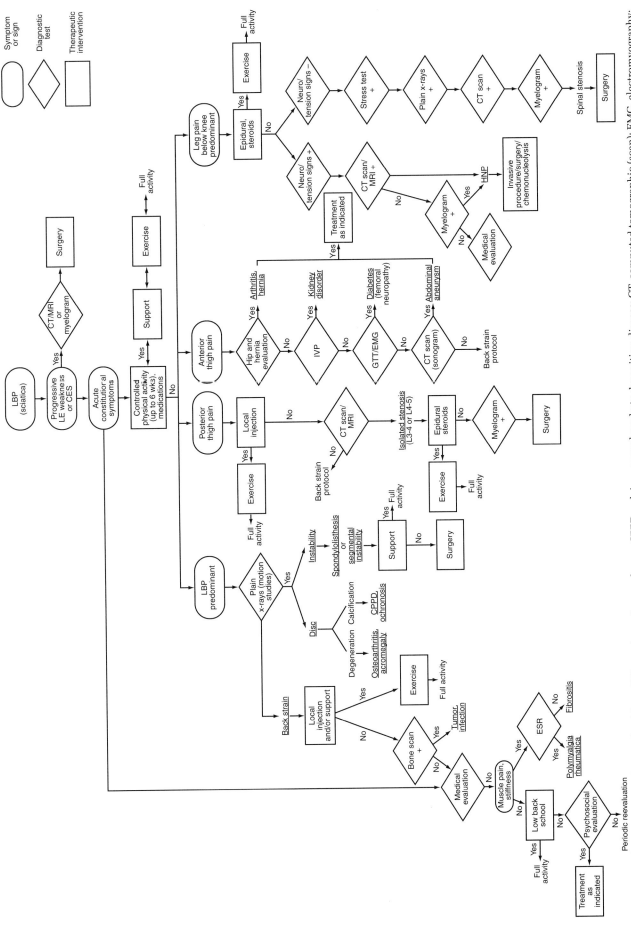

Figure 15–24 ■ Lower back pain algorithm. CES, cauda equina syndrome; CPPD, calcium pyrophosphate deposition disease; CT, computed tomographic (scan); EMG, electromyography; ESR, erythrocyte sedimentation rate; GTT, glucose tolerance test; HNP, herniated nucleus pulposus; IVP, intravenous pyelogram; LBP, low back pain; LE, lower extremity; MRI, magnetic resonance imaging. (From Boden S, Wiesel SW, Laws E, et al: The Aging Spine. Philadelphia, WB Saunders, 1991.)

The Adult Pelvis, Acetabulum, Sacrum, Coccyx

PELVIC ANATOMY

Bones (Fig. 16–1)

Innominate bone
  Two innominate bones make up the pelvis
  Each innominate bone is made up of three units—ilium, ischium, pubis
Sacrum

Joints (Fig. 16–2)

Sacroiliac (SI) joint
  Diarthrodial gliding joint
  Posterior SI ligaments provide stability
Pubic symphysis
Other ligaments—sacrospinous, sacrotuberous

Muscles (Fig. 16–3)

Individual muscle function is discussed in Chapter 17

Nerves (Fig. 16–4)

Lumbosacral plexus (L1-S4)
  Lumbar plexus (L1-L4)
  Sacral plexus (L4-S4)

Vessels (Fig. 16–5)

The aorta bifurcates into the common iliac arteries at the L4 level
The common iliac arteries, in turn, branch into the external iliac and internal iliac arteries
The external iliac arteries give off a few branches in the pelvis and then continue as the femoral arteries
Important branches of the internal iliac (hypogastric) arteries include
  Obturator artery—supplies the transverse acetabular ligament and the artery of the ligamentum teres
  Superior gluteal artery—runs through the greater sciatic foramen
  Inferior gluteal artery—supplies the gluteus maximus muscle

Superior circumflex iliac artery—runs with the lateral femoral cutaneous nerve

Important Anatomic Relationships (Fig. 16–6)

Greater sciatic foramen
  The piriformis muscle is the key to understanding the contents of the greater sciatic foramen
  Eleven structures (including the piriformis muscle) pass from the pelvis, through the greater sciatic foramen, and into the gluteal region

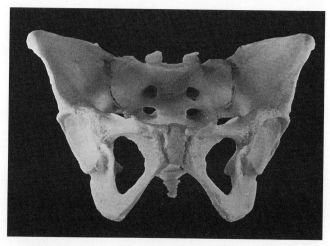

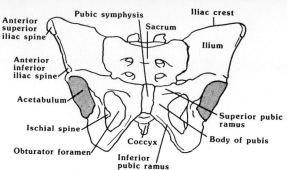

Figure 16–1 ■ Anatomy of the bones of the pelvis. (From Weissman BNW, Sledge CB: Orthopedic Radiology. Philadelphia, WB Saunders, 1987, p 336.)

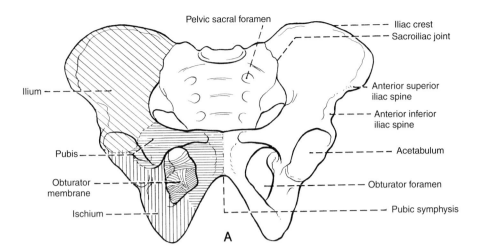

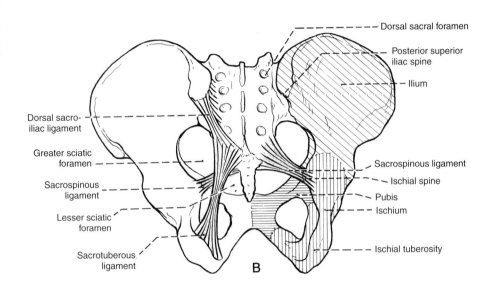

Figure 16–2 ■ Anterior (*A*) and posterior (*B*) view of the pelvic articulations. Without their strong ligamentous attachments, the bones themselves provide no inherent stability. (From Jenkins DB: Hollinshead's Functional Anatomy of the Limbs and Back, 6th ed. Philadelphia, WB Saunders, 1991, p 226.)

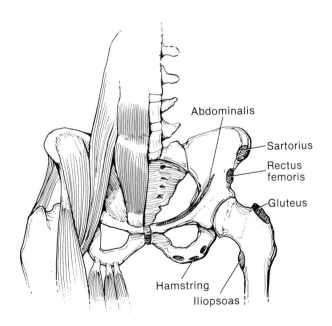

Figure 16–3 ■ Origins and insertions of the muscles of the pelvis. (From Gross ML, Nasser S, Finerman GAM: Hip and pelvis. *In* DeLee JC, Drez D Jr. [eds]: Orthopaedic Sports Medicine: Principles and Practice. Philadelphia, WB Saunders, 1994, p 1069. By permission of Mayo Foundation.)

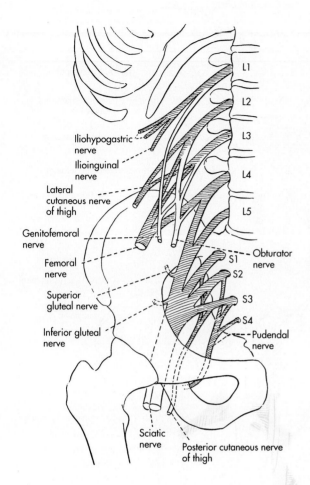

Iliohypogastric nerve

Ilioinguinal nerve

Lateral cutaneous nerve of thigh

Genitofemoral nerve

Femoral nerve

Superior gluteal nerve

Inferior gluteal nerve

Sciatic nerve

Posterior cutaneous nerve of thigh

L1

L2

L3

L4

L5

Obturator nerve

S1

S2

S3

S4

Pudendal nerve

Figure 16–4 ■ Lumbosacral plexus. (Redrawn from the Section of Neurology and the Section of Physiology and Biophysics, Mayo Clinic and Foundation: Clinical Examinations in Neurology, 3rd ed. Philadelphia, WB Saunders, 1971, p 156. From Jenkins DB: Hollinshead's Functional Anatomy of the Limbs and Back, 6th ed. Philadelphia, WB Saunders, 1991, p 239.)

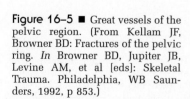

Figure 16–5 ■ Great vessels of the pelvic region. (From Kellam JF, Browner BD: Fractures of the pelvic ring. *In* Browner BD, Jupiter JB, Levine AM, et al [eds]: Skeletal Trauma. Philadelphia, WB Saunders, 1992, p 853.)

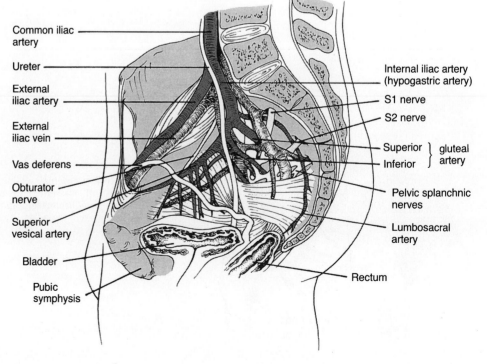

Common iliac artery

Ureter

External iliac artery

External iliac vein

Vas deferens

Obturator nerve

Superior vesical artery

Bladder

Pubic symphysis

Internal iliac artery (hypogastric artery)

S1 nerve

S2 nerve

Superior } gluteal
Inferior } artery

Pelvic splanchnic nerves

Lumbosacral artery

Rectum

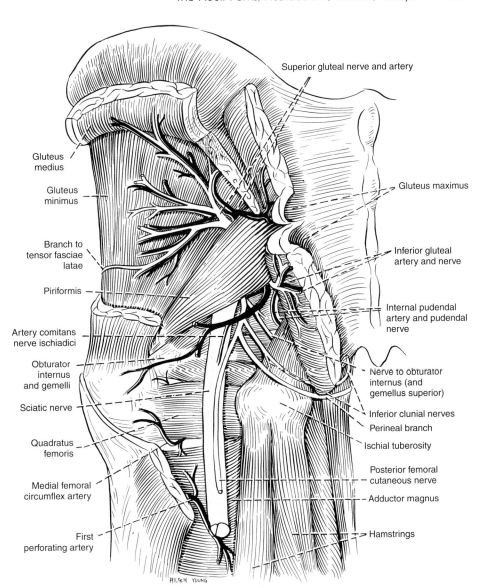

Figure 16–6 ■ Nerves (*white*) and arteries (*black*) and their relationship in the greater sciatic foramen. (From Jenkins DB: Hollinshead's Functional Anatomy of the Limbs and Back, 6th ed. Philadelphia, WB Saunders, 1991, p 260.)

Structures that pass through the greater sciatic foramen *above* the piriformis
   Superior gluteal artery
   Superior gluteal nerve
Structures that pass through the greater sciatic foramen *below* the piriformis
   Inferior gluteal artery
   Inferior gluteal nerve
   Sciatic nerve
   Posterior femoral cutaneous nerve
   Internal pudendal artery
   Pudendal nerve
   Nerve to obturator internus
   Nerve to quadratus femoris
"POPS IQ" is a useful mnemonic that describes the orientation (from medial to lateral) of the nerves that exit the greater sciatic foramen below the piriformis
   Pudendal nerve
   Obturator internus (nerve to)
   Posterior femoral cutaneous nerve

Sciatic nerve
Inferior gluteal nerve
Quadratus femoris (nerve to)

SURGICAL APPROACHES TO THE PELVIS

Ilioinguinal Approach

External oblique aponeurosis is reflected
Incision is along the inguinal ligament
Abdominal muscles and transversalis fascia are detached
Iliopectineal fascia is divided
Exposure of the pelvis through three "anatomic windows"

Extended Iliofemoral Approach

Gluteal muscles are reflected from the lateral iliac wing

Lateral femoral circumflex vessels are ligated
Gluteus medius and minimus tendons are incised at their insertions

Kocher-Langenbeck Approach

Posterior reflection of the gluteus maximus
Gluteus maximus and medius are incised at their insertions
Piriformis and obturator internus are transected at their trochanteric insertions

HISTORY AND PHYSICAL EXAMINATION OF THE PELVIS

History

Age
Mechanism of injury
  Direct blow—contusion
  High hurdles—hamstring avulsion
Chronicity
  Overuse injuries (bursitis, tendinitis)
  Degenerative joint disease

Physical Examination

Observation
  Skin abnormalities
  Pelvic obliquity
Palpation
  Bones
    Anterior superior iliac spine
    Iliac crest
    Iliac tubercle
    Posterior superior iliac spine
    SI joint
  Soft tissues
    Inguinal ligament
    Femoral vessels
    Sartorius muscle
    Adductor longus muscle
    Sciatic nerve
Neurovascular examination
  Sensation (see Fig. 2–5)
Strength testing
  Hip flexors—iliopsoas, sartorius, rectus femoris
  Hip adductors—gracilis, pectineus, adductor longus, adductor brevis, adductor magnus
  Hip abductors—gluteus medius
  Hip extensors—gluteus maximus, hamstrings
Special testing
  SI joint pain
    Patrick's (FABER) test—Flexion, ABduction and External Rotation ("figure 4" position) of the hip can cause SI joint pain, but it is not a very specific test
    Pelvic compression test—anterior to posterior and medial/lateral directed force to test for stability of the pelvis

DIAGNOSTIC TESTS FOR THE PELVIS

Radiographic Evaluation of the Pelvis

AP view
Inlet view (60-degree caudal tilt)—visualizes displacement of the pelvis in the AP plane
Outlet view (45-degree cephalic tilt)—visualizes vertical displacement of the pelvis
Judet iliac oblique (acetabulum is rotated away from the x-ray tube)—visualizes the posterior column and the anterior acetabular wall
Judet obturator oblique (acetabulum is rotated toward the x-ray tube)—visualizes the anterior column and the posterior acetabular wall

Computed Tomography

Very helpful in the management of pelvic/acetabular fractures (preoperative planning)
Three-dimensional CT scan reconstructions are often helpful

Magnetic Resonance Imaging

Helpful in the evaluation of pelvic tumors

COMMON ADULT CONDITIONS OF THE PELVIS

Contusions

Iliac crest contusion (hip pointer)
  Caused by direct trauma
  Treatment is supportive care

Muscle Strains

Significant strains can result in ruptures
Groin pull
  Caused by an overstretch injury of the hip adductors
  Treatment is supportive care
  Common injury in soccer players
  May be confused with an inguinal hernia
Rectus femoris strain
  Caused by an overstretch injury
  Treatment is supportive care

Sacroiliitis

Represents an inflammation of the SI joint
May be associated with the spondyloarthropathies
The patient presents with pain in the region of the SI joint
Patrick's (FABER) test may be helpful in making the diagnosis
Local injections may be useful for symptomatic relief and also for the diagnostic work-up
Treatment
  Nonsteroidal anti-inflammatory drugs (NSAIDs), physical therapy, SI belt

Fusion for severe pain refractory to conservative treatment (or after SI joint infections)

SI Joint Infections

More common in intravenous (IV) drug abusers and immunocompromised individuals

The patient presents with severe and constitutional signs and symptoms (of infection)

Treatment is IV antibiotics

Operative débridement is typically not indicated

Piriformis Syndrome

A myofascial pain syndrome involving the piriformis muscle

The patient presents with buttock pain and may complain of radicular-type symptoms

Pain may be increased on physical examination by passive maximal internal rotation of the hip or resisted active external rotation of the hip (the examiner resists the patient's attempt to externally rotate the hip)

Treatment is supportive care

Coccygodynia

Coccygeal pain

May be related to trauma or abnormal coccyx morphology

Treatment is supportive care

A donut seat cushion (which unloads the coccyx) is often helpful in eliminating painful symptoms

Occasionally, coccygectomy is a last resort for significant pain refractory to conservative management

FRACTURES AND DISLOCATIONS OF THE PELVIS

Overview (Tables 16–1 and 16–2)

Pelvic fractures (Figs. 16–7 to 16–9)

Pelvic fractures are high-energy injuries that can be

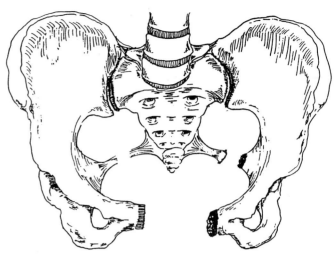

Figure 16–8 ■ AP compression fracture displaying an open-book injury pattern with the pubic symphysis diastasis. (From Kozin SH, Berlet AC: Handbook of Common Orthopaedic Fractures, 3rd ed. West Chester, PA, Medical Surveillance, 1997, p 89.)

associated with significant visceral injuries and intrapelvic/intra-abdominal hemorrhage (often the result of an injury to the superior gluteal artery)

Fluid resuscitation and early stabilization of the pelvis can be lifesaving

Urologic injuries are not uncommon

The pelvis is a bony ring

Single breaks in the ring usually result in a stable fracture pattern

Multiple breaks in the ring may result in an unstable fracture pattern (with pelvic instability)

Acetabular fractures (Fig. 16–10)

Proper treatment of acetabular fractures requires a thorough understanding of the complex bony anatomy of the region

These injuries are intra-articular fractures and commonly require open reduction and internal fixation

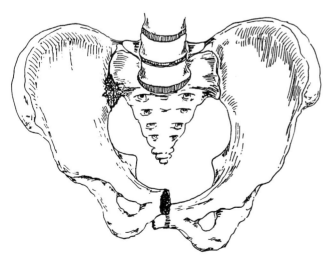

Figure 16–7 ■ Lateral compression fracture. (From Kozin SH, Berlet AC: Handbook of Common Orthopaedic Fractures, 3rd ed. West Chester, PA, Medical Surveillance, 1997, p 89.)

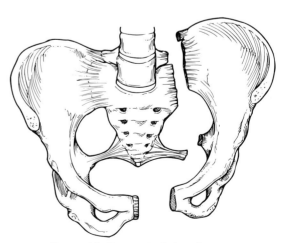

Figure 16–9 ■ Vertical shear fracture.

TUMORS OF THE PELVIS, ACETABULUM, SACRUM, COCCYX

Bone

Paget's disease
Aneurysmal bone cyst

Multiple myeloma
Hemangioma
Angiosarcoma
Metastatic lesions
Giant cell tumor
Chordoma (midline sacral mass)
Chondrosarcoma (pelvis)
Hemangiopericytoma (pelvis)

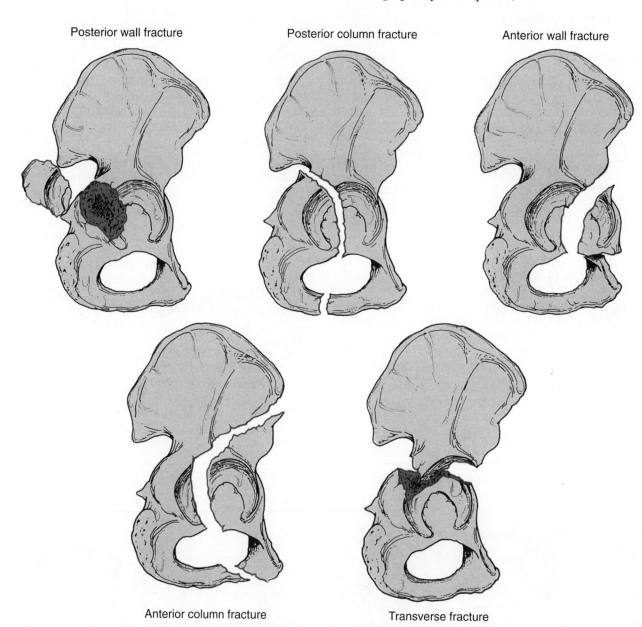

Posterior wall fracture

Posterior column fracture

Anterior wall fracture

Anterior column fracture

Transverse fracture

Figure 16–10 ■ *See legend on opposite page*

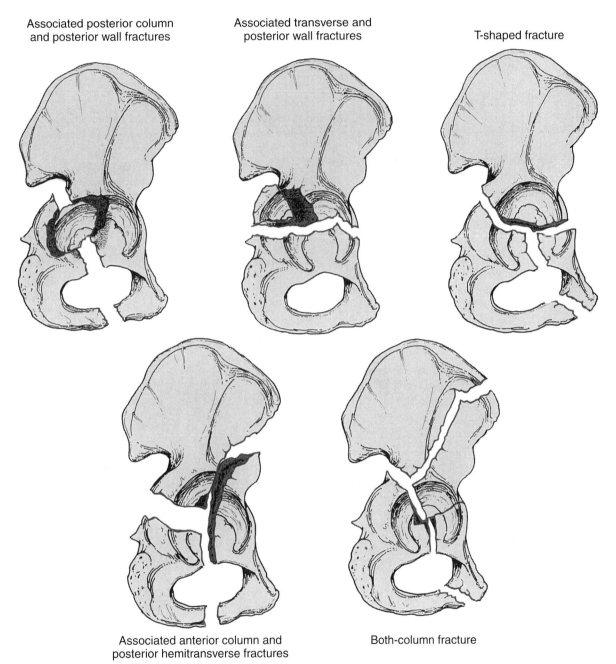

Associated posterior column
and posterior wall fractures

Associated transverse and
posterior wall fractures

T-shaped fracture

Associated anterior column and
posterior hemitransverse fractures

Both-column fracture

Figure 16–10 ■ Types of acetabular fractures. (From Mata J: Surgical treatment of acetabulum fractures. *In* Browner BD, Jupiter JB, Levine AM, et al [eds]: Skeletal Trauma. Philadelphia, WB Saunders, 1992, pp 902–903.)

Table 16–1
FRACTURES OF THE ADULT PELVIS

Fracture	Eponym or Other Name	Classification	Treatment	Most Common Complications of the Injury
Lateral compression (see Fig. 16–7)			Bed rest (occasionally requires delayed ORIF)	Life-threatening hemorrhage, GI injuries, GU injuries (bladder, urethra), neurologic injury, nonunion, malunion, post-traumatic arthritis, pain, sepsis, DVT, heterotopic bone formation, vascular injuries
Anteroposterior compression (see Fig. 16–8)	Open-book injury	Without symphysis diastasis or SI joint disruption	Bed rest	Same as above
		With symphysis diastasis and SI joint disruption	Acute operative stabilization	Same as above
Vertical shear (see Fig. 16–9)	Malgaigne		Acute operative stabilization	Same as above

Acetabulum (see Fig. 16–10)		Letournel
		Simple
		  Posterior wall
		  Posterior column
		  Anterior wall
		  Anterior column
		  Transverse
		Combined
		  Posterior column with posterior wall
		  Transverse with posterior wall
		  "T" fracture
		  Anterior column with posterior hemitransverse
		  Both-column
			Nonoperative
			  <2 mm step-off
			Operative
			  Incongruous or unstable hip joint
				Nerve injury (sciatic, femoral, superior gluteal), vascular injury, heterotopic bone formation, avascular necrosis, post-traumatic arthritis, chondrolysis

ORIF, open reduction with internal fixation; GI, gastrointestinal; GU, genitourinary; DVT, deep venous thrombosis; SI, sacroiliac.

Table 16–2
FRACTURES OF THE ADULT SACRUM AND COCCYX

Fracture	Classification	Treatment	Most Common Complications of the Injury

Sacral fractures	Denis
	  Zone 1—ala
	  Zone 2—foramina
	  Zone 3—central canal involvement
		Bracing for stable fracture patterns without neurologic injury
		Indications for surgical fixation
		  Unstable fracture pattern
		  Neurologic deficit
		  Severe disruption of sacral/pelvic alignment
			Sciatic nerve injury, nerve root injuries (L5, S1, or S2)

Coccyx fractures		Symptomatic (donut seat cushion for sitting unloads the coccyx); operative excision for nonunion or for pain refractory to conservative treatment	

CHAPTER 17

The Adult Hip

HIP ANATOMY

Bones (Fig. 17–1; see Figs. 16–1 and 18–1)

Proximal femur
Femoral head (articulates with the acetabulum)
Femoral neck
Greater trochanter (insertion site for the gluteus medius and gluteus minimus)
Lesser trochanter (iliopsoas insertion site)

Acetabulum
At the confluence of the ilium, ischium, and pubis

Joints (Fig. 17–2)

Hip joint
Femoral head and acetabulum
Ball-and-socket joint
The anterior capsule of the hip is the strongest and

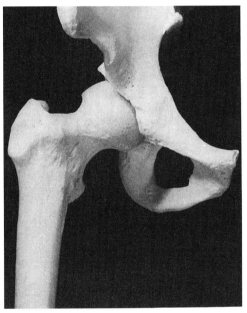

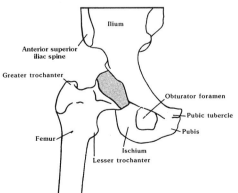

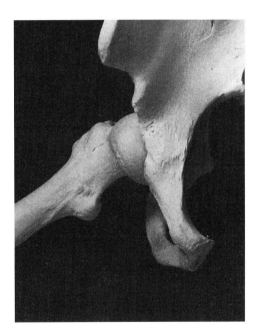

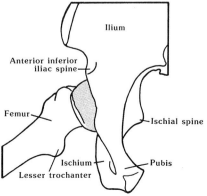

Figure 17–1 ■ Photographic and diagrammatic anatomy of the bones of the hip. (From Weissman BNW, Sledge CB: Orthopedic Radiology. Philadelphia, WB Saunders, 1986, p 386.)

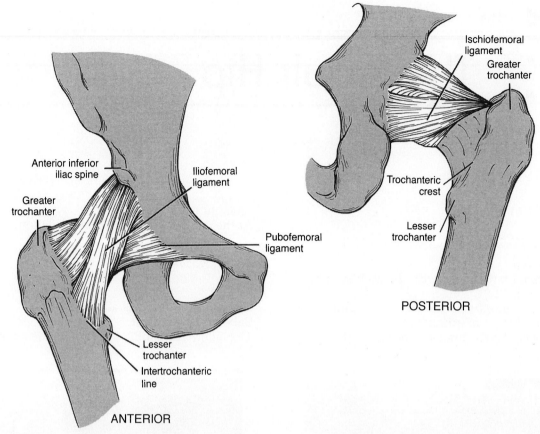

Figure 17–2 ■ Ligaments of the hip joint. (From Levin P: Hip dislocations. *In* Browner BD, Jupiter JB, Levine AM, et al [eds]: Skeletal Trauma. Philadelphia, WB Saunders, 1992, p 1331.)

thickest portion; the capsule is composed of three ligaments
Iliofemoral (Y ligament of Bigelow)—strongest
Ischiofemoral
Pubofemoral

Muscles (Fig. 17–3)

Hip flexors
  Iliacus (femoral nerve)
  Psoas (femoral nerve)
  Pectineus (femoral nerve)
  Rectus femoris (femoral nerve)
  Sartorius (femoral nerve)
Hip adductors
  Adductor magnus (obturator [posterior division] and sciatic nerves)
  Adductor brevis (obturator nerve—posterior division)
  Adductor longus (obturator nerve—anterior division)
  Gracilis (obturator nerve—anterior division)
Hip external rotators
  Gluteus maximus (inferior gluteal nerve)
  Piriformis (nerve to piriformis)
  Obturator externus (obturator nerve)
  Obturator internus (nerve to obturator internus)
  Gemellus superior (nerve to obturator internus)
  Gemellus inferior (nerve to quadratus femoris)
Quadratus femoris (nerve to quadratus femoris)
Hip abductors
  Gluteus medius (superior gluteal nerve)
  Gluteus minimus (superior gluteal nerve)
  Tensor fascia lata (superior gluteal nerve)

Nerves

Discussed in Chapters 16 and 18

Vessels

Blood supply to the femoral head (from three sources) (Fig. 17–4)
  Medial femoral circumflex artery
    The most important source of blood
    A branch of the profunda femoris artery
  Lateral femoral circumflex artery
    Supplies the inferior portion of the femoral head
    A branch of the profunda femoris artery
  Artery of the ligamentum teres
    Minor blood supply in the adult
    A posterior branch of the obturator artery
Other vessels of the hip and pelvis are discussed in Chapter 16

Important Anatomic Relationships
(Fig. 17–5)

Femoral triangle
  Boundaries

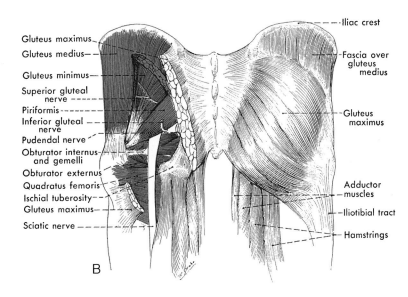

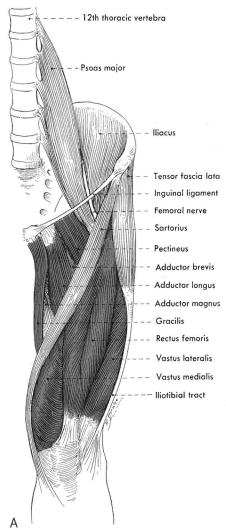

Figure 17–3 ■ Anterior (*A*) and posterior (*B*) muscles of the hip region. (From Jenkins DB: Hollinshead's Functional Anatomy of the Limbs and Back. Philadelphia, WB Saunders, 1991, pp 241, 258.)

Inguinal ligament (superior), sartorius (lateral), adductor longus (medial)

Floor

Lateral to medial: iliacus, psoas, pectineus, adductor longus

Contents

Lateral to medial: femoral **N**erve, **A**rtery, **V**ein, **L**ymphatics (NAVL)

The external iliac arteries become the femoral arteries as they enter the femoral triangle under the inguinal ligament

SURGICAL APPROACHES TO THE HIP

Anterolateral (Watson-Jones) Approach

Fascia lata is split
Anterior third of the gluteus medius is detached
Hip capsule is exposed and incised

Posterior (Moore/Southern) Approach

Gluteus maximus is split
Short external rotators are reflected
Posterior capsule is exposed and incised

Medial (Ludloff) Approach

Adductus longus and gracilis interval (superficial)
Adductus brevis and adductor magnus interval (deep)
Capsule is exposed and incised

HISTORY AND PHYSICAL EXAMINATION OF THE HIP

History

Age
Younger patients—developmental dysplasia of the hip, osteonecrosis, traumatic injuries

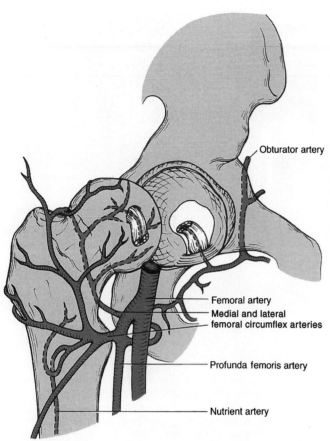

Figure 17–4 ■ Vascular supply to the femoral head. (From Levin P: Hip dislocations. *In* Browner BD, Jupiter JB, Levine AM, et al [eds]: Skeletal Trauma. Philadelphia, WB Saunders, 1992, p 1332.)

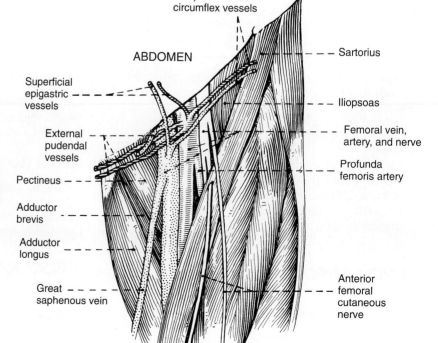

Figure 17–5 ■ Femoral triangle. (From Jenkins DB: Hollinshead's Functional Anatomy of the Limbs and Back. Philadelphia, WB Saunders, 1991, p 243.)

Older patients—osteoarthritis, hip fractures
Mechanism of injury/onset of symptoms
Chronicity of complaints

Physical Examination

Observation
  Gait
    Trendelenburg gait (Fig. 17–6)—patient with glu-
      teus medius weakness may "lurch" toward the
      involved (weak) side to place the center of grav-
      ity toward the weak hip during the stance phase
      of gait
  Contours
  Leg length discrepancies
Palpation
  Greater trochanter
  Trochanteric bursa
  Rectus femoris muscle
Motion (Fig. 17–7)
  Flexion (normal, 125 degrees)
  Extension (normal, 30 degrees)
  Abduction (normal, 45 degrees)
  Adduction (normal, 20 degrees)
  External rotation (normal, 45 degrees)
  Internal rotation (normal, 35 degrees)
Neurovascular examination
  Pulses—femoral artery
  Sensation (see Fig. 2–5)
  Strength testing (Table 17–1)
    Hip flexors—iliopsoas, sartorius, rectus femoris
    Hip adductors—gracilis, pectineus, adductor lon-
      gus, adductor brevis, and adductor magnus
    Hip abductors—gluteus medius
    Hip extensors—gluteus maximus, hamstrings
Special testing
  Leg length discrepancy—the two lower extremities
    should be measured and their lengths compared
    True leg length discrepancy (Fig. 17–8)—**tests for
      bone length inequality**; measured from the ante-
      rior superior iliac spine (ASIS) to the tip of
      the medial malleolus; when a true leg length
      discrepancy exists, the physician is obligated to
      determine the etiology (which bone[s] is [are]
      shortened and why)
    Apparent leg length discrepancy—if the true leg
      lengths of both lower extremities are equal, the
      apparent leg length measures for pelvic obliq-
      uity or hip joint contractures; measured from
      the umbilicus to the tip of the medial malleolus
  Gluteus medius weakness
    Trendelenburg test (Fig. 17–9)—the patient is ob-
      served from behind and asked to stand on one
      leg; upon standing on one leg, the gluteus me-
      dius muscle of the side of the leg on the ground
      (supported side) will contract to elevate the
      hemipelvis on the side of the leg that is not
      touching the ground (unsupported side); if the
      patient is able to stand erect, this indicates nor-
      mal strength of the gluteus medius muscle of
      the leg of the supported side (the hemipelvis on
      the unsupported side will be elevated by the
      normal gluteus medius muscle of the supported

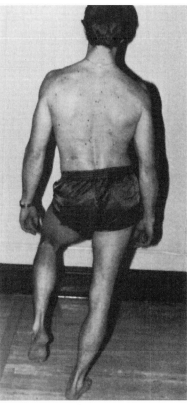

Figure 17–6 ■ Trendelenburg gait. In this example, the patient
has been photographed from behind while he is walking. Note that
the patient "lurches" toward the right side to place his center of
gravity toward the right hip (which has a weak gluteus medius
muscle) during the stance phase of gait. (From Magee DJ: Orthopedic Physical Assessment, 2nd ed. Philadelphia, WB Saunders,
1992, p 575.)

side) and is considered a negative Trendelenburg test; if, however, there is weakness of the
gluteus medius muscle, the patient will be unable to stand erect, the hemipelvis on the unsupported side will not be elevated or will drop
(positive Trendelenburg test), and the patient
may even have to lean over the supported side
(the one with the weak gluteus medius muscle)
to prevent from falling toward the unsupported
side
Hip flexion contracture
  Thomas's test (Fig. 17–10)—the patient lies supine
    and the hip not being tested is passively flexed
    as far as possible; if there is no flexion con-
    tracture, the hip being tested (the straight leg)
    will remain flat on the exam table; if a con-
    tracture is present, the patient's straight leg will
    rise off the table
Iliotibial band contracture
  Ober's test—the patient lies on his or her side
    with the affected leg up; the examiner passively
    abducts the leg as far as possible and flexes the
    knee to 90 degrees; the examiner next releases
    the abducted leg; if the iliotibial band is normal,
    the thigh should drop to the adducted position;
    if there is an iliotibial band contracture, the thigh
    will remain abducted when the leg is released

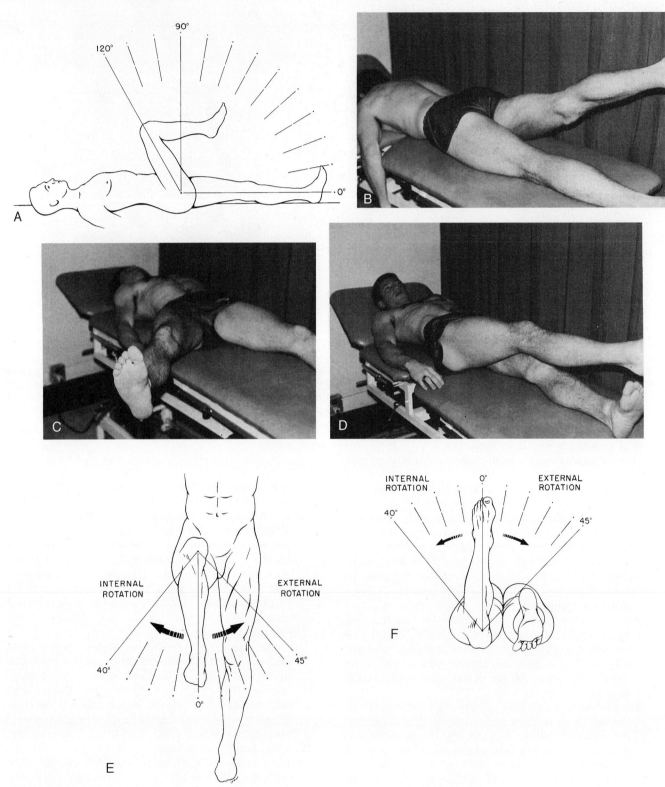

Figure 17-7 ■ Hip motion. *A*, Flexion. *B*, Extension. *C*, Abduction. *D*, Adduction. *E*, Rotation in the supine position. *F*, Rotation in the prone position. (*A, E,* and *F* from Beetham WP, et al: Physical Examination of the Joints. Philadelphia, WB Saunders, 1965, pp 134, 137, 138. *B, C,* and *D* from Magee DJ: Orthopedic Physical Assessment, 2nd ed. Philadelphia, WB Saunders, 1992, p 336.)

Table 17–1
MUSCLES OF THE HIP: THEIR ACTION, INNERVATION, AND NERVE ROOT DERIVATION

Action	Muscles Involved	Innervation	Nerve Root Derivation
Flexion of hip	1. Psoas	Femoral	L1-3
	2. Iliacus	Femoral	L2-3
	3. Rectus femoris	Femoral	L2-4
	4. Sartorius	Femoral	L2-3
	5. Pectineus	Femoral	L2-3
	6. Adductor longus	Obturator	L2-4
	7. Adductor brevis	Obturator	L2-3, L5
	8. Gracilis	Obturator	L2-3
Extension of hip	1. Biceps femoris	Sciatic	L5, S1-2
	2. Semimembranosus	Sciatic	L5, S1-2
	3. Semitendinosus	Sciatic	L5, S1-2
	4. Gluteus maximus	Inferior gluteal	L5, S1-2
	5. Gluteus medius (posterior part)	Superior gluteal	L5, S1
	6. Adductor magnus (ischiocondylar part)	Sciatic	L2-4
Abduction of hip	1. Tensor fascia lata	Superior gluteal	L4-5
	2. Gluteus minimus	Superior gluteal	L5, S1
	3. Gluteus medius	Superior gluteal	L5, S1
	4. Gluteus maximus	Inferior gluteal	L5, S1-2
	5. Sartorius	Femoral	L2-3
Adduction of hip	1. Adductor longus	Obturator	L2-4
	2. Adductor brevis	Obturator	L2-4
	3. Adductor magnus (ischiofomoral portion)	Obturator	L2-4
	4. Gracilis	Obturator	L2-3
	5. Pectineus	Femoral	L2-3
Internal rotation of hip	1. Adductor longus	Obturator	L2-4
	2. Adductor brevis	Obturator	L2-4
	3. Adductor magnus	Obturator and sciatic	L2-4
	4. Gluteus medius (anterior part)	Superior gluteal	L5, S1
	5. Gluteus minimus (anterior part)	Superior gluteal	L5, S1
	6. Tensor fascia lata	Superior gluteal	L4-5
	7. Pectineus	Femoral	L2-3
	8. Gracilis	Obturator	L2-3
External rotation of hip	1. Gluteus maximus	Inferior gluteal	L5, S1-2
	2. Obturator internus	Nerve to obturator internus	L5, S1
	3. Obturator externus	Obturator	L3-4
	4. Quadratus femoris	Nerve to quadratus femoris	L5, S1
	5. Piriformis	Nerve to piriformis	L5, S1-2
	6. Gemellus superior	Nerve to obturator internus	L5, S1
	7. Gemellus inferior	Nerve to quadratus femoris	L5, S1
	8. Sartorius	Femoral	L2-3
	9. Gluteus medius (posterior part)	Superior gluteal	L5, S1

Modified from Magee DJ: Orthopedic Physical Assessment, 2nd ed. Philadelphia, WB Saunders, 1992, p 338.

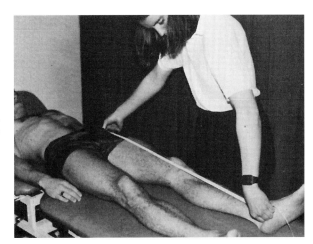

Figure 17–8 ■ Technique of measurement for true leg length discrepancy. (From Magee DJ: Orthopedic Physical Assessment, 2nd ed. Philadelphia, WB Saunders, 1992, p 605.)

NEGATIVE TEST

POSITIVE TEST

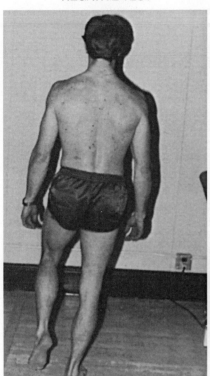
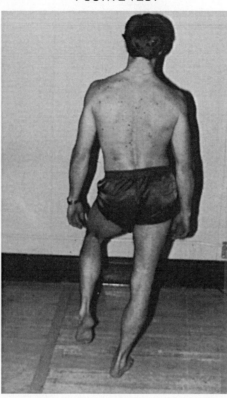

Figure 17–9 ■ Trendelenburg test. Note that the gluteus medius muscle of the *right* hip is being tested in both photographs. A positive test for weakness of the right gluteus medius muscle is characterized by a drop of the left hemipelvis and the patient's leaning to the right to place his center of gravity toward the weak right hip to prevent falling toward the left (unsupported) side. (From Magee DJ: Orthopedic Physical Assessment, 2nd ed. Philadelphia, WB Saunders, 1992, p 324.)

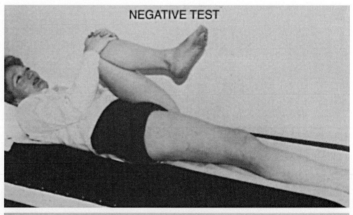

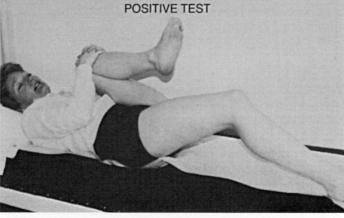

Figure 17–10 ■ Thomas's test. In these photographs the right hip is being tested. (From Magee DJ: Orthopedic Physical Assessment, 2nd ed. Philadelphia, WB Saunders, 1992, p 353.)

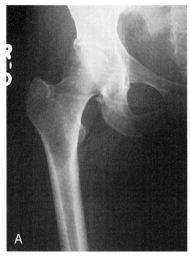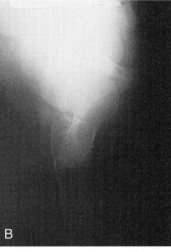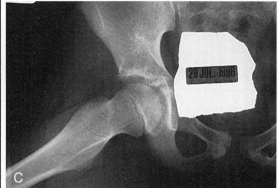

Figure 17–11 ■ Radiographic views of the hip. *A,* AP; *B,* surgical lateral; and *C,* frog-leg lateral of the hip. (Courtesy of Fondren Orthopedic Group LLP, Texas Orthopedic Hospital, Houston, Texas.)

DIAGNOSTIC TESTS FOR THE HIP

Plain Radiographs (Fig. 17–11)

Anteroposterior (AP)
Lateral
   Surgical
   Frog-leg

Bone Scan

Helpful in identifying subtle fractures

Computed Tomography

May be helpful for complex fractures/dislocations

Magnetic Resonance Imaging (Fig. 17–12)

Useful in the evaluation for osteonecrosis and occult
   hip pain

Arthroscopy

Indications
   Loose bodies
   Labral tears (difficult to identify preoperatively)
   Articular cartilage lesions
   Synovitis

COMMON ADULT CONDITIONS OF THE HIP

Osteonecrosis (See Chapter 1)

Death of subchondral bone (caused by a vascular insult)
Risk factors
   Steroid use
   Alcohol abuse
   Dysbarism (caisson disease)
   Excessive radiation
   Blood dyscrasias (Gaucher's disease, etc)
   Trauma

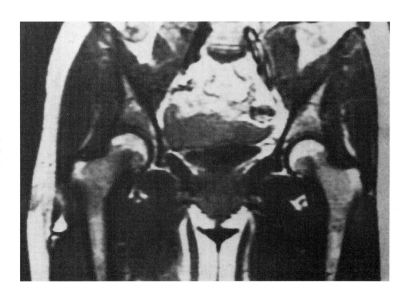

Figure 17–12 ■ Normal MRI of the hips. (From Dalinka MK, Neustadter LM: Radiology of the hip. *In* Steinberg ME [ed]: The Hip and Its Disorders. Philadelphia, WB Saunders, 1991, p 68.)

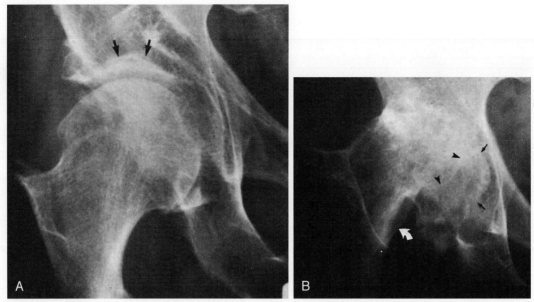

Figure 17–13 ■ Osteoarthritis. *A,* Early disease. *B,* Late disease with complete obliteration of the joint space. (From Weissman BNW, Sledge CB: Orthopedic Radiology. Philadelphia, WB Saunders, 1986, p 403.)

Pathologic changes
  Necrotic bone leads to collapse of subchondral bone
    and the overlying (normal) articular cartilage
Clinical findings
  Pain
  Limited hip range of motion
Diagnosis
  Early diagnosis requires a high index of suspicion
  Magnetic resonance imaging (MRI) is positive earli-
    est, even before the appearance of symptoms
  Bone scan is also useful but less sensitive than MRI
  X-rays are often normal until late in the disease
  Laboratory tests are typically normal
Treatment options
  Early disease—core decompression, vascularized
    bone graft, hip osteotomy
  Late disease—total hip arthroplasty

Arthritis

Etiologies (discussed in greater detail in Chapters 3
    and 5)
  Osteoarthritis
  Rheumatoid arthritis
  Post-traumatic arthritis
  Following an infection of the hip joint
  Late effects of congenital/pediatric hip disorders
  Others (crystal deposition diseases, spondyloarthro-
    pathies, storage diseases, collagen vascular dis-
    eases)
Clinical findings
  Activity-related pain
  Loss of hip motion (internal rotation is lost earliest
    in the disease process)
  Crepitus
  Radiographic changes (Fig. 17–13)
    Loss of joint space
    Bony sclerosis
    Osteophytes (bone spurs)

Treatment options
  Nonoperative—nonsteroidal anti-inflammatory
    drugs, activity modification, physical therapy,
    cane (held in the contralateral hand)
  Operative
    Total hip arthroplasty (see Fig. 7–14)
      Femoral component—stem and head
      Acetabular component—metal shell and poly-
        ethylene liner
      Complications—osteolysis (from polyethylene
        wear debris), loosening of components, dislo-
        cation, implant failure, heterotopic bone for-

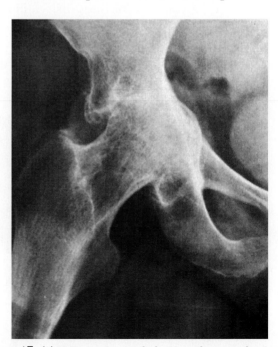

Figure 17–14 ■ Protrusio acetabuli. Note the central migration of the femoral head into the pelvis in this patient with rheumatoid arthritis. (From Weissman BNW, Sledge CB: Orthopedic Radiology. Philadelphia, WB Saunders, 1986, p 404.)

mation, thromboembolic disease, infection, neurovascular injuries
Intrapelvic structures can be injured during the placement of acetabular screws used to fix the metal acetabular shell to the bony acetabulum; screws should be placed only in the posterior quadrants of the acetabulum; screws placed in the anterior superior quadrant risk injury to the external iliac vein; screws placed in the anterior inferior quadrant risk injury to the obturator artery and nerve
Hip arthrodesis
Hip osteotomy

Other Hip Problems

Greater trochanteric bursitis
Localized tenderness to palpation over the greater trochanter
Pain with resisted abduction
Local injection, stretching programs are helpful
Iliopsoas bursitis

Localized pain and snapping upon active flexion of the hip against resistance or upon passive hyperextension of the hip
Treatment is supportive care
Protrusio acetabuli (Fig. 17–14)
Intrapelvic protrusion of the femoral head (through the acetabulum)
Etiologies
Rheumatoid arthritis
Ankylosing spondylitis
Paget's disease
Metabolic bone diseases
Marfan syndrome
Otto's pelvis
Others

FRACTURES AND DISLOCATIONS OF THE HIP

General Overview

Fractures of the hip (Table 17–2) include
Femoral neck fractures (Fig. 17–15)

Table 17–2
FRACTURES OF THE ADULT HIP

Fracture	Classification	Treatment	Most Common Complications of the Injury

Femoral neck (see Fig. 17–15)	Garden (I–IV)
	   I. Incomplete/valgus impaction
	   II. Complete, undisplaced
	   III. Complete, partial displacement
	   IV. Complete, total displacement
		ORIF
		 ORIF
		 ORIF in young patients; arthroplasty for elderly patients (physiologic age >70 years)
		 ORIF in young patients; arthroplasty for elderly patients (physiologic age >70 years)
		
		 Prosthetic replacement for
		   1. Elderly
		   2. Chronically ill
		   3. Pathologic fracture
		   4. Parkinson's disease patients (with hip fracture)
		   5. Rheumatoid arthritis patients (with hip fracture)
			Malunion, nonunion, avascular necrosis of the femoral head, pulmonary embolism, DVT, infection, death (one third of all elderly patients die within 1 year of injury)

Stress fracture of the femoral neck	Nondisplaced Displaced	Bed rest, progressive weight bearing Operative treatment	Malunion, nonunion, avascular necrosis of the femoral head, pulmonary embolism, DVT, infection, death (one third of all elderly patients die within 1 year of injury), completion of fracture

Intertrochanteric (see Fig. 17–16)	Boyd and Griffin (I–IV)
	   I. Nondisplaced
	   II. Displaced
	   III. Reverse obliquity
	   IV. Subtrochanteric extension
		Operative reduction and stabilization	Varus deformity, hardware migration/cutout, infection

Greater trochanter		ORIF if displaced >1 cm in younger patients	
Lesser trochanter		ORIF if displaced >2 cm in younger patients	

Subtrochanteric (less than 5 cm below the top of the lesser trochanter; distal to this would be a femoral shaft fracture) (see Fig. 17–17)	Seinsheimer (I–V)
	   I. Nondisplaced/minimally displaced
	   II. Two-part
	   III. Three-part
	   IV. Comminuted
	   V. Peritrochanteric (combined subtrochanteric and intertrochanteric fractures)
		Operative treatment	Malunion, nonunion, avascular necrosis of the femoral head, pulmonary embolism, DVT, infection

ORIF, open reduction with internal fixation; DVT, deep venous thrombosis.

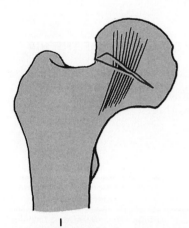

I

Incomplete / valgus impaction

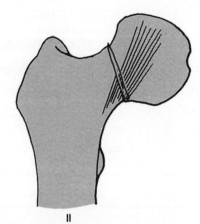

II

Complete, undisplaced

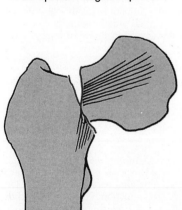

III

Complete, partial displacement

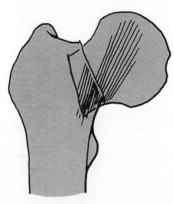

IV

Complete, total displacement

Figure 17–15 ■ Garden classification of femoral neck fractures. (From Swiontkowski MF: Intracapsular hip fractures. *In* Browner BD, Jupiter JB, Levine AM, et al [eds]: Skeletal Trauma. Philadelphia, WB Saunders, 1992, p 1390.)

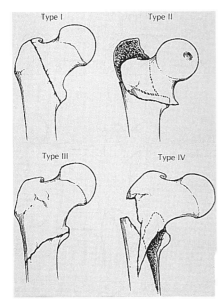

Figure 17-16 ■ Intertrochanteric hip fractures—Boyd and Griffin classification. (From DeLee JC: Fractures and dislocations of the hip. *In* Rockwood CA, Green DP [eds]: Fractures in Adults, 2nd ed. Philadelphia, JB Lippincott, 1984, p 1261.)

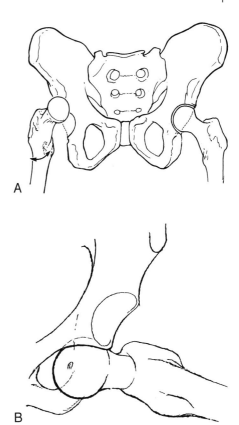

Figure 17-18 ■ Anterior hip dislocations can be (*A*) superior (Epstein I [pubic or subspinous—more common]) or (*B*) inferior (Epstein II [obturator—rare]). (From Connolly JF: DePalma's The Management of Fractures and Dislocations: An Atlas. Philadelphia, WB Saunders, 1981.)

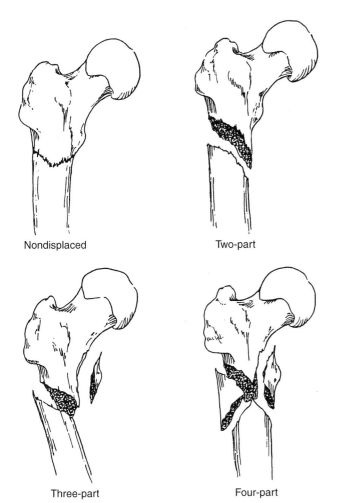

Nondisplaced   Two-part

Three-part   Four-part

Figure 17-17 ■ Subtrochanteric fractures. (Modified from Kozin SH, Berlet AC: Handbook of Common Orthopaedic Fractures, 3rd ed. West Chester, PA, Medical Surveillance, 1997, pp 117, 119.)

Intertrochanteric hip fractures (Fig. 17–16)
Fractures of the greater and lesser trochanter
Subtrochanteric fractures (Fig. 17–17)
Dislocations of the hip (Table 17–3) include
   Anterior dislocations (with or without an associated fracture) (Fig. 17–18)
   Posterior dislocations (with or without an associated fracture) (Fig. 17–19)
Femoral neck fractures (see Fig. 17–15)
   Classification is based on the degree of displacement and is prognostic for development of late post-traumatic osteonecrosis, which develops most commonly in older patients with displaced fractures and is caused by disruption of the blood supply to the femoral head
   The classic presentation of a femoral neck fracture is acute onset of hip pain, inability to bear weight, and a shortened and externally rotated lower extremity
   Treatment is based on the degree of displacement and the physiologic age of the patient
Intertrochanteric hip fractures (see Fig. 17–16)
   Typically do not develop osteonecrosis because the fracture is distal to the blood supply of the femoral head
   Treatment is operative reduction and stabilization
Subtrochanteric fractures (see Fig. 17–17)
   Require operative stabilization

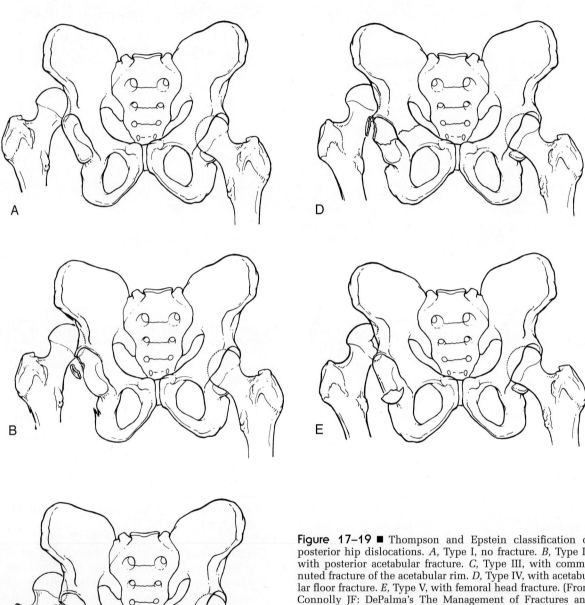

Figure 17–19 ■ Thompson and Epstein classification of posterior hip dislocations. *A*, Type I, no fracture. *B*, Type II, with posterior acetabular fracture. *C*, Type III, with comminuted fracture of the acetabular rim. *D*, Type IV, with acetabular floor fracture. *E*, Type V, with femoral head fracture. (From Connolly JF: DePalma's The Management of Fractures and Dislocations: An Atlas. Philadelphia, WB Saunders, 1981.)

Table 17–3
DISLOCATIONS OF THE ADULT HIP

Dislocation	Classification	Treatment	Most Common Complications of the Injury
Anterior (see Fig. 17–18)	Epstein (I and II) IA. Anterior/superior dislocation, no fracture of acetabulum IB. Anterior/superior dislocation with femoral head fracture IC. Anterior/superior dislocation with acetabular fracture IIA. Anterior/inferior dislocation, no fracture of acetabulum IIB. Anterior/inferior dislocation with femoral head fracture IIC. Anterior/inferior dislocation with acetabular fracture	Closed reduction Open reduction for 1. Irreducible (interposed fragment or soft tissue) 2. Unstable hip exam after closed reduction	Injury to femoral artery or nerve, injury to sciatic nerve, avascular necrosis (risk related to delay in closed reduction), post-traumatic arthritis, hip instability
Posterior (see Fig. 17–19)	Thompson and Epstein (I–V) I. With no or minimal fracture of acetabulum II. With fracture of posterior acetabular rim III. With comminuted acetabular rim fracture IV. With fracture of acetabular floor V. With femoral head fracture Pipkin subdivided posterior hip dislocations with femoral head fractures (Thompson and Epstein V) into four types I. Femoral head fracture caudal to ligamentum teres II. Femoral head fracture cephalad to ligamentum teres III. Femoral head and neck fracture IV. Associated with an acetabular fracture	Traction ORIF Traction vs. operative treatment Traction vs. operative treatment Traction vs. operative treatment Traction vs. ORIF Traction vs. ORIF ORIF in younger patients; arthroplasty in older patients ORIF in younger patients; arthroplasty in older patients	Injury to femoral artery or nerve, injury to sciatic nerve, avascular necrosis (risk related to delay in closed reduction), post-traumatic arthritis, hip instability

ORIF, open reduction with internal fixation.

Hip dislocations (see Figs. 17–18 and 17–19) (see Table 17–3)
High-energy injuries
Good results are difficult to achieve
Osteonecrosis is an unfortunate common sequela of the injury and is related to the time interval that the hip is dislocated
Post-traumatic arthritis is common
Sciatic nerve injuries are not uncommon
Anterior dislocations present with the lower extremity shortened and externally rotated; closed reduction may be accomplished using the **Allis reduction maneuver** (Fig. 17–20)
Posterior dislocations present with the lower extremity internally rotated; closed reduction may be accomplished using **Bigelow's maneuver** (Fig. 17–21)
Failure of closed reduction of a hip dislocation suggests entrapment of a bony fragment or interposition of soft tissue and requires open reduction

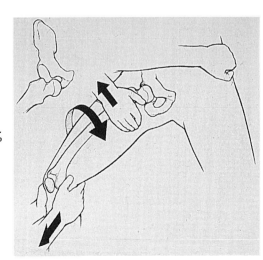

Figure 17–20 ■ The Allis maneuver for reduction of an anterior hip dislocation. (From DeLee JC: Fractures and dislocations of the hip. In Rockwood CA, Green DP [eds]: Fractures in Adults, 2nd ed. Philadelphia, JB Lippincott, 1984, p 1302.)

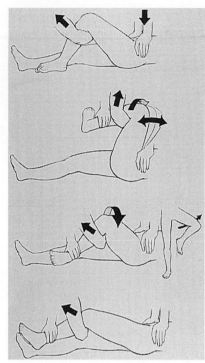

Figure 17–21 ■ The Bigelow maneuver for reduction of a posterior hip dislocation. (From DeLee JC: Fractures and dislocations of the hip. *In* Rockwood CA, Green DP [eds]: Fractures in Adults, 2nd ed. Philadelphia, JB Lippincott, 1984, p 1308.)

Fracture-dislocations
    High-energy injuries that usually require operative treatment

TUMORS OF THE HIP

Bone

Clear cell chondrosarcoma
Metastatic lesions

Soft Tissue

Synovial chondromatosis
Synovial sarcoma

DIFFERENTIAL DIAGNOSIS OF COMMON HIP COMPLAINTS

Pain

Muscle strains
Greater trochanteric bursitis
Fractures
Dislocations
Arthritis
Rheumatologic conditions
Osteonecrosis
Infections
Tumors

Loss of Motion

Arthritis
Rheumatologic conditions
Osteonecrosis
Fractures
Dislocations
Infections
Tumors

PEARLS AND PITFALLS

The earliest hip motion that is lost in arthritic conditions is internal rotation
Presentation of a patient with hip pain with a shortened and externally rotated lower extremity is consistent with a hip fracture
Presentation of a patient with a flexed hip who refuses to move the joint is consistent with a hip infection

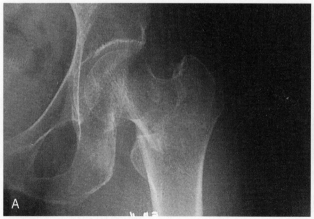
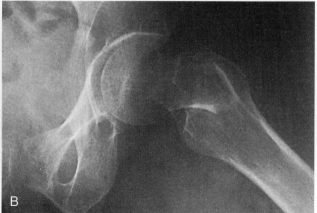

Figure 17–22 ■ *A,* This femoral neck fracture appears to be nondisplaced on the AP view. *B,* The lateral view shows displacement of the proximal femoral shaft on the femoral head and neck. This case shows the importance of obtaining *at least* two radiographic views of *all fractures.* As this case illustrates, this is particularly important when assessing fractures around the hip. (Courtesy of Fondren Orthopedic Group LLP, Texas Orthopedic Hospital, Houston, Texas.)

Beware of the patient with a painful total hip arthroplasty; an infected total joint may not always be obvious

When evaluating a hip fracture, it is important to carefully examine the lateral radiograph; a fracture that appears to be nondisplaced or minimally displaced on the AP view can be significantly displaced on the lateral view (Fig. 17–22)

CHAPTER 18

The Adult Thigh

THIGH ANATOMY

Bone (Fig. 18–1)

Femur

Muscles (Fig. 18–2; see Fig. 17–3)

Anterior thigh (quadriceps muscles)
  Vastus lateralis (femoral nerve)

Vastus medialis (femoral nerve)
Vastus intermedius (femoral nerve)
Rectus femoris (femoral nerve)
Posterior thigh (hamstrings)
  Biceps femoris
    Long head (origin on the ischium) (tibial nerve)
    Short head (origin on the femur) (peroneal nerve)
  Semitendinosus (tibial nerve)
  Semimembranosus (tibial nerve)

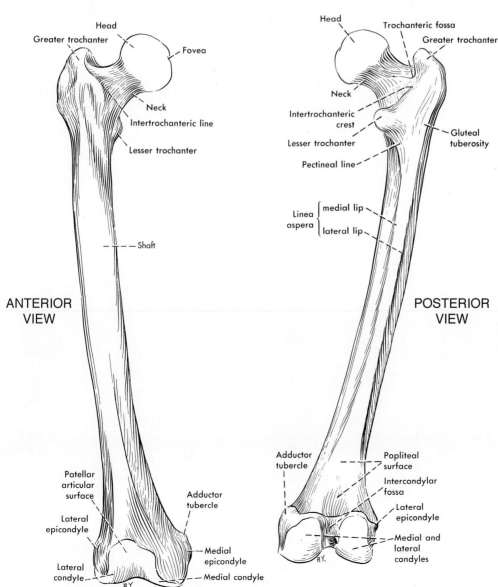

ANTERIOR VIEW

POSTERIOR VIEW

Figure 18–1 ■ Anterior and posterior views of the femur. (From Jenkins DB: Hollinshead's Functional Anatomy of the Limbs and Back, 6th ed. Philadelphia, WB Saunders, 1991, p 228.)

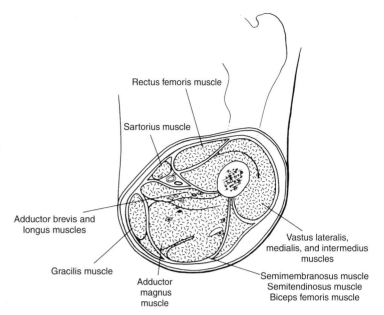

Figure 18–2 ■ Cross-sectional anatomy of the thigh. (From Brunet ME, Hontas RB: The thigh. *In* DeLee JC, Drez D Jr [eds]: Orthopaedic Sports Medicine: Principles and Practice. Philadelphia, WB Saunders, 1994, p 1109.)

Medial thigh (adductors)
  Adductor magnus (obturator and tibial nerves)
  Adductor longus (obturator nerve)
  Adductor brevis (obturator nerve)
  Gracilis (obturator nerve)
Tensor fascia lata (superior gluteal nerve)

Nerves (Fig. 18–3)

Sciatic nerve
  Runs between the biceps femoris and the semimembranosus
  Tibial portion (supplies the hamstrings)
  Peroneal portion (supplies the short head of the biceps)
Femoral nerve
  Supplies the quadriceps muscles after exiting the femoral triangle (see Fig. 17–5)

Vessels (Fig. 18–4)

Femoral artery
  Deep branch (profunda femoris artery)—supplies the nutrient segmental vessels (perforators) to the femur (at the lateral intermuscular septum)
  Superficial branch
    Runs medially (deep to the sartorius)
    Becomes the popliteal artery proximal to the knee

SURGICAL APPROACHES TO THE THIGH

Lateral Approach

Fascia lata is split
Vastus lateralis is reflected off the lateral intermuscular septum or is split along its fibers

Anteromedial Approach

Between the rectus femoris and the vastus medialis
Vastus intermedius is split

Posterior Approach

Between the biceps femoris and the vastus lateralis

HISTORY AND PHYSICAL EXAMINATION OF THE THIGH

History

Mechanism of injury
Referred pain (from back or hip pathology)
Chronicity

Physical Examination

Observation
  Abnormal contours
Palpation
  Femur
  Muscles (quadriceps, hamstrings)
  Defects, tenderness
Neurovascular exam
  Distal muscle function
  Sensation (see Fig. 2–5)
  Strength testing (hip and knee flexors and extensors)

DIAGNOSTIC TESTS FOR THE THIGH

Radiographs

Anteroposterior
Lateral

Imaging

Computed tomography/magnetic resonance imaging for the work-up of a tumor (mass)

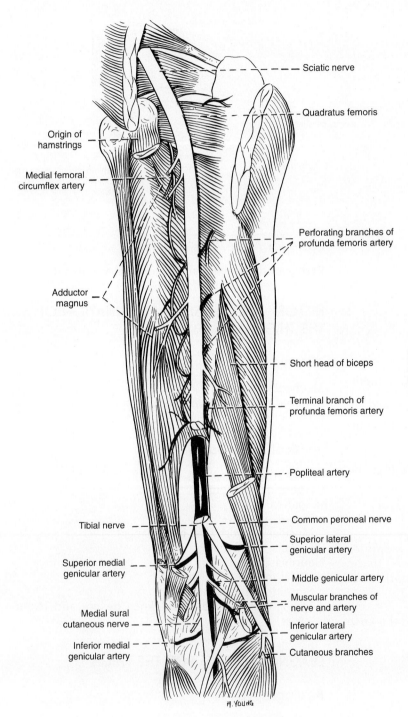

Origin of
hamstrings

Medial femoral
circumflex artery

Adductor
magnus

Tibial nerve

Superior medial
genicular artery

Medial sural
cutaneous nerve

Inferior medial
genicular artery

Sciatic nerve

Quadratus femoris

Perforating branches of
profunda femoris artery

Short head of biceps

Terminal branch of
profunda femoris artery

Popliteal artery

Common peroneal nerve

Superior lateral
genicular artery

Middle genicular artery

Muscular branches of
nerve and artery

Inferior lateral
genicular artery

Cutaneous branches

A. YOUNG

Figure 18–3 ■ Sciatic nerve. (From Jenkins DB: Hollinshead's Functional Anatomy of the Limbs and Back, 6th ed. Philadelphia, WB Saunders, 1991, p 266.)

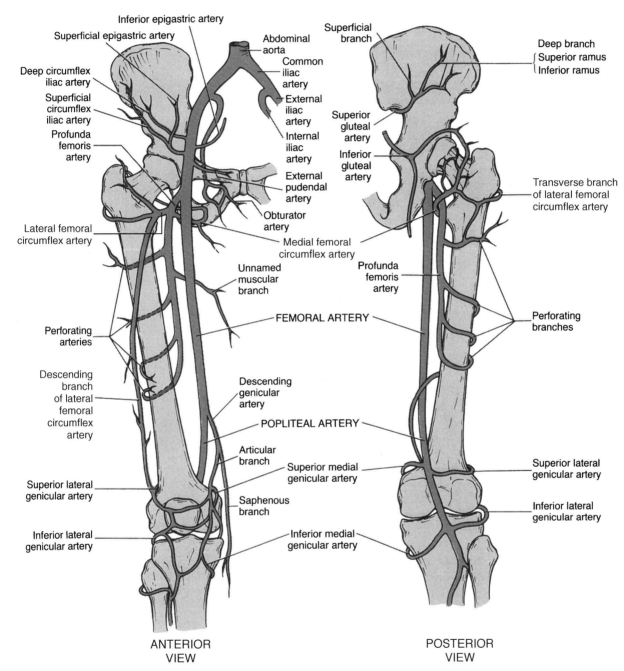

Figure 18–4 ■ Blood supply to the thigh. (From Johnson KD: Femoral shaft fractures. *In* Browner BD, Jupiter JB, Levine AM, et al [eds]: Skeletal Trauma. Philadelphia, WB Saunders, 1992, p 1529.)

COMMON ADULT CONDITIONS OF THE THIGH

Quadriceps Contusion

Common in contact sports from direct trauma
Treatment
  Acute—cold, compression, and rest with the knee immobilized (elastic wrap) in flexion
  Later—range-of-motion exercises, quadriceps rehabilitation
Late sequelae
  Myositis ossificans (Fig. 18–5)—bone formation in the soft tissues
    Symptomatic treatment
    Late excision of symptomatic cases of ectopic bone only after it has matured (takes about 12 to 18 months)

Hamstring Strain

Common injury in athletes
Mechanism of injury—sudden forceful change in the length of the muscle (such as during sprinting, while the hip is flexed and the knee is extended)
Symptoms (proportional to the degree of the strain)—spasm, loss of knee extension, swelling, pain
Treatment—ice, elevation, compression (such as with an elastic wrap), stretching exercises

Iliotibial Band Friction Syndrome

Represents abrasion of the iliotibial band on the lateral femoral condyle
Common in cyclists

Localized tenderness, especially with the knee flexed 30 degrees
Treatment is supportive; occasionally operative decompression is required

Meralgia Paresthetica

Compression injury of the lateral femoral cutaneous nerve within the soft tissue tunnel it traverses as it passes deep to the inguinal ligament
Presents as anterolateral thigh pain with loss of sensation
Arises as a result of direct trauma or constrictive clothing or equipment
Diagnosis
  Positive Tinel's sign over the area of nerve compression
  Electromyography and nerve conduction studies to rule out other etiologies (lumbar radiculopathy, lumbar plexopathy, femoral neuropathy)
Treatment is supportive

FRACTURES AND DISLOCATIONS OF THE THIGH

Overview (Table 18–1)

Femoral shaft fracture (Fig. 18–6)
Adult femoral shaft fractures require operative stabilization
Operative stabilization should be performed as early as possible (within 24 hours) to minimize the risk of complications (fat embolism syndrome, acute respiratory distress syndrome, deep venous throm-

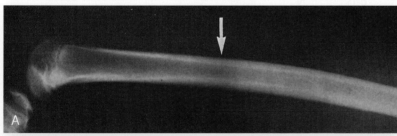
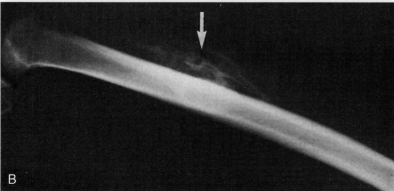

Figure 18–5 ■ *A,* Early (<3 weeks) and *B,* late (>6 weeks) radiographs of myositis ossificans (*arrows*) of the thigh related to a thigh contusion. (From Brunet ME, Hontas RB: The thigh. *In* DeLee JC, Drez D Jr [eds]: Orthopaedic Sports Medicine: Principles and Practice. Philadelphia, WB Saunders, 1994, p 1107.)

Table 18–1
FRACTURES OF THE ADULT FEMUR

Fracture	Eponym or Other Name	Classification	Treatment	Most Common Complications of the Injury
Femoral shaft (5 cm below the top of the lesser trochanter to 8 cm above the knee joint) (see Fig. 18–6)		Winquist and Hansen (O–IV) O. No comminution I. Transverse, butterfly fragment <25% of fracture surface area II. Transverse, butterfly fragment 25–50% III. Comminuted, butterfly fragment >50%, unstable fracture pattern IV. Extensive comminution, no cortical contact	Operative treatment (most commonly intramedullary rod fixation)	Nonunion, malunion (shortening, rotation), missed diagnosis of knee ligament injury, other fractures, neurovascular injuries, knee stiffness, DVT, PE, fat embolism
Femoral shaft fracture associated with ipsilateral femoral neck fracture			ORIF	Malunion, nonunion, avascular necrosis of the femoral head, DVT, PE, fat embolism, death (one third of all elderly patients die within 1 year of injury), missed diagnosis of knee ligament injury, other fractures, neurovascular injuries, knee stiffness
Femoral shaft fracture associated with ipsilateral tibial shaft fracture	Floating knee			Nonunion, malunion (shortening, rotation), delayed union, missed diagnosis of knee ligament injury, other fractures, neurovascular injuries, knee stiffness, DVT, PE, fat embolism

DVT, deep venous thrombosis; PE, pulmonary embolism; ORIF, open reduction with internal fixation.

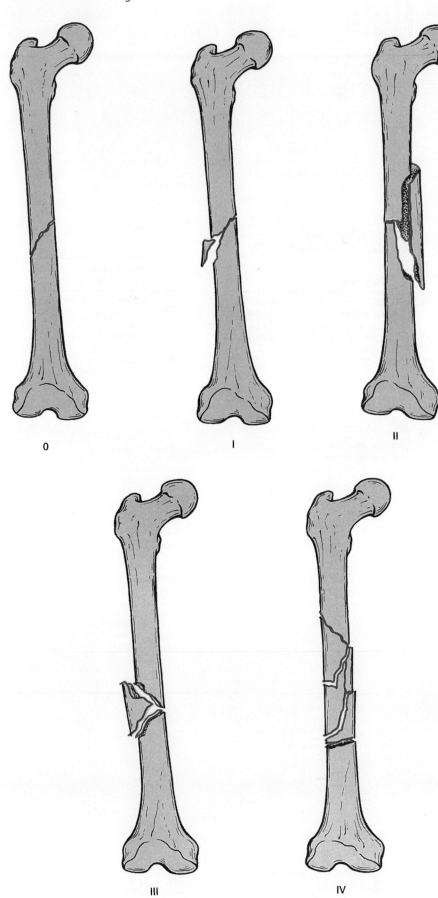

0

I

II

III

IV

Figure 18–6 ■ Femoral shaft fracture classification (Winquist and Hansen). (From Johnson KD: Femoral shaft fractures. *In* Browner BD, Jupiter JB, Levine AM, et al [eds]: Skeletal Trauma. Philadelphia, WB Saunders, 1992, p 1537.)

bosis, pneumonia, and others) and allow mobilization of the patient as early as possible

Approximately 20% of patients with a femoral shaft fracture have an associated knee ligament injury; therefore, it is important to examine the knee after operative stabilization of the femur fracture

The most common method of operative stabilization of a femoral shaft fracture is an intramedullary rod (nail) (see Figs. 7–11 and 7–12)

Every patient with a femoral shaft fracture should be evaluated with hip x-rays to look for a hip fracture (which should not be missed)

A floating knee injury consists of an ipsilateral femoral and tibial shaft fracture; the knee is said to be "floating" because it is not connected to the rest of the skeleton

TUMORS OF THE THIGH

Bone

Paget's disease
Chondrosarcoma
Aneurysmal bone cyst
Fibrous dysplasia
Malignant lymphoma
Angiosarcoma

Soft Tissue

Lipoma
Hemangioma
Malignant fibrous histiocytoma
Fibrosarcoma
Liposarcoma

CHAPTER 19

The Adult Knee

KNEE ANATOMY

Bones (Fig. 19–1)

Distal femur
  Medial femoral condyle (larger than the lateral femoral condyle)
  Lateral femoral condyle
Proximal tibia (tibial plateau)
  Medial condyle is concave

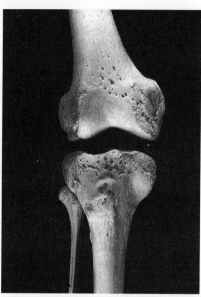

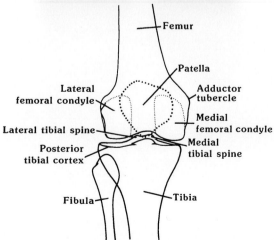

Figure 19–1 ■ Anterior view and drawing demonstrating the bones of the knee. (From Weissman BNW, Sledge CB: Orthopedic Radiology. Philadelphia, WB Saunders, 1986, p 498.)

Lateral condyle is convex
Intercondylar eminence (anterior cruciate ligament [ACL] attachment site anteriorly, posterior cruciate ligament (PCL) attachment site posteriorly)
Tubercles
  Tibial tubercle—patellar tendon insertion site
  Gerdy's tubercle—iliotibial band insertion site (on the proximal tibia)
Proximal fibula
Patella
  Largest sesamoid bone in the body
  Thickest articular cartilage in the body
  Lateral facets larger than medial facets
  Three functions
    Protects the knee joint
    Acts as a fulcrum for the quadriceps (to increase their mechanical advantage)
    Enhances knee joint lubrication and nutrition

Joints

Tibiofemoral joint (Fig. 19–2)
  Combination of a hinge, a sliding, and a gliding joint
  Ligaments
    ACL—resists anterior displacement of the tibia on the femur
    PCL—resists posterior displacement of the tibia on the femur
    Lateral collateral ligament (LCL) (also known as the fibular collateral ligament)—resists varus angulation
    Medial collateral ligament (MCL)—resists valgus angulation
    Meniscofemoral ligaments—ligament of Humphry (courses anterior to the PCL) and ligament of Wrisberg (courses posterior to the PCL)
    Meniscotibial (coronary) ligament
    Posterolateral corner—resists external rotation
    Posteromedial corner—resists internal rotation
  Menisci (Fig. 19–3)
    Medial—"C" shaped
    Lateral—circular
    Each meniscus has an anterior, a middle, and a posterior horn
    Peripheral 25% of the meniscus is vascularized; the central 75% is avascular
    Function
      Deepens the articular surfaces for load transmission

The Adult Knee ■ 295

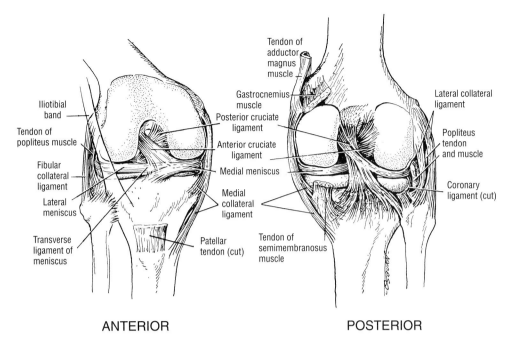

ANTERIOR   POSTERIOR

Figure 19–2 ■ Ligaments of the knee. Note that the posterior cruciate ligament originates below the level of the tibial plateau. (From O'Donoghue DH: Treatment of Injuries to Athletes. Philadelphia, WB Saunders, 1976, p 559.)

Reduces stresses on the joint surfaces
Enhances joint stability by acting as a secondary
stabilizer
Patellofemoral joint
Transmits loads of up to three times body weight

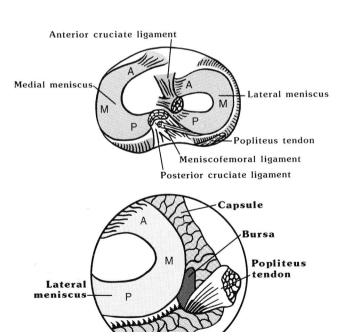

Figure 19–3 ■ Menisci. The medial meniscus is attached to the capsule throughout its periphery and is "C" shaped. The lateral meniscus is more circular in shape, and its periphery is interrupted posteriorly by the popliteus tendon. Each meniscus has an anterior (A), a middle (M), and a posterior (P) horn. (Modified from Weissman BNW, Sledge CB: Orthopedic Radiology. Philadelphia, WB Saunders, 1986, p 506.)

Proximal tibiofibular joint
Gliding joint

Muscles (Fig. 19–4)

Quadriceps (extend the knee)
Vastus intermedius
Vastus medialis
Vastus lateralis
Rectus femoris
Medial hamstrings (flex and internally rotate the knee)
Gracilis
Semimembranosus
Semitendinosus
Lateral hamstrings (flex and externally rotate the knee)
Biceps femoris
Posterior muscles (flex the knee)
Gastrocnemius
Plantaris
Popliteus

Nerves (Fig. 19–5)

Tibial nerve
Lies medially in the popliteal fossa
Splits the two heads of the gastrocnemius
Common peroneal nerve
Lies laterally in the popliteal fossa
Splits the biceps femoris and winds around the fibular neck

Vessels (Fig. 19–6)

Popliteal artery
Genicular branches (medial, lateral, middle)

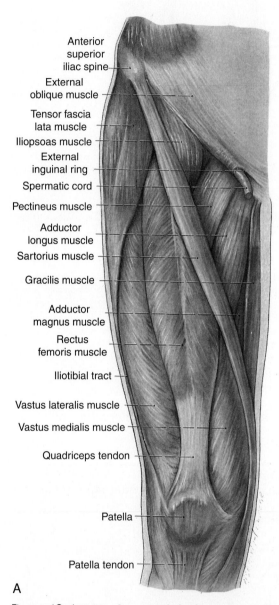

Anterior superior iliac spine
External oblique muscle
Tensor fascia lata muscle
Iliopsoas muscle
External inguinal ring
Spermatic cord
Pectineus muscle
Adductor longus muscle
Sartorius muscle
Gracilis muscle
Adductor magnus muscle
Rectus femoris muscle
Iliotibial tract
Vastus lateralis muscle
Vastus medialis muscle
Quadriceps tendon
Patella
Patella tendon

A

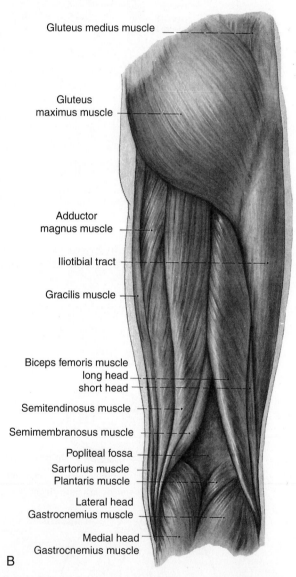

Gluteus medius muscle
Gluteus maximus muscle
Adductor magnus muscle
Iliotibial tract
Gracilis muscle
Biceps femoris muscle long head
short head
Semitendinosus muscle
Semimembranosus muscle
Popliteal fossa
Sartorius muscle
Plantaris muscle
Lateral head Gastrocnemius muscle
Medial head Gastrocnemius muscle

B

Figure 19–4 ■ Muscles around the knee. *A,* Anterior muscles include the quadriceps (vastus intermedius, vastus medialis, vastus lateralis, rectus femoris), and sartorius. *B,* Posterior muscles include the hamstrings (biceps femoris, gracilis, semitendinosus, semimembranosus) and calf muscles (not shown). (From Jacob SW, Francone C, Lossow WJ: Structure and Function in Man, 5th ed. Philadelphia, WB Saunders, 1982, p 216.)

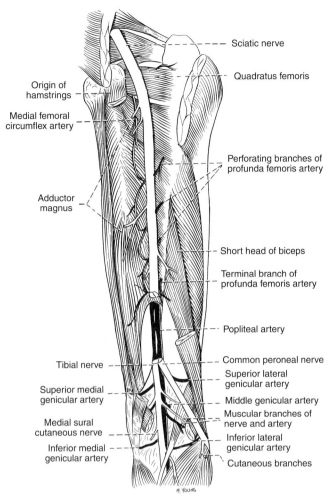

Figure 19-5 ■ The sciatic nerve (white) branches into the tibial and common peroneal nerves at the popliteal hiatus in the posterior aspect of the knee. Note that the sciatic nerve is more superficial than the popliteal artery. (From Jenkins DB: Hollinshead's Functional Anatomy of the Limbs and Back, 6th ed. Philadelphia, WB Saunders, 1991, p 266.)

Anterior tibial branch (pierces the interosseous membrane)
Posterior tibial branch
"Trifurcation" vessels
  Anterior tibial artery (branch of the popliteal artery)
  Posterior tibial artery (continuation of the popliteal artery)
  Peroneal artery (branch of the posterior tibial artery or less commonly the popliteal artery)

Important Anatomic Relationships

Medial layers of the knee (Fig. 19-7)
  Layer I—sartorius and patellar retinaculum
  Layer II—superficial MCL and the medial hamstrings
  Layer III—deep MCL and joint capsule
Lateral layers of the knee (Fig. 19-8)
  Layer I—prepatellar bursa, iliotibial tract, and biceps tendon

Layer II—patellar retinaculum
Layer III—joint capsule, LCL, arcuate ligament, and fabellofibular ligament
Popliteal fossa (Fig. 19-9)
  Borders—semimembranosus, biceps, gastrocnemius
  Floor—plantaris (medial)
  Neurovascular contents (lateral to medial)—common peroneal nerve, tibial nerve, popliteal vein, popliteal artery

SURGICAL APPROACHES TO THE KNEE

Medial Parapatellar Approach

Incision along the medial border of the quadriceps tendon, the patella, and the patellar tendon
Patella can be everted

Medial Approach

Between the sartorius and the medial patellar retinaculum
Superficial MCL is exposed
Incision posterior to the MCL for exposure of the posteromedial corner

Lateral Approach

Between the iliotibial band and the biceps femoris
LCL is exposed

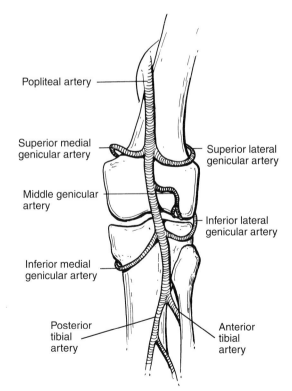

Figure 19-6 ■ The popliteal artery has several genicular branches and terminates as the anterior and posterior tibial arteries. The middle genicular artery supplies the cruciate ligaments. (From DeLee JC, Bergfeld JA, Drez D, et al: The posterior cruciate ligament. In DeLee JC, Drez D Jr [eds]: Orthopaedic Sports Medicine: Principles and Practice. Philadelphia, WB Saunders, 1994, p 1376.)

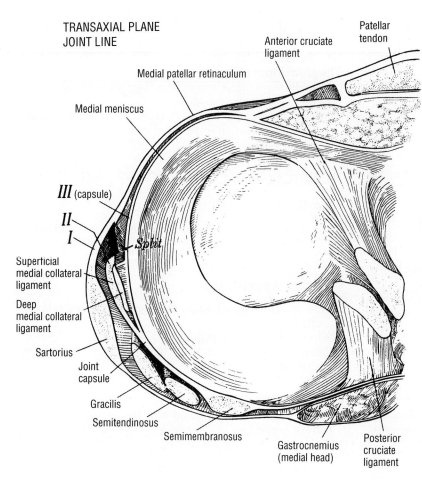

TRANSAXIAL PLANE
JOINT LINE

Anterior cruciate ligament

Patellar tendon

Medial patellar retinaculum

Medial meniscus

III (capsule)

II

I

Split

Superficial medial collateral ligament

Deep medial collateral ligament

Sartorius

Joint capsule

Gracilis

Semitendinosus

Semimembranosus

Gastrocnemius (medial head)

Posterior cruciate ligament

Figure 19–7 ■ Cross-section through the medial knee joint. Medial structures of the knee include the sartorius and the patellar retinaculum (layer I); the hamstring tendons and superficial medial collateral ligament (MCL) (layer II); and the deep MCL and joint capsule (layer III). (From Warren LF, Marshall JL: The supporting structures and layers of the medial side of the knee. J Bone Joint Surg 61A:56–62, 1979.)

Incision posterior to the LCL for exposure of the posterolateral corner

Posterior Approach

Through the popliteal fossa

Alternative approach is in the interval between the semimembranosus and the medial head of the gastrocnemius

Medial head of the gastrocnemius is retracted medially to expose the tibial insertion of the PCL

HISTORY AND PHYSICAL EXAMINATION OF THE KNEE

History

Mechanism of injury (key factor)
  Pivoting injury with a "pop" and swelling—ACL injury
  Twisting injury with a history of knee locking—meniscal tear
  Anterior force to the proximal tibia (dashboard injury)—PCL injury
  Valgus force—MCL injury
  Varus force—LCL injury
  External rotation force—posterolateral corner injury

Pain with prolonged sitting or stair climbing—patellofemoral disorders
Age
Chronicity

Physical Examination

Observation
  Gait
  Swelling (extra-articular versus intra-articular)
  Muscle atrophy
  Alignment (5 to 7 degrees of valgus is normal)
  Hyperextension (genu recurvatum)
  Flexion contracture
Palpation
  Bones
    Patella
    Distal femur
    Proximal tibia
    Joint lines (medially and laterally)
    Adductor tubercle
    Tibial tubercle
  Soft tissues
    MCL—inserts on the tibia
    LCL—inserts on the fibula
    Patellar tendon
    Quadriceps
    Menisci

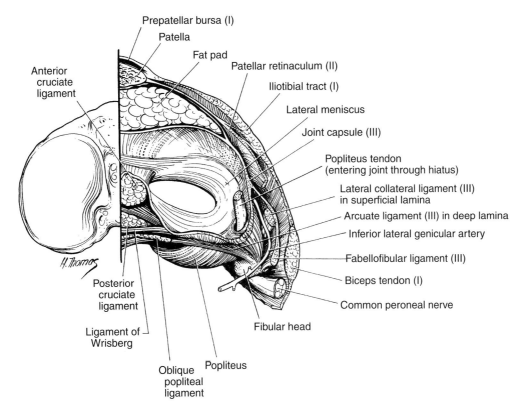

Figure 19–8 ■ Cross-section through the lateral knee joint. Lateral structures of the knee are shown and the layer they course through is indicated in parentheses. (I), layer I; (II), layer II; (III), layer III. (From Seebacher JR, Ingilis AE, Marshall JL, et al: The structure of the posterolateral aspect of the knee. J Bone Joint Surg 64A:536–541, 1982.)

Pes anserinus
Biceps femoris/iliotibial tract
Peroneal nerve
Popliteal fossa
Gastrocnemius muscles

Motion (Fig. 19–10)
  Flexion (normal, 135 degrees)
  Extension (normal, 10 degrees of hyperextension)
  Rotation (normal, 10 degrees of external/internal rotation)

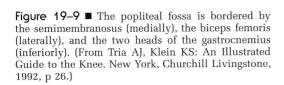

Figure 19–9 ■ The popliteal fossa is bordered by the semimembranosus (medially), the biceps femoris (laterally), and the two heads of the gastrocnemius (inferiorly). (From Tria AJ, Klein KS: An Illustrated Guide to the Knee. New York, Churchill Livingstone, 1992, p 26.)

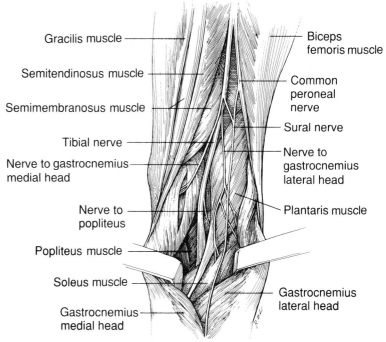

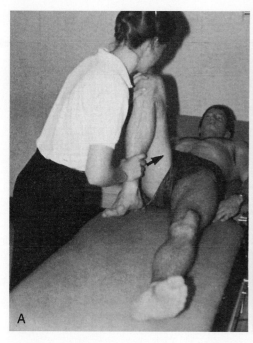 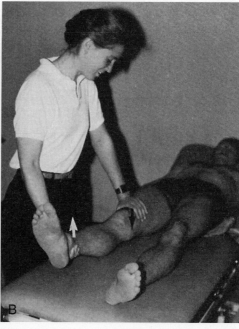

Figure 19-10 ■ Knee motion includes flexion (*A*), extension (*B*), and rotation (not shown). (From Magee DJ: Orthopedic Physical Assessment, 2nd ed. Philadelphia, WB Saunders, 1992, p 383.)

Neurovascular examination
    Pulses—popliteal artery (is palpable in the posterior aspect of the knee in the popliteal fossa)
    Sensation (see Fig. 2–5)
    Reflexes
        Patellar tendon (L4)
    Strength testing (Table 19–1)
        Knee extension (quadriceps)
        Knee flexion (hamstrings, gastrocnemius)

Special testing
    ACL laxity (Fig. 19–11)
        Lachman's test—with the knee flexed 30 degrees, an anterior force (examiner's hand positioned in the posterior calf) is used to attempt to displace the tibia anteriorly on the femur; the injured knee should be compared to the normal contralateral knee
        Anterior draw test—with the knee flexed 90 de-

Table 19-1
MUSCLES ABOUT THE KNEE: THEIR ACTIONS, NERVE SUPPLY, AND NERVE ROOT DERIVATIONS

Action	Muscles Involved	Innervation	Nerve Root Derivation
Flexion of knee	1. Biceps femoris	Sciatic	L5, S1-2
	2. Semimembranosus	Sciatic	L5, S1-2
	3. Semitendinosus	Sciatic	L5, S1-2
	4. Gracilis	Obturator	L2-3
	5. Sartorius	Femoral	L2-3
	6. Popliteus	Tibial	L4-L5, S1
	7. Gastrocnemius	Tibial	S1-2
	8. Tensor fascia lata (in 45 to 145 degrees of flexion)	Superior gluteal	L4-5
	9. Plantaris	Tibial	S1-2
Extension of knee	1. Rectus femoris	Femoral	L2-4
	2. Vastus medialis	Femoral	L2-4
	3. Vastus intermedius	Femoral	L2-4
	4. Vastus lateralis	Femoral	L2-4
	5. Tensor fascia lata (in 0 to 30 degrees of flexion)	Superior gluteal	L4-5
Medial rotation of flexed leg (non–weight bearing)	1. Popliteus	Tibial	L4-5
	2. Semimembranosus	Sciatic	L5, S1-2
	3. Semitendinosus	Sciatic	L5, S1-2
	4. Sartorius	Femoral	L2-3
	5. Gracilis	Obturator	L2-3
Lateral rotation of flexed leg (non–weight bearing)	1. Biceps femoris	Sciatic	L5, S1-2

From Magee DJ: Orthopedic Physical Assessment, 2nd ed. Philadelphia, WB Saunders, 1992, p 385.

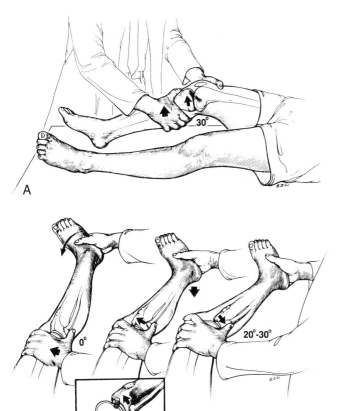

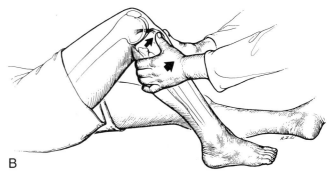

A

B

C

Figure 19–11 ■ Tests for anterior cruciate ligament laxity. *A,* Lachman's test—anterior displacement of the tibia (on the femur) with the knee flexed 30 degrees (this is the most sensitive test for anterior instability). *B,* Anterior draw test—anterior displacement of the tibia (on the femur) with the knee flexed 90 degrees. *C,* Pivot shift test—valgus and internal rotation force is applied to the knee as it is slowly flexed from the fully extended position. The knee will reduce (from its subluxed position) with a clunk (palpable, audible, visible) as the knee moves from full extension to 20 to 30 degrees of flexion. (From Tria AJ, Klein KS: An Illustrated Guide to the Knee. New York, Churchill Livingstone, 1992, pp 50–52.)

grees, an anterior force (examiner's hand positioned in the posterior calf) is used to attempt to displace the tibia anteriorly on the femur; the injured knee should be compared to the normal contralateral knee

Pivot shift test—flexion and valgus force on the extended knee with the foot in internal rotation results in reduction of the knee with a "clunk" at 20 to 30 degrees of flexion in the patient with an ACL injury

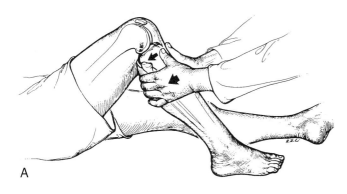

A

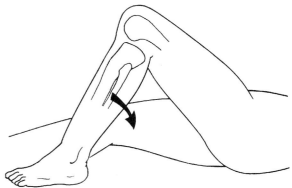

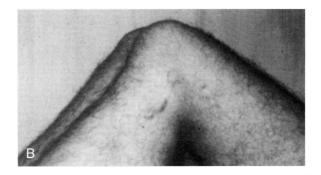

B

Figure 19–12 ■ Tests for posterior cruciate ligament laxity. *A,* Posterior draw test—posterior displacement of the tibia (on the femur) with the knee flexed 90 degrees (this is the most sensitive test for posterior instability). *B,* Posterior sag sign. Note posterior displacement of left tibia on the femur. (*A* from Tria AJ, Klein KS: An Illustrated Guide to the Knee. New York, Churchill Livingstone, 1992, p 53; *B* from O'Donoghue DH: Treatment of Injuries to Athletes, 4th ed. Philadelphia, WB Saunders, 1984, p 450.)

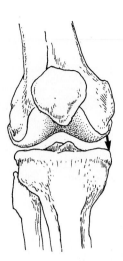

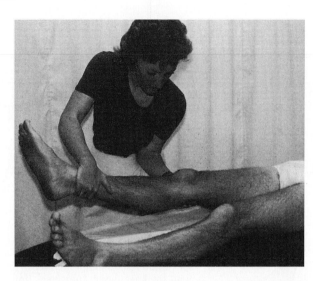

Figure 19–13 ■ Test for medial collateral ligament laxity (valgus stress test). This test must be performed with the knee positioned in 30 degrees of flexion (see explanation in text). (From Magee DJ: Orthopedic Physical Assessment, 2nd ed. Philadelphia, WB Saunders, 1992, p 396.)

PCL laxity (Fig. 19–12)

Posterior draw test—with the knee flexed 90 degrees, a posterior force displaces the tibia beyond the neutral step-off of the tibia in relation to the femur at the medial joint line in the patient with a PCL injury

Posterior sag sign—with the patient lying supine, the hip and knee are flexed 90 degrees; posterior subluxation of the tibia in relation to the femur is a positive sign

MCL laxity (Fig. 19–13)

Valgus stress test—with the knee in 30 degrees of flexion, medial joint opening of more than 5 to 10 mm is abnormal

LCL laxity (Fig. 19–14)

Varus stress test—with the knee in 30 degrees of flexion, lateral joint opening of more than 5 to 10 mm is abnormal

Note: When testing the knee for varus or valgus instability, the knee must be stressed while at 30 degrees of flexion and *not* in full extension; in full extension the PCL becomes tight and will mask an MCL or LCL tear (the knee joint will not open to varus or valgus stress in full extension even if there is a complete MCL or LCL tear); flexing the knee 30 degrees takes the tension off the PCL and allows direct examination of the collateral ligaments (MCL and LCL)

Posterolateral corner injury

Excessive external rotation of the involved leg occurs, as compared to the uninvolved leg, when the foot/ankle/tibia are stressed with an external rotation force (by the examiner) with the knee in 30 degrees of flexion

Posterolateral draw test—the foot is positioned in external rotation for a posterior draw examination; an isolated PCL injury will have diminished translation with the foot positioned in external rotation, as compared to a combined LCL and PCL injury, which will have increased translation

Reversed pivot shift test—with the foot externally rotated, the leg is brought from flexion to extension while a valgus force is applied; the shift occurs with a "clunk" as the abnormally posteriorly subluxated lateral side of the tibia reduces with the knee in 20 to 30 degrees of flexion

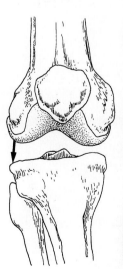

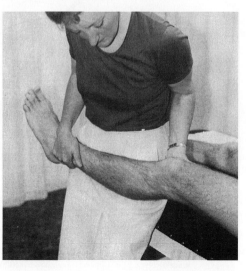

Figure 19–14 ■ Test for lateral laxity (varus stress test). This test must be performed with the knee positioned in 30 degrees of flexion (see explanation in text). (From Magee DJ: Orthopedic Physical Assessment, 2nd ed. Philadelphia, WB Saunders, 1992, p 397.)

External rotation recurvatum test—the feet are passively lifted off a flat surface with the patient supine; the injured knee falls into varus and hyperextension, and the tibia rotates externally

Meniscal injury

Joint line tenderness

McMurray's test (Fig. 19–15)—flexion of the hip and knee and rotation of tibia can result in a painful "clunk" with a displaced meniscal tear as the torn meniscus is trapped with this maneuver

Squat test/duck walk (exacerbates symptoms)

Patellofemoral pathology

Patellar tilt

Patellar glide

Patella apprehension—pain with passive lateral displacement of the patella is associated with patella instability

Q angle (Fig. 19–16)—measured from the anterior superior iliac spine to the patella to the tibial

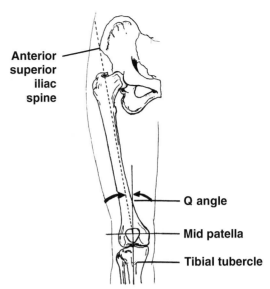

Figure 19–16 ■ Measurement of the Q angle. (From Garth WP, Fagan KM: Knee injuries in sports. *In* Masear VR [ed]: Primary Care Orthopaedics. Philadelphia, WB Saunders, 1996, p 98.)

tubercle) (normal Q angle is less than 15 degrees)

J sign—lateral deviation of the patella as the knee moves into terminal extension

DIAGNOSTIC TESTS FOR THE KNEE

Radiographic Evaluation

Standard radiographs (Fig. 19–17)

Anteroposterior (AP)

Lateral

Patellar (sunrise) view

Special findings on AP radiographs (Fig. 19–18)

Fairbank's signs (postmeniscectomy arthritis)—squaring, ridge (osteophytes), narrowing

Segond fracture (lateral capsular sign)—avulsion fracture of the proximal lateral tibial cortex associated with an ACL (and usually an MCL) injury

Pellegrini-Stieda—chronic ossification or an old avulsion fracture off the femoral side of an injured MCL

Tibial eminence avulsion fracture

Osteochondritis dissecans

Discoid meniscus

Bipartite patella—failure of ossification of the superolateral facet of the patella can be normal and may not represent a fracture

Fabella—normal sesamoid bone located in the lateral head of the gastrocnemius; can be mistaken for an avulsion fracture or loose body

Special radiographs

Flexion weight-bearing PA (Rosenberg) view (for detecting subtle arthritis) (Fig. 19–19)

Long (51-inch) cassette lower extremity view—useful for measurement of the lower extremity **mechanical and anatomic axes**

Stress views (can confirm ligamentous injuries)

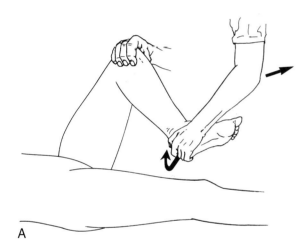

A

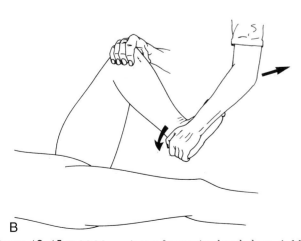

B

Figure 19–15 ■ McMurray's test for meniscal pathology. *A,* Medial meniscus. *B,* Lateral meniscus. (From Magee DJ: Orthopedic Physical Assessment, 2nd ed. Philadelphia, WB Saunders, 1992, p 413.)

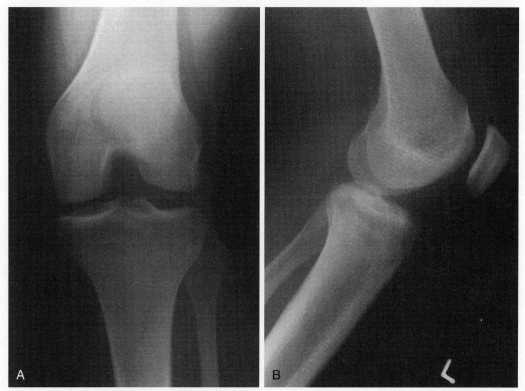

Figure 19–17 ■ AP (*A*) and lateral (*B*) radiographs of the knee. (From Garth WP, Fagan KM: Knee injuries in sports. *In* Masear VR [ed]: Primary Care Orthopaedics. Philadelphia, WB Saunders, 1996, p 89.)

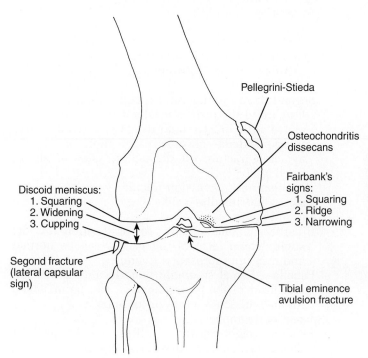

Figure 19–18 ■ Special findings that can be seen for certain conditions on the AP radiograph include Fairbank's signs (post-meniscectomy), Segond fracture (anterior cruciate ligament injury), Pellegrini-Stieda (chronic medial collateral ligament injury), and tibial eminence avulsion fracture.

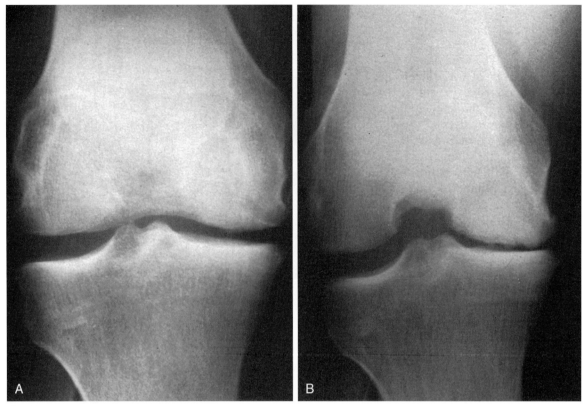

Figure 19–19 ■ Weight-bearing radiographs are essential in evaluating a patient with suspected degenerative changes. *A,* A supine AP radiograph. *B,* A standing flexion weight-bearing PA radiograph (Rosenberg view) of the same patient. Note obvious degenerative joint disease seen in *B,* but not *A.* (From Sisk TD: Knee realignment and replacement in the recreational athlete. *In* DeLee JC, Drez D Jr [eds]: Orthopaedic Sports Medicine: Principles and Practice. Philadelphia, WB Saunders, 1994, p 1479.)

Nuclear Imaging

Detects subtle arthritis and is useful in determining the extent of arthritic involvement in the individual knee compartments

Computed Tomography (CT)

Can be helpful in the evaluation of patella malalignment and for intra-articular fractures

Magnetic Resonance Imaging (MRI)
(Fig. 19–20)

Helpful in the diagnosis of injuries to the ACL, PCL, MCL, menisci, and other structures

Diagnostic Injection

Intra-articular lidocaine injection may be helpful in the evaluation of knee pain; pain from knee pathology resolves after injection, whereas referred pain will not resolve; aspiration of blood with fat droplets suggests that there is an intra-articular fracture

Arthroscopy (Fig. 19–21)

Rarely used for purely diagnostic purposes
Can confirm a diagnosis
Useful therapeutic (operative) tool

COMMON ADULT CONDITIONS OF THE KNEE

Meniscal Pathology

Meniscal tears—injury to the fibrocartilaginous meniscus
  Medial tears are three times more common than lateral tears
  Traumatic, longitudinal tears are common in younger patients
  Chronic, degenerative tears are more common in older patients
  Classification of meniscal tears (Fig. 19–22)
  Treatment options
    Partial meniscectomy
    Meniscal repair—performed only for peripheral tears (risk injury to the saphenous nerve for repair of the medial meniscus and the peroneal nerve for repair of the lateral meniscus)
Baker's (popliteal) cyst—can be associated with a meniscal tear or another intra-articular process; rarely requires treatment other than addressing the etiologic factor
Meniscal cyst—fluid-filled cyst projecting subcutaneously from a meniscal tear
  Typically the lateral meniscus is involved
  Horizontal cleavage tear of the meniscus is usually present

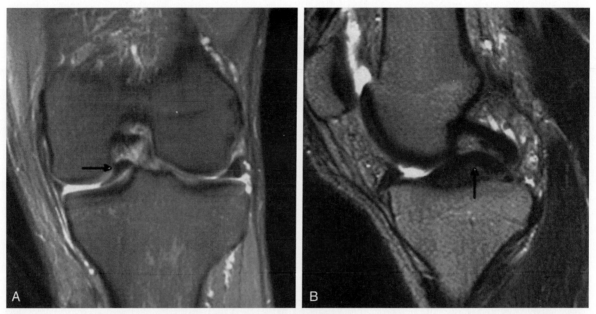

Figure 19–20 ■ MRI of the knee. *Arrows* show the displaced bucket-handle tear of the medial meniscus. ACL tear. (From Miller MD, Osborne JR, Warner JJP, et al: MRI-Arthroscopy Correlative Atlas. Philadelphia, WB Saunders, 1997, p 55.)

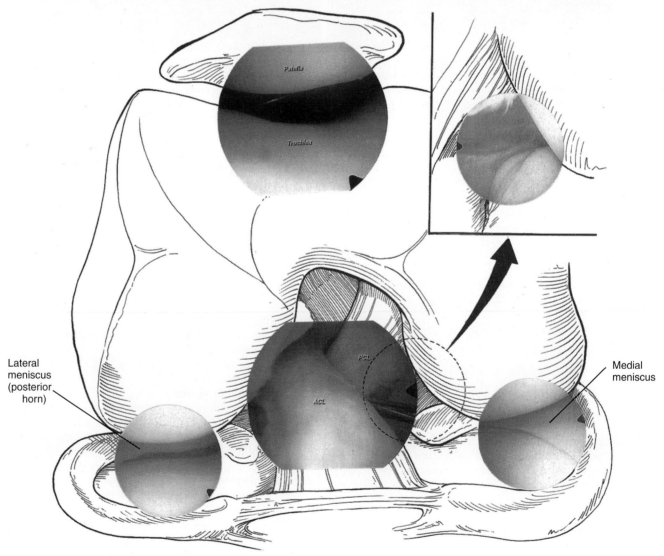

Figure 19–21 ■ Arthroscopic anatomy of the knee. ACL, anterior cruciate ligament; PCL, posterior cruciate ligament. (From Miller MD, Osborne JR, Warner JJP, et al: MRI-Arthroscopy Correlative Atlas. Philadelphia, WB Saunders, 1997, p 51.)

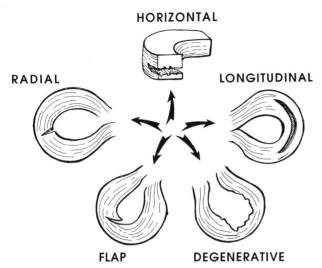

Figure 19–22 ■ The five basic types of meniscal tears. (From Fu FH, Baratz M: Meniscal injuries. *In* DeLee JC, Drez D Jr [eds]: Orthopaedic Sports Medicine: Principles and Practice. Philadelphia, WB Saunders, 1994, p 1149.)

Treatment—arthroscopic partial meniscectomy and decompression of the cyst
Discoid meniscus—thickened, incompletely developed meniscus that can involve (cover) the entire tibial plateau
Typically the lateral meniscus is involved
Plain radiographs (see Fig. 19–18)
   Widened knee joint space
   Squaring of the lateral femoral condyle
   Cupping of the lateral tibial plateau
   Hypoplastic lateral intercondylar spine
Classification
   Incomplete
   Complete
   Wrisberg (snapping) variant—no peripheral (capsular) attachments to the discoid meniscus are present
Meniscal transplantation—replacement of a damaged meniscus with a donor graft
Controversial
Investigational
Indications unclear

Osteochondral Lesions

Osteochondritis dissicans (OCD) (Fig. 19–23)—separation of cartilage and subchondral bone
   Etiology—occult trauma (vascular insult?)
   Location—usually involves the **lateral aspect of the medial femoral condyle**
   Treatment—operative excision or fixation
Articular cartilage injury
   Delaminating injury of the articular cartilage from the subchondral bone
   Typically involves the medial femoral condyle
   Usually from a shearing injury
   Treatment—operative débridement/chondroplasty
Loose bodies

Can occur from fractures or other injuries
Usually require removal

Synovial Lesions

Pigmented villonodular synovitis (PVNS) (Fig. 19–24)—proliferation of diseased synovium in the knee joint
   Symptoms—pain, swelling, mass
   Treatment—operative synovectomy
Other forms of synovitis
   Rheumatoid, osteochondromatosis, hemophilia
   Treatment—operative synovectomy
Synovial plica—thickened band of synovial tissue
   Medial patellar plica (synovial shelf)
   The plica can abrade the medial femoral condyle
   Occasionally may require operative resection
   Diagnosis is overused

Ligamentous Injuries

ACL
   Noncontact pivoting injury
   A "pop" is felt by the patient
   Acute knee swelling (hemarthrosis)
   Examination
      Lachman's test is the most sensitive for an acute injury

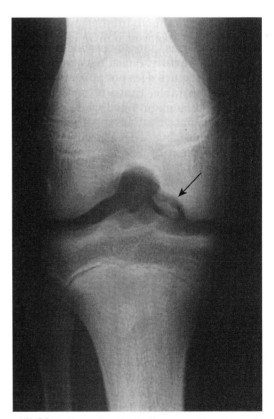

Figure 19–23 ■ Osteochondritis dissecans. Note loose fragment on the lateral aspect of the medial femoral condyle (*arrow*). (From Garth WP, Fagan KM: Knee injuries in sports. *In* Masear VR [ed]: Primary Care Orthopaedics. Philadelphia, WB Saunders, 1996, p 92.)

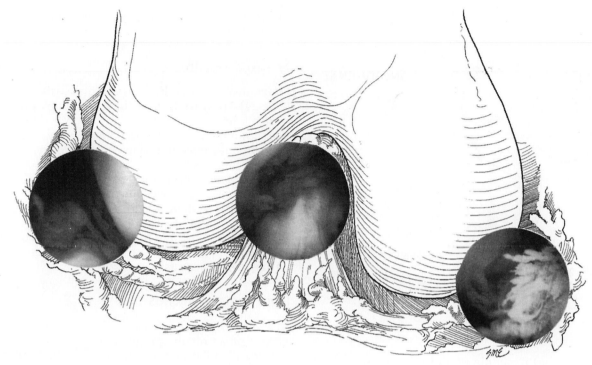

Figure 19–24 ■ Arthroscopic appearance of pigmented villonodular synovitis. (From Miller MD, Osborne JR, Warner JJP, et al: MRI-Arthroscopy Correlative Atlas. Philadelphia, WB Saunders, 1997.)

Pivot shift test is a sensitive examination under anesthesia

Treatment options

Nonoperative—quadriceps rehabilitation, functional bracing

Operative—arthroscopically assisted ACL reconstruction (patellar tendon or hamstring graft is commonly used to reconstruct the ACL)

PCL

Mechanism of injury

Blow to the anterior tibia with the knee flexed (dashboard injury)

Examination

Posterior draw is the most sensitive examination

Treatment options

Nonoperative—quadriceps rehabilitation; recent reports suggest that nonoperative management may result in late chondrosis (degenerative changes) of the patella and the medial femoral condyle

Operative—arthroscopically assisted PCL reconstruction

MCL

Mechanism of injury

Valgus (contact) stress

Examination

Valgus stress opening of the medial side of the knee (with the knee examined in a position of 30 degrees of flexion) (see Fig. 19–13)

Joint laxity is graded in millimeters of opening

Grade 1   1–5 mm
Grade 2   6–10 mm
Grade 3   >10 mm

Treatment options

Nonoperative—hinged knee brace for 6 to 8 weeks

Operative—only for failure of nonoperative management

LCL

Mechanism of injury

Varus stress

Examination

Varus stress opening of the lateral side of the knee (with the knee examined in a position of 30 degrees of flexion) (see Fig. 19–14)

Joint laxity is graded in millimeters of opening (same method as used for MCL injuries)

Treatment options

Nonoperative—hinged knee brace for 6 to 8 weeks

Operative repair/reconstruction

Posterolateral corner of the knee

Components

LCL

Arcuate ligament

Popliteus tendon

Lateral head of the gastrocnemius

Popliteofibular ligament

Short lateral ligament

Fabellofibular ligament

Posterolateral capsule

"Arcuate ligament complex"—historical term used to describe the arcuate ligament, the LCL, the popliteus, and the lateral head of the gastrocnemius; this term has been largely replaced with the individual terms described above or the "posterolateral corner" to describe all of the structures in this area

Injuries are usually combined with other ligamentous injuries (especially the PCL)

Mechanism of injury

Excessive external rotation force

Examination

Excessive external rotation (as compared to the opposite normal side)

Other (less consistent) tests

External rotation recurvatum

Posterolateral draw

Reversed pivot shift

Treatment

Acute repair offers the most consistent results

Delayed reconstructions are less predictable

Multiple ligament injury

Likely to be associated with a knee (tibiofemoral) dislocation

An arteriogram to assess vascular status is mandatory in the patient with a knee dislocation

Note: **A knee dislocation refers to dislocation of the tibia on the femur; this is a much more severe injury than a patella dislocation, which is not commonly referred to as a "knee dislocation"**

Diagnosis

Clinical examination and radiographs

Classification—based on the direction of displacement of the tibia (Fig. 19–25)

Treatment

Reduction

Delayed reconstruction of the torn ligaments at 5 to 7 days after injury

Primary repair of bony avulsions

Reconstruction of intrasubstance ligament injuries

Anterior Knee Pain

Quadriceps tendon rupture

More common in patients over 40 years of age

Palpable defect in the quadriceps tendon

Inability of the patient to actively extend the knee

Primary operative repair is favored

Patellar tendon rupture

More common in younger patients

Palpable defect in the patellar tendon

Inability of the patient to actively extend the knee

Primary operative repair favored

Patellar tendinitis (jumper's knee)

Common in athletes who participate in jumping sports (volleyball/basketball)

Pain at the inferior pole of the patella; pain becomes worse with the knee in extension

Nonoperative treatment—stretching/strengthening, ultrasound, orthoses

Operative treatment—operative excision of necrotic fibers

Quadriceps tendinitis

Painful clicking, localized pain

Supportive treatment

Prepatellar bursitis (housemaid's knee)

History of prolonged kneeling (on prepatellar bursa)

Pain to palpation over **swollen** prepatellar bursa

Supportive treatment

Pes anserinus bursitis

Painful swelling at the insertion of the sartorius, gracilis, and semitendinosus muscles at the anteromedial aspect of the proximal tibia (approximately 5 cm below the anteromedial joint line)

Treatment includes application of heat, NSAIDs, and activity restriction; judicious use of steroid injections can also be helpful

Synovial plica (discussed above)

Anterior fat pad syndrome (Hoffa's syndrome)

Fibrosis of the anterior fat pad

Diagnosis aided by local injection (relieves symptoms)

Arthroscopic excision sometimes necessary

Patellofemoral disorders

Lateral patellar compression syndrome

Tight lateral retinaculum with lateral tilting of the patella

Treatment

Nonoperative—activity modification, NSAIDs, strengthening of the vastus medialis obliquus (VMO) muscle

Operative—lateral retinacular release

Patellar instability

Etiology—abnormal alignment of the lower extremity, excessive Q angle, patella alta, poorly developed vastus medialis musculature, and

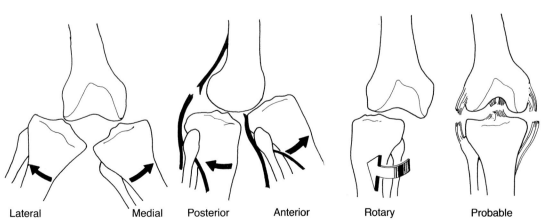

Figure 19–25 ■ Classification of knee dislocations is based on the direction of the displaced tibia. (From Miller MD, Cooper DE, Warner JJP: Review of Sports Medicine and Arthroscopy. Philadelphia, WB Saunders, 1995, p 51.)

systemic ligamentous laxity are all related to the development of patellar instability

Diagnosis—excessive lateral mobility of the patella, apprehension (to the examiner's attempt to push the patella laterally); radiographs and CT can be helpful in evaluating patellar tracking

Rehabilitation—the mainstay of treatment; emphasize closed-chain quadriceps rehabilitation

Proximal and/or distal operative realignment for cases that fail to improve with rehabilitation

Chondromalacia
  "Softening" or degeneration of the articular cartilage on the undersurface of the patella; classification is based on four stages (Outerbridge)
  Pathologic diagnosis
  Treatment options limited

Abnormalities of patellar height (Fig. 19–26)
  Patella alta—high-riding patella; may be associated with patellar instability
  Patella baja—low-riding patella; may be associated with arthrofibrosis (stiff knee)

Patellofemoral arthritis
  Injuries and malalignment contribute
  Supportive treatment/VMO strengthening
  Late—anteromedial tibial tubercle transfer

Other Causes of Knee Pain

Iliotibial band friction syndrome
  Common in runners and cyclists
  Localized tenderness over the iliotibial band with the knee in 30 degrees of flexion
  Treatment is rehabilitation (occasional surgery)

Semimembranosus tendinitis
  Common in male athletes in their 30s
  Localized tenderness over the semimembranosus tendon
  MRI scan may be helpful for making the diagnosis
  Treatment is stretching and strengthening

Tibiofemoral arthritis

Etiology
  Trauma
    After surgery (meniscectomy)
  Genetic?

Diagnosis
  Pain, crepitus
  Loss of knee range of motion
  Radiographic findings
    Fairbank's signs (see Fig. 19–18)
    Squaring of the condyles
    Osteophyte formation and sclerosis
    Narrowing of the joint space
    Flexion weight-bearing PA (Rosenberg view) may be helpful (see Fig. 19–19)

Treatment options
  Nonoperative—NSAIDs, activity modification, cane, physical therapy
  Operative
    Arthroscopic débridement—questionable efficacy, only short-term relief
    Proximal tibial osteotomy or distal femoral osteotomy—performed to alter the mechanical axis of the lower extremity and thereby shift the line of force away from the arthritic portion of the tibiofemoral articulation; it is best used in cases where only one compartment of the knee joint is primarily involved (for example, arthritis of the medial compartment of the tibiofemoral articulation could be treated with a valgus-forming osteotomy that would shift the mechanical axis of the lower extremity laterally [into the lateral compartment], which would unload the arthritic medial compartment)
  Total knee arthroplasty
    Contraindications to total knee arthroplasty
      Nonfunctioning knee extensors
      Active sepsis
      Prior knee fusion
      Neuropathic knee joint

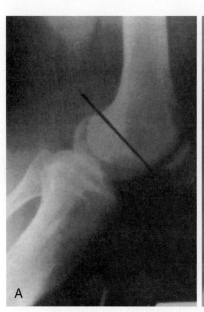
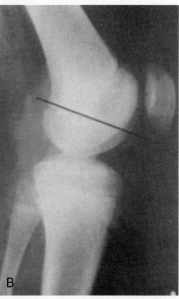

Figure 19–26 ■ Lateral radiographs taken at 30 to 45 degrees of knee flexion can be used to estimate patellar height. *A,* Normally the inferior pole of the patella will intersect the intercondylar (Blumensaat's) line of the femur. *B,* Patella alta—the inferior pole of the patella is well superior to this line. (From Hughston JC, et al: Patellar Subluxation and Dislocation. Philadelphia, WB Saunders, 1984, p 52.)

Technique challenges of total knee arthroplasty

Ensure that the knee joint is horizontal (parallel to the ankle joint and floor) in the stance phase of gait

Restore the anatomic and mechanical axes of the lower extremity (Fig. 19–27)

Ensure that the flexion gap is equal to the extension gap so that the knee ligaments are well balanced

Proper soft tissue balancing

Proper patella placement and alignment

Complications of total knee arthroplasty

Infection

Patella fracture

Patella dislocation

Component loosening

Tibial tray (polyethylene) wear

Peroneal nerve palsy

Supracondylar femur fracture

Wound problems and skin slough

Decreased knee range of motion

Reflex Sympathetic Dystrophy (RSD)

Pain out of proportion to the physical findings

Aggravated response to an injury

Three stages

Swelling, warmth, hyperhidrosis

Brawny edema, trophic skin changes

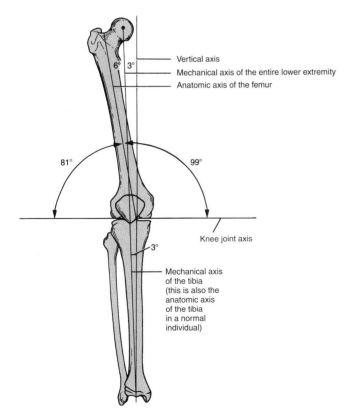

Figure 19–27 ■ Lower extremity axes. (Modified from Helfet DL: Fractures of the distal femur. *In* Browner BD, Jupiter JB, Levine AM, et al [eds]: Skeletal Trauma. Philadelphia, WB Saunders, 1992, p 1645.)

Glossy, cool, dry skin and stiffness

Treatment

Aggressive physical therapy

Nerve stimulation

NSAIDs

Sympathetic block (also diagnostic)

For more information on RSD, see Chapter 3

Osteonecrosis

Death of bone cells as a result of ischemia

Associated with fractures, thrombosis, and vascular injury

Commonly involves the medial femoral condyle (Fig. 19–28)

"Bone infarct" is a localized area of osteonecrosis away from the joint (usually at the metaphyseal-diaphyseal junction)

Plain radiographs are usually diagnostic; MRI can be helpful in the early stages

Treatment can include osteotomies or unicompartmental arthroplasty

Nonunion/Malunion of Fractures

Management can be difficult and must be individualized based on the fracture, alignment, and patient activity demands

FRACTURES AND DISLOCATIONS OF THE KNEE

Overview (Tables 19–2 and 19–3)

Supracondylar femur fractures (Fig. 19–29) are usually treated with a blade plate, a dynamic compression screw, or a retrograde intramedullary nail; anatomic alignment of intra-articular components is key

Patella fractures (Fig. 19–30) can be treated with immobilization in extension only if the patient can perform a straight leg raise and the fracture fragments are minimally displaced; tension band wiring is usually successful for displaced fractures; articular fragments and those that occur as a result of a patella dislocation are best removed arthroscopically

Fractures of the tibial plateau (Fig. 19–31) require precise reduction and fixation; adjunctive arthroscopy is often helpful in achieving reduction; these fractures often require a side plate for "buttressing" the fracture

Tibial spine (eminence) fractures (Fig. 19–32) can often be reduced with extension casting; operative repair of a bony avulsion is favored if the fragment remains displaced

Displaced avulsion fractures of the tibial tubercle and proximal fibula often require operative reduction and fixation

Tendon avulsions require operative treatment

Patella dislocations are usually treated with immobilization in extension; arthroscopic removal of asso-

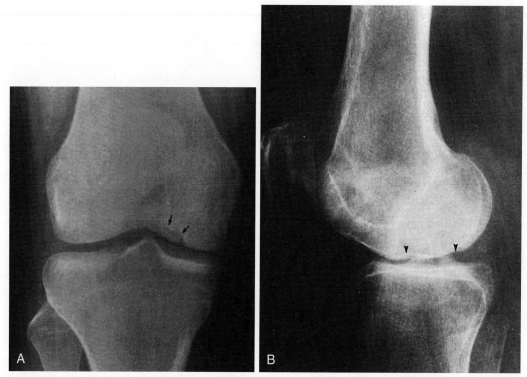

Figure 19–28 ■ AP (*A*) and lateral (*B*) radiographs showing osteonecrosis of the medial femoral condyle. Note flattening of the medial femoral condyle on AP and lateral views (*arrowheads*). (From Weissman BNW, Sledge CB: Orthopedic Radiology. Philadelphia, WB Saunders, 1986, p 551.)

Table 19–2
FRACTURES OF THE ADULT KNEE

Fracture	Classification	Treatment	Most Common Complications of the Injury
Supracondylar femur (less than 8 cm above the knee joint; proximal to this would be a femoral shaft fracture) (see Fig. 19–29)	Descriptive	Operative treatment	Knee stiffness, post-traumatic arthritis, popliteal artery injury, malunion, nonunion, DVT, PE
Patella (see Fig. 19–30)	Descriptive Undisplaced Displaced	Cylinder cast ORIF (fragment excision for highly comminuted fractures)	Avascular necrosis, post-traumatic arthritis
Chondral/osteochondral fractures (distal femur, proximal tibia, patella)		Athroscopic examination with fixation and débridement as needed	Post-traumatic arthritis
Tibial plateau (see Fig. 19–31)	Hohl; Shatzker; AO group; descriptive (medial vs. lateral plateau, extent of displacement and comminution, etc.)	Anatomic reduction; operative treatment most commonly required (internal and/or external fixation)	Post-traumatic arthritis, knee stiffness, avascular necrosis
Tibial spine (eminence) (see Fig. 19–32)	Meyers and McKeever (I–III)	Closed reduction of fracture by placing knee in full extension, place in long leg cast × 6 weeks; ORIF if fracture is unreducible using closed manipulation	Decreased ROM
Tibial tubercle		Operative fixation (most commonly screw or staple)	Extensor mechanism weakness or malalignment
Proximal fibular		Closed treatment (ORIF if knee is unstable)	

AO, Arbeitgemeinschaft für Osteosynthesefragen; DVT, deep venous thrombosis; ORIF, open reduction with internal fixation; PE, pulmonary embolism; ROM, range of motion.

Table 19–3
DISLOCATIONS AND SOFT TISSUE INJURIES OF THE ADULT KNEE

Injury	Classification	Treatment	Most Common Complications of the Injury
Quadriceps rupture		Operative repair	
Patellar tendon rupture		Operative repair	Missed diagnosis
Patella dislocation (almost always dislocates laterally)	Acute, recurrent, subluxation	Cylinder cast × 4 weeks followed by rehabilitation; operative treatment for acute dislocation with associated fractures or recurrent subluxations or dislocations despite full rehab trial	Recurrence
Knee (tibiofemoral) dislocation (see Fig. 19–33)	Descriptive	Reduce emergently, arteriogram mandatory; closed immobilization vs. operative stabilization depending on exact nature of ligamentous (and vascular) injuries	Popliteal artery injury, ACL injury, tibial and peroneal nerve injuries
Proximal tibiofibular dislocation	Descriptive	Closed reduction (flex knee to 90 degrees); ORIF for failed closed reduction or knee instability	

ACL, anterior cruciate ligament; ORIF, open reduction with internal fixation.

ciated loose bodies is appropriate when they are identified; recurrent instability may require proximal and/or distal realignment procedures

Knee dislocations (Fig. 19–33) are a true orthopaedic emergency; reduction and vascular evaluation (with arteriography) are essential; timing of surgical repair (of the ligaments) is controversial

Proximal tibiofibular dislocation is unusual but can be treated with closed reduction in most cases

TUMORS OF THE KNEE

Bone

Osteosarcoma (parosteal)
Malignant fibrous histiocytoma

Fibrosarcoma
Giant cell tumor
Chondromyxoid fibroma

Soft Tissue

Pigmented villonodular synovitis
Synovial chondromatosis
Synovial sarcoma

DIFFERENTIAL DIAGNOSIS OF COMMON KNEE COMPLAINTS

Pain

Ligamentous injuries
Meniscal tears
Osteochondral lesions
Synovial lesions
Fractures
Dislocations
Arthritis
Rheumatologic conditions
Bursitis
Tumors
Infection

Instability

Ligamentous injury
Patellofemoral laxity

Weakness

Tendon injury/rupture
Neuromuscular abnormalities
Traumatic nerve injuries
Fractures
Tumors

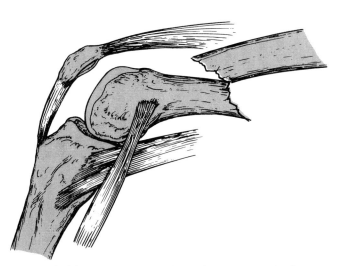

Figure 19–29 ■ Supracondylar femur fractures occur in the zone between the distal diaphysis and the articular condyles. These fractures are displaced by the quadriceps, posterior hamstrings, and gastrocnemius. (From Helfet DL: Fractures of the distal femur. *In* Browner BD, Jupiter JB, Levine AM, et al [eds]: Skeletal Trauma. Philadelphia, WB Saunders, 1992, p 1644.)

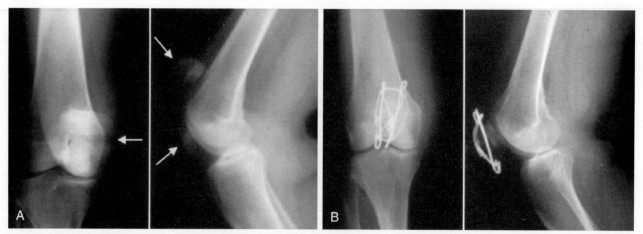

Figure 19–30 ■ *A*, AP and lateral radiographs of a displaced patella fracture (*arrow* shows the fracture line on the AP view; *arrows* show the two major fracture fragments on the lateral view). *B*, AP and lateral radiographs following ORIF with a tension band wire technique. (Courtesy of Robert H. Fain Jr., Fondren Orthopedic Group LLP, Texas Orthopedic Hospital, Houston, Texas.)

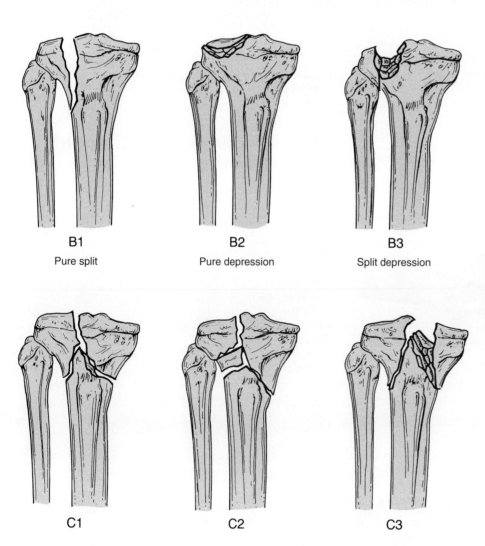

B1
Pure split

B2
Pure depression

B3
Split depression

C1

C2

C3

Figure 19–31 ■ AO (Arbeitgemeinschaft für Osteosynthesefragen) classification of tibial plateau fractures. (From Schatzker J: Tibial plateau fractures. *In* Browner BD, Jupiter JB, Levine AM, et al [eds]: Skeletal Trauma. Philadelphia, WB Saunders, 1992, p 1750.)

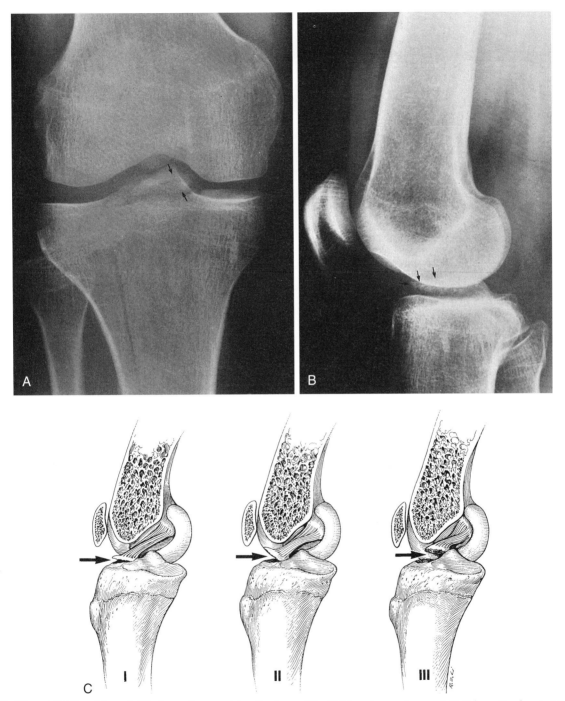

Figure 19–32 ■ AP (*A*) and lateral (*B*) views of an avulsion fracture of the tibial eminence (*arrows*). *C,* Schematic showing Meyers and McKeever classification of tibial eminence fractures. (*A* and *B* from Weissman BNW, Sledge CB: Orthopedic Radiology. Philadelphia, WB Saunders, 1986, p 513; *C* from Tria AJ, Klein KS: An Illustrated Guide to The Knee. New York, Churchill Livingstone, 1992, p 108.)

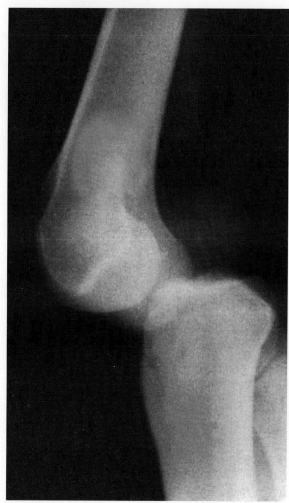

Figure 19–33 ■ Posterior knee dislocation as seen on a lateral x-ray of the knee. (From Leffers D: Dislocations and soft tissue injuries of the knee. *In* Browner BD, Jupiter JB, Levine AM, et al [eds]: Skeletal Trauma. Philadelphia, WB Saunders, 1992, p 1726.)

Tingling/Loss of Sensation

Lumbosacral plexus injury
Peripheral nerve injuries or entrapments

Effusion

Ligamentous injuries
Meniscal tears
Osteochondral lesions
Synovial lesions
Arthritis
Rheumatologic conditions
Fractures
Dislocations

Deformity

Patella dislocation
Knee (tibiofemoral) dislocation
Arthritis
Rheumatologic conditions
Fractures (and fracture malunions)
Soft tissue ruptures
Tumors/cysts

Catching/Locking

Meniscal tears
Osteochondral lesions
Loose bodies

Loss of Motion

Effusion
Locked meniscal tear
Loose bodies
Tendon injury/rupture
Arthritis
Rheumatologic conditions
Fractures
Dislocations
Infection
Tumors
Nerve injuries

PEARLS AND PITFALLS

An acute knee effusion after an injury is usually caused by a meniscal or an ACL injury
The medial meniscus is more commonly injured than the lateral meniscus
A valgus stress injury to the knee may result in the "unhappy triad"; injury to the ACL, the MCL, and one of the menisci
Key diagnostic examination techniques for the knee include
  Lachman's test—ACL injury
  Posterior draw test—PCL injury
  Valgus/varus stress testing at 30 degrees flexion—MCL or LCL injury
  Asymmetric external rotation—posterolateral corner injury
  Joint line tenderness (especially in flexion)—meniscal injuries
Knee dislocations mandate an arteriogram
Standing flexion weight-bearing views are helpful in the identification of early arthritis
Displaced intra-articular fractures around the knee generally require operative treatment

CHAPTER 20

The Adult Leg

LEG ANATOMY

Bones (Fig. 20–1)

Tibia
Fibula

Muscles (Four Compartments of the Leg)
(Fig. 20–2)

Anterior compartment
  Tibialis anterior (TA) (deep peroneal nerve)
  Extensor hallucis longus (EHL) (deep peroneal nerve)
  Extensor digitorum longus (EDL) (deep peroneal nerve)
  Peroneus tertius (deep peroneal nerve)
Lateral compartment
  Peroneus longus (PL) (superficial peroneal nerve)
  Peroneus brevis (PB) (superficial peroneal nerve)
Superficial posterior compartment
  Gastrocnemius (tibial nerve)
  Soleus (tibial nerve)
  Plantaris (tibial nerve)
Deep posterior compartment
  Popliteus (tibial nerve)
  Flexor hallucis longus (FHL) (tibial nerve)
  Flexor digitorum longus (FDL) (tibial nerve)
  Tibialis posterior (TP) (tibial nerve)
    Sometimes considered as a separate (fifth) compartment

Nerves (Fig. 20–3)

Tibial nerve (posterior leg)
Common peroneal nerve
  Superficial branch—lateral compartment
  Deep branch—anterior compartment

Vessels (see Fig. 20–3)

Anterior tibial artery—runs between the TA and the EHL
Posterior tibial artery—runs medially in the leg
Peroneal artery—branches from the posterior tibial artery (or less commonly from the popliteal artery)

SURGICAL APPROACHES TO THE LEG

Anterior Approach

Subperiosteal dissection of the tibialis anterior off the tibia

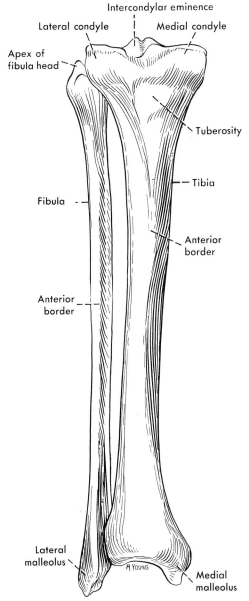

Figure 20–1 ■ Bones of the leg include the tibia and fibula. (From Jenkins DB: Hollinshead's Functional Anatomy of the Limbs and Back, 6th ed. Philadelphia, WB Saunders, 1991, p 285.)

Posterolateral Approach

Between the FHL and the peroneal muscles
FHL is detached from its origin on the fibula; the

317

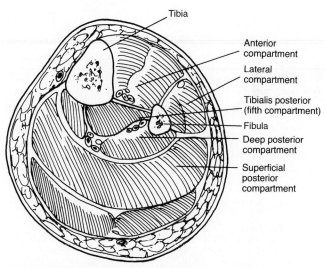

Figure 20–2 ■ Cross-sectional diagram showing the compartments of the leg. (From Andrish JT: The leg. *In* DeLee JC, Drez D Jr [eds]: *Orthopaedic Sports Medicine: Principles and Practice.* Philadelphia, WB Saunders, 1994, p 1605.)

TP is reflected to expose the posterior surface of the tibia

HISTORY AND PHYSICAL EXAMINATION OF THE LEG

History

Mechanism of injury
Referred pain to the leg may be from the lumbar spine, hip, or knee
Chronicity of symptoms

Physical Examination

Observation
  Abnormal contours
Palpation (for pain, defects)
  Tibia
  Fibula
  Muscles (four compartments)
Neurovascular exam
  Distal function (tibial nerve, peroneal nerve)
  Pulses—dorsalis pedis and posterior tibial
  Sensation (see Fig. 2–5)
  Strength testing—ankle and foot

DIAGNOSTIC TESTS FOR THE LEG

Radiographs

Anteroposterior
Lateral

Imaging

Computed tomography
  Helps define the fracture pattern in high-energy distal tibia (pilon) fractures (Fig. 20–4)

Magnetic resonance imaging
  Work-up of a tumor (mass)

COMMON ADULT CONDITIONS OF THE LEG

Gastrocnemius-Soleus Strain or Rupture

"Tennis leg"
Mechanism of injury

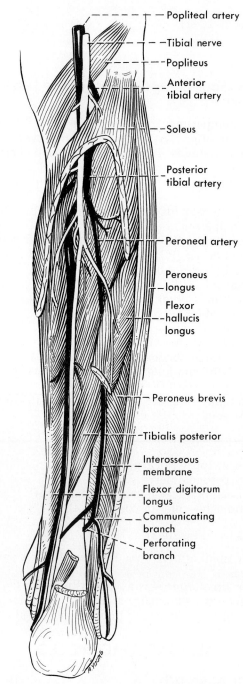

Figure 20–3 ■ Nerves (*white*) and arteries (*black*) of the posterior leg. (From Jenkins DB: Hollinshead's Functional Anatomy of the Limbs and Back, 6th ed. Philadelphia, WB Saunders, 1991, p 292.)

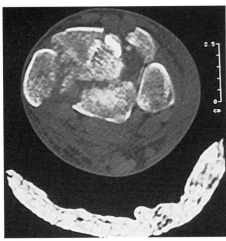

Figure 20–4 ■ CT scan of an intra-articular distal tibial (pilon) fracture. (Courtesy of Fondren Orthopedic Group LLP, Texas Orthopedic Hospital, Houston, Texas.)

Forced plantar flexion of the ankle while pushing off
Diagnosis
    Localized pain and swelling of the calf
Treatment
    Nonoperative—rest, ice, immobilization

Shin Splints

Exercise-related periostitis of the tibialis posterior origin in the posterior aspect of the mid to distal tibial shaft
Pain and tenderness are common
X-rays may demonstrate periosteal changes
Treatment is supportive

Stress Fracture of the Tibia

Associated with overuse, amenorrhea, and osteoporosis
A bone scan can be helpful in making the diagnosis (Fig. 20–5)
Treatment—activity modification, non–weight bearing (crutches)

Exertional Compartment Syndrome

Elevated pressures in a confined fascial space after exercise
Diagnosis
    Exercise-related pain
    Compartment pressures are measured before, dur-

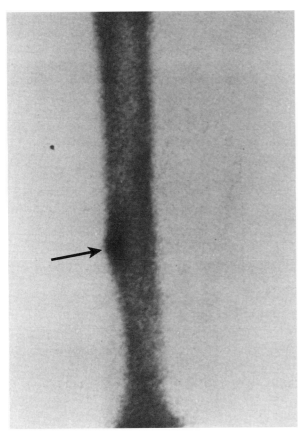

Figure 20–5 ■ Bone scan demonstrating a tibial stress fracture. *Arrow* shows the area of increased uptake. (From Andrish JT: The leg. *In* DeLee JC, Drez D Jr [eds]: Orthopaedic Sports Medicine: Principles and Practice. Philadelphia, WB Saunders, 1994, p 1611.)

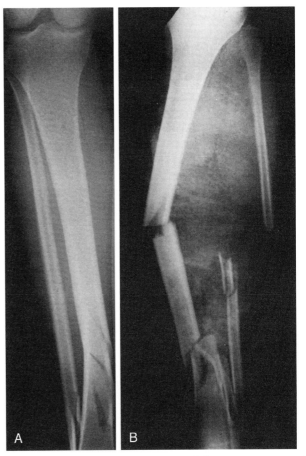

Figure 20–6 ■ Tibial shaft fractures of different severity. *A,* Minor severity. *B,* Major severity (high-energy segmental fracture). (From Trafton PG: Tibial shaft fractures. *In* Browner BD, Jupiter JB, Levine AM, et al [eds]: Skeletal Trauma. Philadelphia, WB Saunders, 1992, p 1786.)

ing, and after exercise as measured in an acute compartment syndrome (see Chapter 3)

Resting compartment pressure greater than 15 mm Hg is abnormal

Delay in normalization of compartment pressures to less than 20 mm Hg 5 minutes after exercise is also abnormal

Treatment

Activity modification

Surgical release (fasciotomy) for refractory cases with significant painful symptoms

Nerve Entrapment Syndromes

Common

Present with localized pain, tenderness, paresthesias in the dermatomal distribution of the nerve, and a positive Tinel's at the site of entrapment

Examples

Saphenous nerve

Common peroneal nerve

Superficial peroneal nerve

FRACTURES AND DISLOCATIONS OF THE LEG

Overview

Tibial shaft fractures (Fig. 20–6)

Tibial shaft fractures (see Fig. 20–6)—the most common fracture of the long bones

Can result from direct trauma or rotational injuries

Every patient with a tibial shaft fracture should be closely monitored (admitted for at least 24 hours) for the development of a compartment syndrome

The type of treatment is based on the stability of the fracture pattern and a number of other clinical factors (Table 20–1)

Because of the subcutaneous position of the tibia, open fractures are not uncommon; aggressive débridement is important to avoid the development of a deep infection

Soft tissue loss in open fractures can also be a challenging problem

Table 20–1
FRACTURES OF THE ADULT TIBIA AND FIBULA

Fracture	Eponym or Other Name	Classification	Treatment	Most Common Complications of the Injury

Tibial shaft (see Fig. 20–6)		Descriptive	Most can be treated with long leg cast for 6 weeks followed by patella tendon–bearing cast
			Indications for operative treatment (most commonly intramedullary rod fixation for closed fractures and lesser open fractures [type I or II] or external fixation for severe [type III] open fractures) include
			  1. Unstable fracture pattern
			  2. Inability to maintain reduction in cast
			  3. Associated vascular injuries
			  4. Open fractures
			  5. Pathologic fractures
			  6. Polytrauma patient
			  7. Segmental fractures
			  8. Bilateral tibia fractures
			  9. Associated ipsilateral lower-extremity fractures
			  10. Floating knee injuries (ipsilateral tibia and femur fractures)
			  11. Severe knee ligamentous injuries
			Consider amputation for
			  1. Type IIIC injury
			  2. Tibial nerve injury (insensate foot)
			  3. Ischemia >8 hours
			  4. Severe ipsilateral foot injury
				Delayed union, nonunion, malunion, infection

Stress fracture tibial shaft (see Fig. 20–5)			Activity modification, symptomatic casting, avoidance of athletic activity for 6–12 weeks	Progression to a complete fracture
Fibular shaft			Short leg cast	
Tibial plafond (distal tibia) (see Figs. 20–4 and 20–7)	Pilon	Reudi and Allgower (I–III)		Post-traumatic arthritis, malunion, nonunion
		I. Minimally displaced	Long leg cast (non–weight bearing)	
		II. Incongruous	Operative stabilization (internal and/or external fixation)	Post-traumatic arthritis
		III. Comminuted	Operative stabilization (external fixation best because of tenuous soft tissue envelope overlying the distal tibia)	Post-traumatic arthritis

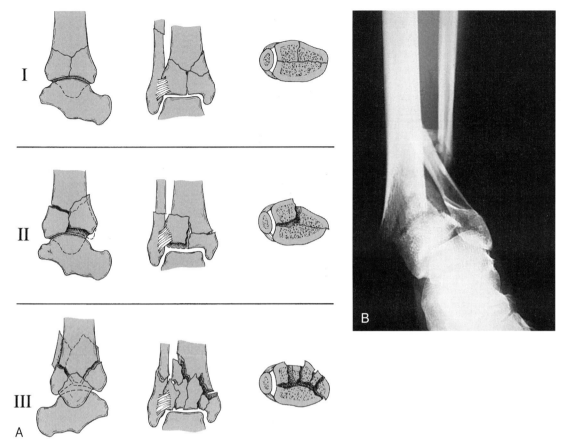

Figure 20–7 ■ *A*, Classification of tibial pilon fractures is based on the degree of comminution and displacement. *B*, AP radiograph of the tibial pilon fracture shown in Figure 20–4. This is a high-energy injury that typically results from an axial (vertical) load. (*A* from Trafton PG, Bray TJ, Simpson LA: Fractures and soft tissue injuries of the ankle. *In* Browner BD, Jupiter JB, Levine AM, et al [eds]: Skeletal Trauma. Philadelphia, WB Saunders, 1992, p 1932; *B* courtesy of Fondren Orthopedic Group LLP, Texas Orthopedic Hospital, Houston, Texas.)

Nonunion of a tibial shaft fracture is an unfortunate, challenging problem that commonly occurs

Tibial pilon fractures (Fig. 20–7)

Tibial pilon fractures (see Fig. 20–7)—result from either a high-energy axial load (fall from height) or a lower-energy rotational injury (skiing injury)

Soft tissue problems are common in injuries of the distal tibia, even those without an open wound

Most tibial pilon fractures require operative stabilization (see Table 20–1)

TUMORS OF THE LEG

Bone

Adamantinoma (tibia)
Chondromyxoid fibroma (tibia)
Osteoma (tibia)
Aneurysmal bone cyst (tibia/fibula)
Malignant fibrous histiocytoma (tibia/fibula)
Angiosarcoma (tibia)

CHAPTER 21

The Adult Ankle

ANKLE ANATOMY

Bones (Fig. 21–1)

Distal tibia
  Inferior quadrilateral surface—articulates with the talus
  Medial malleolus—pyramid shaped
Distal fibula (lateral malleolus)
  Extends distal to the medial malleolus
  The key to the ankle mortise

Talus (Fig. 21–2)
  No muscles are attached to the talus (no origins or insertions)
  Parts
    Body
    Neck
    Head
    Dome—covered in cartilage; the anterior portion of the dome is wider than the posterior portion
  Has a tenuous blood supply

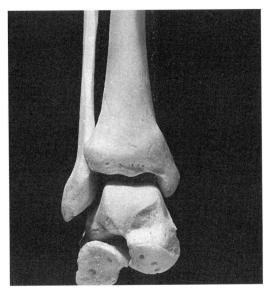
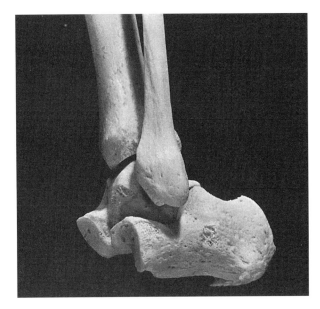
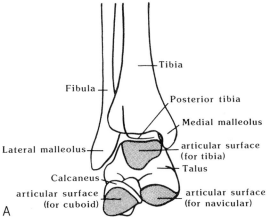
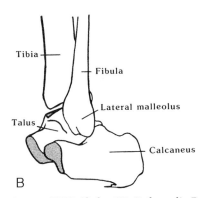

Figure 21–1 ■ The bones of the ankle. *A*, AP view; *B*, lateral view. (From Weissman BNW, Sledge CB: Orthopedic Radiology. Philadelphia, WB Saunders, 1986, p 590.)

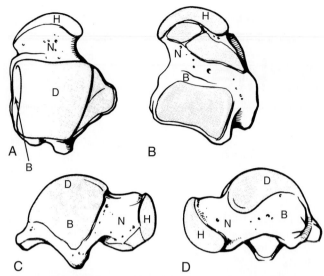

Figure 21–2 ■ Anatomy of the talus. *A*, superior; *B*, inferior; *C*, lateral; and *D*, medial projections. H, head; N, neck; B, body; D, dome. (From King RE, Powell DF: Injury to the talus. *In* Jahss MH [ed]: Disorders of the Foot and Ankle, 2nd ed. Philadelphia, WB Saunders, 1991, p 2293.)

Joints

Ankle joint
  Hinge joint
  Ligaments
    Medial ankle ligaments (Fig. 21–3)
      Deltoid ligament—consists of a deep (most important) and a superficial portion
    Lateral ankle ligaments (Fig. 21–4)
      Anterior talofibular ligament (ATFL)—the key lateral ligamentous stabilizer of the ankle
      Calcaneofibular ligament (CFL)
      Posterior talofibular ligament (PTFL)
    Syndesmotic ligaments (Fig. 21–5)—responsible for maintaining the stability of the distal tibiofibular articulation
      Anterior inferior tibiofibular ligament
      Posterior inferior tibiofibular ligament

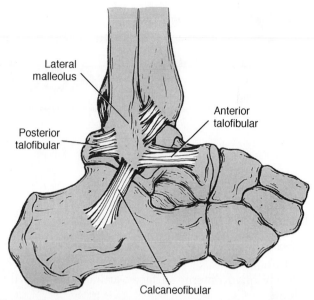

Figure 21–4 ■ The lateral ankle ligaments include the anterior talofibular (the most important stabilizer and the most commonly injured), the calcaneofibular, and the posterior talofibular. (From Trafton PG, Bray TJ, Simpson LA: Fractures and soft tissue injuries of the ankle. *In* Browner BD, Jupiter JB, Levine AM, et al [eds]: Skeletal Trauma. Philadelphia, WB Saunders, 1992, p 1874.)

      Inferior transverse ligament
      Interosseous ligament

Muscles

See Chapter 20

Nerves (Fig. 21–6)

Tibial nerve
  Passes behind the medial malleolus, courses deep to the flexor retinaculum, and divides into the medial and lateral plantar nerves (sensory and motor to the foot) and the medial calcaneal branches (sensory to the heel)
Deep peroneal nerve

Figure 21–3 ■ The medial collateral (deltoid) ligament of the ankle includes both superficial and deep components. *A*, The superficial components include the superficial talotibial, naviculotibial, and calcaneotibial components. *B*, The deep deltoid ligament fibers run transversely from the posterior colliculus of the tibia to the talus. (From Trafton PG, Bray TJ, Simpson LA: Fractures and soft tissue injuries of the ankle. *In* Browner BD, Jupiter JB, Levine AM, et al [eds]: Skeletal Trauma. Philadelphia, WB Saunders, 1992, p 1872.)

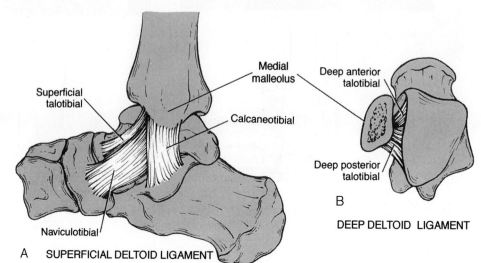

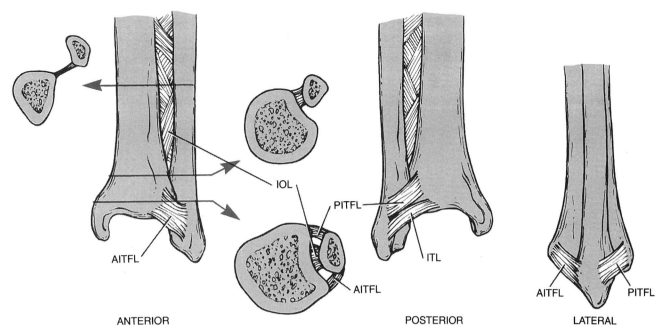

Figure 21–5 ■ The syndesmotic ligaments include the anterior inferior tibiofibular ligament (AITFL), the posterior inferior tibiofibular ligament (PITFL), the inferior transverse ligament (ITL), and the interosseous ligament (IOL). (From Trafton PG, Bray TJ, Simpson LA: Fractures and soft tissue injuries of the ankle. *In* Browner BD, Jupiter JB, Levine AM, et al [eds]: Skeletal Trauma. Philadelphia, WB Saunders, 1992, p 1874. Redrawn from Hamilton WC: Traumatic Disorders of the Ankle. New York, Springer-Verlag, 1989.)

Crosses under the extensor hallucis longus (EHL) at the ankle mortise (with the dorsalis pedis artery) and supplies sensation to the dorsal first web space of the foot and motor to the extensor digitorum brevis

Vessels (see Fig. 21–6)

Posterior tibial artery
  Divides into the medial and lateral plantar arteries behind the medial malleolus
Anterior tibial artery
  Courses deep to the EHL
  Becomes the dorsalis pedis artery as it courses deep to the extensor retinaculum

Important Anatomic Relationships
(Figs. 21–6 to 21–8)

Structures that course behind the medial malleolus—mnemonic to remember the order from anterior to posterior: **T**om, **D**ick, **A**nd **V**ery **N**ervous **H**arry
  Tibialis posterior (TP) (most anterior)
  Flexor **D**igitorum longus (FDL)
  Posterior tibial **A**rtery
  Posterior tibial **V**ein
  Tibial **N**erve
  Flexor **H**allucis longus (FHL) (most posterior)
Structures that course behind the lateral malleolus
  Peroneus longus is superficial and posterior to the peroneus brevis
Anterior structures (medial to lateral)—mnemonic: **THE**
  Tibialis anterior (TA)
  Extensor **H**allucis longus

Extensor digitorum longus (EDL)

SURGICAL APPROACHES TO THE ANKLE

Anterior (Dorsal) Approach to the Ankle

Between the EHL and the EDL
Protect the anterior tibial artery and the deep peroneal nerve, both of which course medial to the EHL

Approach to the Medial Malleolus

Direct approach
Protect the long saphenous vein and the saphenous nerve, both of which run anterior to the medial malleolus
Medial malleolus can be osteotomized to expose the talar dome (alternative is an incision through the tibialis posterior tendon sheath)

Approach to the Lateral Malleolus

Direct approach

Posteromedial Approach to the Ankle

Between the Achilles tendon and the FHL
  The FHL is the only tendon medially with muscle fibers this distal in the leg
  Avoid neurovascular structures coursing medial to the FHL

Posterolateral Approach to the Ankle

Between the Achilles tendon and the peroneus brevis
Deeper dissection between the FHL and the peroneus brevis

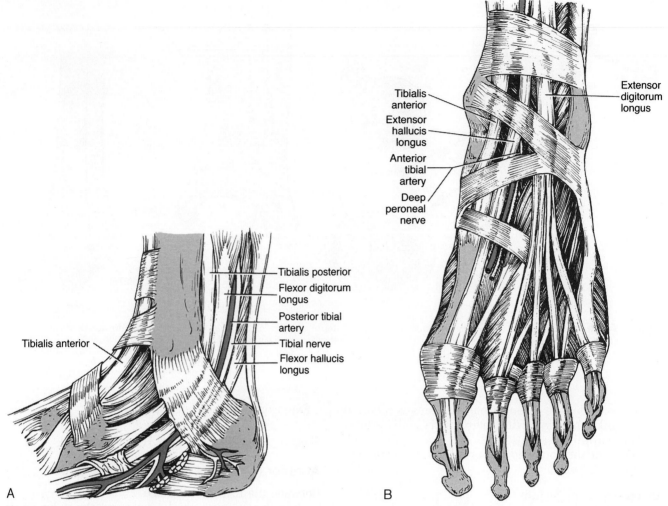

Figure 21–6 ■ *A*, Medial and *B*, anterior views of the ankle. The posterior tibial artery and tibial nerve are shown in *A*, and the anterior tibial artery and deep peroneal nerve are shown in *B*. (From Trafton PG, Bray TJ, Simpson LA: Fractures and soft tissue injuries of the ankle. *In* Browner BD, Jupiter JB, Levine AM, et al [eds]: Skeletal Trauma. Philadelphia, WB Saunders, 1992, pp 1875, 1876.)

Peroneus brevis is the only tendon laterally with muscle fibers this distal in the leg

Stay close to the Achilles tendon to avoid the sural nerve

The FHL can be subperiosteally dissected off the fibula/tibia

HISTORY AND PHYSICAL EXAMINATION OF THE ANKLE

History

Age
  Older patients—arthritis most common
  Middle-aged patients—tendinitis, Achilles tendon rupture most common
  Younger patients—ankle sprains most common
Mechanism of injury
Chronicity

Physical Examination

Observation
  Gait
  Skin changes
  Abnormal contours
  Swelling
Palpation
  Bones
    Medial malleolus (tibia)
    Lateral malleolus (fibula)
    Talus
  Soft tissues
    Lateral
      ATFL
      CFL
      Peroneal tendons
    Medial
      Deltoid ligament
      Tendons (TP, FDL, FHL)
    Posterior
      Achilles tendon
      Petrocalcaneal bursa
    Anterior
      Talar head
      Talar dome
Motion (Fig. 21–9)

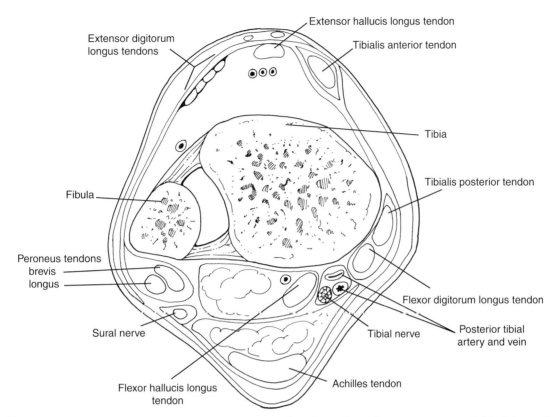

Figure 21–7 ■ Cross-section at the level of the ankle demonstrating the relationships of structures coursing behind the medial malleolus (tibialis posterior, flexor digitorum longus, posterior tibial artery and vein, tibial nerve, flexor hallucis longus); the lateral malleolus (peroneus longus, which is superficial and posterior to peroneus brevis); and the anterior structures (medial to lateral: tibialis anterior, extensor hallucis longus, extensor digitorum longus).

Figure 21–8 ■ Lateral view of the ankle demonstrating the relationship of the peroneus longus and brevis. (From Trafton PG, Bray TJ, Simpson LA: Fractures and soft tissue injuries of the ankle. *In* Browner BD, Jupiter JB, Levine AM, et al [eds]: Skeletal Trauma. Philadelphia, WB Saunders, 1992, p 1875.)

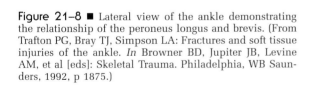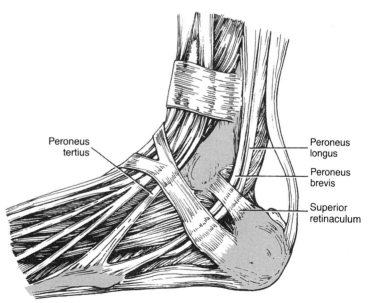

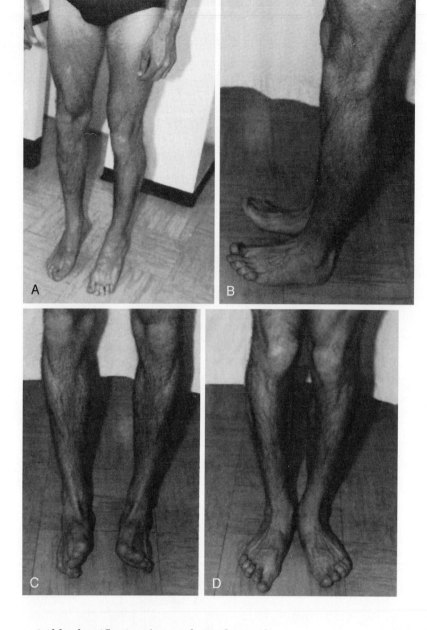

Figure 21–9 ■ Active motion of the ankle. *A,* Plantar flexion. *B,* Dorsiflexion. *C,* Supination. *D,* Pronation. (From Magee DJ: Orthopedic Physical Assessment, 2nd ed. Philadelphia, WB Saunders, 1992, p 469.)

Ankle dorsiflexion (normal, 20 degrees)
Ankle plantar flexion (normal, 50 degrees)
Supination
Pronation
Neurovascular examination
  Pulses
    Posterior tibial artery
    Dorsalis pedis artery
  Sensation (see Fig. 2–5)
  Reflexes
    Achilles (S1)
  Strength testing (Table 21–1)
    Ankle dorsiflexors (TA, EHL, EDL)
    Ankle plantar flexors (peroneus longus, peroneus brevis, gastrocnemius, soleus, FHL, FDL, TP)
Special testing (condition specific)
  Lateral ankle instability
    Anterior draw test (Fig. 21–10)—useful to test the integrity of the ATFL; this test must be performed with the ankle held in plantar flexion because in this position the effect of the CFL is eliminated (the CFL is lax when the ankle is in plantar flexion) and therefore the integrity of the ATFL can be tested
    Talar tilt test (Fig. 21–11)—useful to test the integrity of *both* the ATFL and the CFL; both ligaments must be torn for a positive talar tilt test
  Syndesmotic injury (Fig. 21–12)
    Squeeze test—squeezing the calf causes ankle pain in the patient with a disruption of the syndesmotic ligaments because of instability of the distal tibiofibular articulation
    Abduction external rotation stress test—increased pain upon passive abduction and external rotation of the ankle (with the knee stabilized) in the patient with a syndesmotic injury

Table 21-1
MUSCLES OF THE ANKLE: THEIR ACTION, INNERVATION, AND NERVE ROOT DERIVATION

Action	Muscles Involved	Innervation	Nerve Root Derivation
Plantar flexion (flexion) of ankle	1. Gastrocnemius*	Tibial	S1-2
	2. Soleus*	Tibial	S1-2
	3. Plantaris	Tibial	S1-2
	4. Flexor digitorum longus	Tibial	S2-3
	5. Peroneus longus	Superficial peroneal	L5, S1-2
	6. Peroneus brevis	Superficial peroneal	L5, S1-2
	7. Flexor hallucis longus	Tibial	S2-3
	8. Tibialis posterior	Tibial	L4-5
Dorsiflexion (extension) of ankle	1. Tibialis anterior	Deep peroneal	L4-5
	2. Extensor digitorum longus	Deep peroneal	L5, S1
	3. Extensor hallucis longus	Deep peroneal	L5, S1
	4. Peroneus tertius	Deep peroneal	L5, S1
Inversion	1. Tibialis posterior	Tibial	L4-5
	2. Flexor digitorum longus	Tibial	S2-3
	3. Flexor hallucis longus	Tibial	S2-3
	4. Tibialis anterior	Deep peroneal	L4-5
	5. Extensor hallucis longus	Deep peroneal	L5, S1
Eversion	1. Peroneus longus	Superficial peroneal	L5, S1-2
	2. Peroneus brevis	Superficial peroneal	L5, S1-2
	3. Peroneus tertius	Deep peroneal	L5, S1
	4. Extensor digitorum longus	Deep peroneal	S5, S1

* The gastrocnemius and soleus muscles are sometimes grouped together as the triceps surae muscles.
From Magee DJ: Orthopaedic Physical Assessment, 2nd ed. Philadelphia, WB Saunders, 1992, p 475.

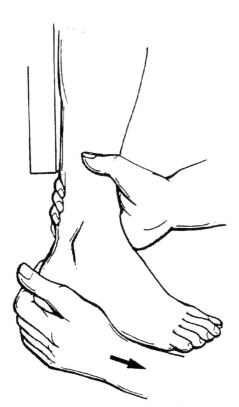

Figure 21-10 ■ Anterior draw test of the ankle (tests the integrity of the anterior talofibular ligament). (Modified from Renstrom PAFH, Kannus P: Injuries of the foot and ankle. *In* DeLee JC, Drez D Jr [eds]: Orthopaedic Sports Medicine: Principles and Practice. Philadelphia, WB Saunders, 1994, p 1709.)

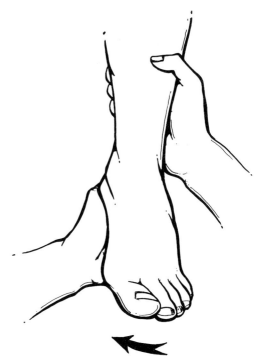

Figure 21-11 ■ Talar tilt test (inversion stress) of the ankle (tests the integrity of the anterior talofibular ligament and the calcaneofibular ligament). (From Renstrom PAFH, Kannus P: Injuries of the foot and ankle. *In* DeLee JC, Drez D Jr [eds]: Orthopaedic Sports Medicine: Principles and Practice. Philadelphia, WB Saunders, 1994, p 1710.)

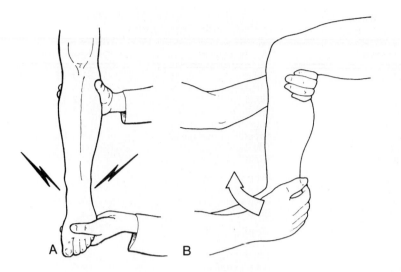
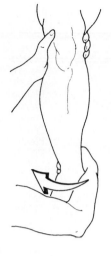

Figure 21-12 ■ *A*, Squeeze test and *B*, abduction external rotation stress test for syndesmotic injuries. (From Miller MD, Cooper DE, Warner JJP: Review of Sports Medicine and Arthroscopy. Philadelphia, WB Saunders, 1995, p 92.)

Achilles tendon injury

Thompson's test (Fig. 21–13)—squeezing the calf causes ankle plantar flexion if the Achilles tendon is intact; a positive Thompson's test is when squeezing of the calf does not cause ankle plantar flexion because the Achilles tendon is torn

DIAGNOSTIC TESTS FOR THE ANKLE

Plain Radiographs

Anteroposterior view (Fig. 21–14)

Taken in line with the long axis of the foot

Useful to evaluate for

Medial malleolus fractures

Lateral malleolus fractures

Osteochondral fractures (distal tibia, talar dome)

Measurements

Tibiofibular clear space—measured 1 cm above the tibial plafond; greater than 5 mm is abnormal and suggests a syndesmotic disruption

Tibiofibular overlap—measured from the lateral edge of the tibia to the medial edge of the fibula; less than 6 mm is abnormal and suggests a syndesmotic disruption

Lateral view (Fig. 21–15)

Taken perpendicular to the long axis of the foot

Useful to evaluate for

Displacement of the talus in the anterior or posterior direction (ankle subluxation or dislocation)

Fractures of the anterior or posterior tibial margins

Talar neck fractures

Fibula fractures

Fibula dislocations

Mortise view (Fig. 21–16)

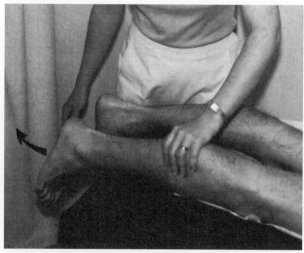

Figure 21–13 ■ Thompson's test for Achilles tendon injury. Squeezing the calf normally causes plantar flexion of the ankle (*arrow*). An abnormal test (Achilles tendon rupture) is when squeezing the calf does not result in plantar flexion of the ankle. (From Magee DJ: Orthopedic Physical Assessment, 2nd ed. Philadelphia, WB Saunders, 1992, p 483.)

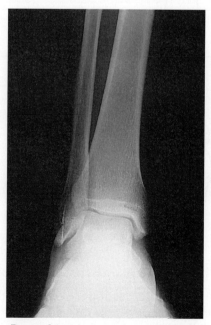

Figure 21–14 ■ AP view of the ankle.

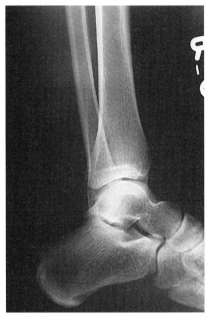

Figure 21–15 ■ Lateral view of the ankle.

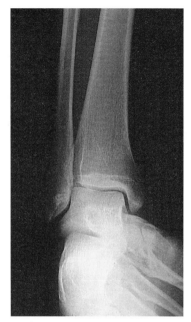

Figure 21–16 ■ Mortise view of the ankle.

Taken with the leg internally rotated 15 to 20 degrees; this brings the fibula (anterior) in line with the tibia (with the leg held in the neutral [AP] position, the fibula is normally posterior to the tibia)

In a properly taken mortise view, the lateral border of the talus should appear to be vertical (it does not appear vertical on an AP view)

Most useful to evaluate for a disruption of the syndesmotic ligaments (seen on x-ray as a widened tibiofibular clear space)

Measurements

Medial and lateral clear spaces—measured at the level of the talar dome; these clear spaces should be equal and are normally less than 4 mm (asymmetry suggests a syndesmotic disruption or an improperly positioned mortise view)

Tibiofibular clear space—measured 1 cm above the tibial plafond; greater than 5 mm is abnormal and suggests a syndesmotic disruption

Tibiofibular overlap—measured from the lateral edge of the tibia to the medial edge of the fibula; less than 1 mm is abnormal and suggests a syndesmotic disruption

Special Radiographs (Fig. 21–17)

Stress radiographs

X-rays taken during stress testing; useful for the evaluation of lateral ligamentous integrity

Anterior draw stress x-ray

Talar tilt stress x-ray

Figure 21–17 ■ *A*, Anterior draw stress radiograph. The anterior talar displacement is recorded by measuring the shortest distance from the most posterior articular surface of the tibia to the talar dome. *B*, Talar tilt (inversion) stress radiograph. The talar tilt angle is measured between the tibial plafond and the talar dome. Comparison between right and left ankles may be helpful. (From Renstrom PAFH, Kannus P: Injuries of the foot and ankle. *In* DeLee JC, Drez D Jr [eds]: Orthopaedic Sports Medicine: Principles and Practice. Philadelphia, WB Saunders, 1994, pp 1711, 1713.)

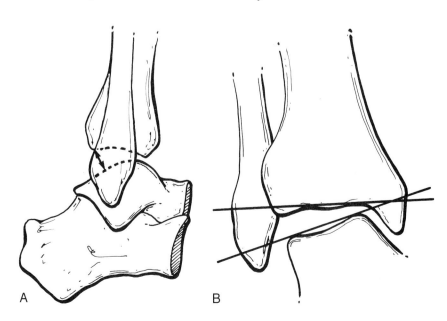

A   B

Imaging

Computed tomography (CT)—condition specific
Magnetic resonance imaging (MRI)—condition specific

Arthroscopy

Indications
   Osteochondral lesions of the talus
   Post-traumatic synovitis
   Osteoarthritis/tibiotalar spurring

COMMON ADULT CONDITIONS

Tendon Problems

Peroneal tendon problems
  Tendinitis/tenosynovitis
    Etiology—prolonged mechanical attrition in a tendon with a tenuous blood supply
    Presentation—painful swelling behind the lateral malleolus in the region of the peroneal tendons
    Treatment—most commonly conservative with nonsteroidal anti-inflammatory drugs (NSAIDs), bracing, splinting or casting, and decreased activity for the acute inflammatory phase; physical therapy and modalities may also be helpful; operative decompression is rarely indicated
  Rupture
    Represents the end stage of tendinitis/tenosynovitis
    Frank rupture of this tendon is relatively uncommon, but longitudinal tears are being recognized with increasing frequency
    Presentation—weakness or inability to actively evert the foot
    Treatment—operative repair
  Subluxation/dislocation (Fig. 21–18)
    Etiology—violent dorsiflexion of the ankle with the foot in an everted position (a common skiing injury); causes the peroneal tendons to become subluxated or dislocated from their fibro-osseous tendon sheath
    Presentation—the patient presents complaining of pain with a popping or snapping sensation to the posterolateral ankle; the patient is unable to resist dorsiflexion at the ankle with the foot positioned (by the examiner) in the plantarflexed and everted position
    Treatment—closed reduction by positioning the ankle in plantar flexion and immobilization for 4 to 6 weeks; chronic cases that do not improve with conservative treatment may require operative reconstruction
Tibialis posterior tendon problems
  Tendinitis/tendinosis
    Etiology—chronic degenerative process most commonly seen in middle-aged women
    Presentation—gradual onset of posteromedial ankle pain that is aggravated by prolonged walking and standing; pain is reproducible with active ankle inversion and passive ankle eversion; MRI is useful in demonstrating inflammatory changes in the tibialis posterior tendon sheath
    Treatment—orthotic shoe inserts, NSAIDs, physical therapy, or immobilization in a cast, splint, or brace for highly symptomatic cases
  Rupture (Fig. 21–19)
    Etiology—represents a continuum of the pathologic process from a long-standing tendinitis

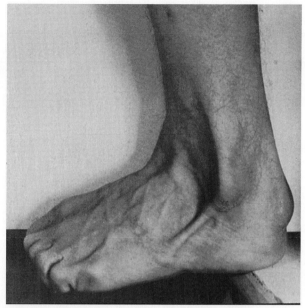

Figure 21–18 ■ Subluxation of the peroneal tendons. Clinical photograph shows anterior subluxation of the peroneal tendons. (From Kelikian H, Kelikian AS: Disorders of the Ankle. Philadelphia, WB Saunders, 1985, p 765.)

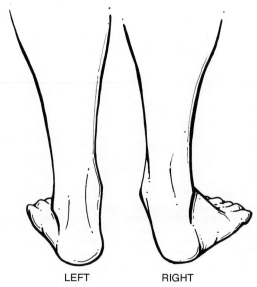

LEFT   RIGHT

Figure 21–19 ■ The "too many toes" sign is associated with tibialis posterior tendon rupture. More toes are visible lateral to the heel on the patient's affected right side. (From Keene JS: Tendon injuries of the foot and ankle. In DeLee JC, Drez D Jr [eds]: Orthopaedic Sports Medicine: Principles and Practice. Philadelphia, WB Saunders, 1994, p 1772.)

Presentation—acquired flatfoot (planovalgus) deformity (normally the tibialis posterior tendon is responsible for supporting the arch); the patient may also demonstrate a lack of hindfoot inversion upon toe rising (in the normal foot, the tibialis posterior tendon will invert the hindfoot on a toe rise; this will be absent if the tendon is ruptured); the patient may also demonstrate the so-called **too many toes sign** (see Fig. 21–19)—when the patient is standing and is viewed from behind, more toes are seen laterally on the involved foot than on the uninvolved foot (because of collapse of the medial arch)

Treatment—individualized based on patient characteristics and functional demands

Achilles tendon problems

Tendinitis

Etiology—cumulative impact loading and repetitive microtrauma to the tendon (commonly seen in runners)

Presentation—posterior ankle pain reproducible with palpation and stretching of the Achilles tendon, soft tissue swelling, or crepitus

Treatment—NSAIDs, heel lift, physical therapy for strengthening and stretching exercises, modalities, and immobilization in a cast, splint, or brace for 7 to 10 days for severely symptomatic cases; **injection of the tendon sheath may be harmful**

Rupture

Etiology—arises as a continuum of a chronic tendinitis or the result of an acute traumatic injury (forced ankle dorsiflexion with the Achilles tendon in a contracted state)

Presentation—the patient presents with a history of a sudden snap in the posterior ankle region with acute onset of pain and swelling (common in basketball players and in racket sport players); there is often a history of a sensation of being shot in the back of the ankle; physical exam reveals a palpable defect in the Achilles tendon and a positive Thompson's test (see Fig. 21–13)

Treatment—**controversial**—operative repair versus prolonged casting with the ankle held in the plantarflexed position; the risk of tendon rerupture is higher in patients treated with casting; the risk of soft tissue problems is greater in those treated operatively

Tibialis anterior tendon problems

Rupture

Etiology—degenerative process most common in patients older than 45 years of age

Presentation—the patient presents with a remote history of vague ankle pain; **the classic presentation is a painless, flatfooted (slapping) gait that is often noted by the patient only after friends and relatives notice the abnormal gait pattern;** on physical exam the patient demonstrates weakness of active ankle dorsiflexion; a palpable defect over the tibialis anterior tendon may also be noted by the examiner

Treatment—individualized based on patient characteristics and functional demands

Ankle Sprains

The most common mechanism of injury for an ankle sprain is ankle inversion (stresses the lateral ligamentous stabilizers)

The lateral ligaments are always injured from anterior to posterior (the ATFL is the most common ankle ligament injured and is always injured first; the CFL is always the next lateral ligament injured; the PTFL is injured last and is the least commonly injured lateral ligament) (see Fig. 21–4)

Presentation—the patient presents with localized tenderness over the lateral ligamentous structures (most commonly the ATFL)

Deltoid ligament injuries present with medial tenderness

Anterior draw testing is positive in patients with an ATFL injury (see Fig. 21–10)

The talar tilt test (see Fig. 21–11) will be positive in a patient with a combined injury of both the ATFL and the CFL

Physical exam should include an assessment for a syndesmotic injury (squeeze test and abduction external rotation stress test [see Fig. 21–12])

A thorough assessment should also be performed to rule out an ankle fracture or a proximal fracture (proximal fibula fractures arise from rotational injuries where force is transmitted proximally through the syndesmotic ligaments, resulting in a proximal fibula (Maisonneuve's) fracture [Fig. 21–20])

The indications for x-raying an acute ankle injury to rule out a fracture are any of the following (Ottawa ankle rules)

Tenderness to palpation at the (posterior) tip of the lateral malleolus

Tenderness to palpation at the (posterior) tip of the medial malleolus

Inability to bear weight at the time of injury or at the time of physical examination

Stress radiographs (anterior draw stress x-ray and talar tilt stress x-ray) are also useful

Treatment

Acute ankle sprains—treated according to the mnemonic **RICE**

Rest—non–weight bearing or protected weight bearing based on resolution of symptoms

Ice

Compression (elastic wrap)

Elevation

Cast immobilization is reserved for patients with severe pain and swelling that prohibits ankle motion

After the acute phase, a course of physical therapy is helpful (range-of-motion exercises, strengthening exercises, proprioceptive training, and other modalities as needed)

Chronic ankle sprains

Muscle-strengthening exercises

Operative reconstruction is indicated for recurrent ankle instability that is refractory to extended nonoperative management

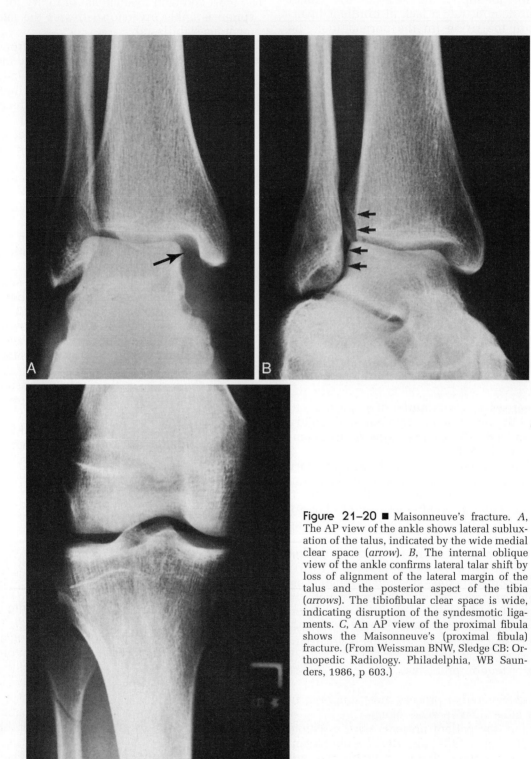

Figure 21–20 ■ Maisonneuve's fracture. *A*, The AP view of the ankle shows lateral subluxation of the talus, indicated by the wide medial clear space (*arrow*). *B*, The internal oblique view of the ankle confirms lateral talar shift by loss of alignment of the lateral margin of the talus and the posterior aspect of the tibia (*arrows*). The tibiofibular clear space is wide, indicating disruption of the syndesmotic ligaments. *C*, An AP view of the proximal fibula shows the Maisonneuve's (proximal fibula) fracture. (From Weissman BNW, Sledge CB: Orthopedic Radiology. Philadelphia, WB Saunders, 1986, p 603.)

Arthritic Conditions of the Ankle

Primary osteoarthritis
  Uncommon
Post-traumatic arthritis (Fig. 21–21)
  Most commonly arises after an ankle fracture or
    dislocation
    May result from a previous articular injury
    May result from a poorly reduced ankle or distal
      tibial fracture
  Presentation
    Ankle pain
    Decreased ankle motion
    X-rays show joint space narrowing, osteophytes,
      sclerosis, deformity
  Treatment
    NSAIDs
    Ankle-foot orthosis (AFO)
    Shoe modification
    Tibiotalar (ankle) arthrodesis for advanced symp-
      tomatic cases
Rheumatoid arthritis (RA)
  The ankle is the least commonly involved of all the
    major weight bearing joints of the body in patients
    with RA
  RA is less of a problem in the ankle than in the
    forefoot and hindfoot
  Presents with boggy, painful ankle synovitis with
    loss of motion
  Synovectomy for advanced cases may be helpful
  Arthrodesis is rarely indicated
Charcot's ankle joint
  Results from a neuropathic condition (such as dia-
    betes)
  X-rays show severe joint destruction (Fig. 21–22)
  Treatment is bracing and avoidance of operative
    procedures

Osteochondral Injuries of the Talus
(Fig. 21–23)

Presentation
  Painful ankle effusion
  Limited ankle motion
  There is often a remote history of an ankle sprain
Plain radiographs
  Mortise view visualizes the lesion best (see Fig. 21–
    23)
CT/MRI—useful to image lesions that are poorly visu-
  alized using plain radiographs
Lesion location and characteristics
  Lateral lesions—anterior talus, shallow lesion
  Medial lesions—posterior talus, deep lesion
Treatment options
  Conservative care
  Arthroscopic débridement

Os Trigonum (Fig. 21–24)

Represents a nonunited lateral tubercle on the posterior talus
**This is most commonly a normal asymptomatic inci-
  dental finding noted on the x-rays of a patient
  being evaluated (such as for an ankle sprain)**
The os trigonum appears with smooth edges on x-ray,
  and this appearance differentiates it from an acute
  fracture (see Fig. 21–24)

Nerve Entrapments

Present with localized pain, tenderness, and paresthesias in the dermatomal distribution of the nerve,
  and with a positive Tinel's sign at the site of entrapment
Examples
  Tarsal tunnel syndrome

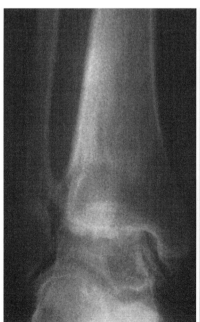
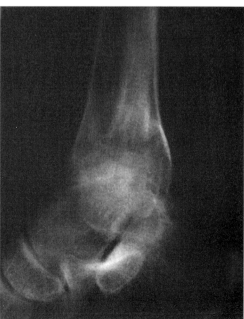

Figure 21–21 ■ Post-traumatic arthritis several years after an ankle fracture. (From Trafton PG, Bray TJ, Simpson LA: Fractures and soft tissue
injuries of the ankle. In Browner BD,
Jupiter JB, Levine AM, et al [eds]: Skeletal Trauma. Philadelphia, WB Saunders, 1992, p 1950.)

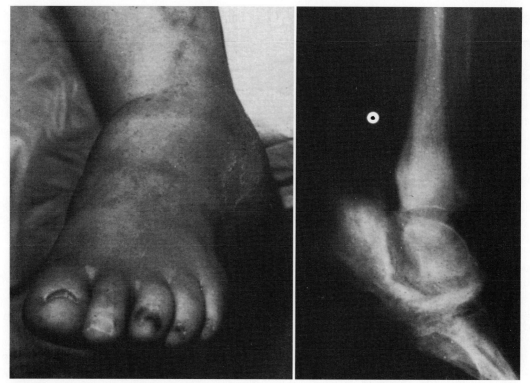

Figure 21-22 ■ Charcot's foot and ankle. Clinical photograph shows marked swelling of the foot and ankle. The lateral radiograph demonstrates severe destruction of the subtalar joint and involvement of the ankle (tibiotalar joint). (From Jacobs RL, Karmody A: The diabetic foot. *In* Jahss MH [ed]: Disorders of the Foot. Philadelphia, WB Saunders, 1982, p 1380.)

Entrapment of the tibial nerve as it passes deep to the flexor retinaculum (lacinate ligament); possible etiologies of nerve compression include (1) bony trauma or exostosis; (2) space-occupying lesions (lipoma, ganglion cyst, synovial cyst);

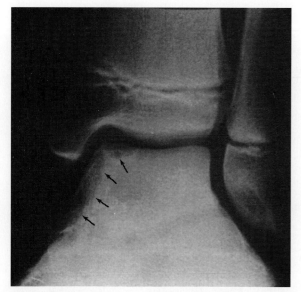

Figure 21-23 ■ Mortise view of the ankle showing an osteochondral lesion of the medial talus (*arrows*). (From Canale ST: Osteochondroses and related problems of the foot and ankle. *In* DeLee JC, Drez D Jr [eds]: Orthopaedic Sports Medicine: Principles and Practice. Philadelphia, WB Saunders, 1994, p 1959.)

(3) tortuous vein compressing the nerve; and (4) severe foot pronation

Presentation—burning pain and paresthesias behind the medial malleolus with radiation into the plantar foot (sole to toes)

Electromyography/nerve conduction studies—sometimes helpful to confirm the diagnosis

Treatment options
  NSAIDs
  Activity limitation
  Arch supports
  Operative release/decompression
Deep peroneal nerve entrapment syndrome
Sural nerve entrapment syndrome

FRACTURES AND DISLOCATION OF THE ANKLE

Overview (Table 21-2)

Ankle fractures include fractures of any of the following bones and may occur with combinations of fractures
  Lateral malleolus
  Medial malleolus
  Posterior malleolus
  Anterior lip of the tibia
The basic mechanism of an ankle fracture can be one of the following

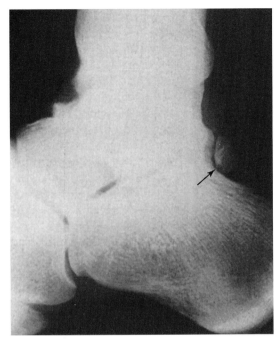

Figure 21–24 ■ Lateral radiograph demonstrating a large os trigonum of the posterior aspect of the talus (*arrow*). (From Renstrom PAFH, Kannus P: Injuries of the foot and ankle. *In* DeLee JC, Drez D Jr [eds]: Orthopaedic Sports Medicine: Principles and Practice. Philadelphia, WB Saunders, 1994, p 1749.)

External rotation (most common)
Adduction
Abduction
Axial loading

The Danis-Weber classification (Fig. 21–25) is a relatively simple scheme based on the level of the fibula fracture and is useful for treatment decision making

Danis-Weber A—the fibula fracture is distal to the ankle mortise; treatment is closed reduction with casting

Danis-Weber B—the fibula fracture is oblique and begins at the level of the ankle mortise and extends proximally; treatment is closed reduction and casting unless examination reveals a syndesmotic disruption

Danis-Weber C—the fibular fracture is proximal to the ankle mortise (high) and the syndesmosis is disrupted; treatment is open reduction with internal fixation (ORIF)

It should be noted that the Danis-Weber classification does not take the medial malleolus into consideration; it is primarily used to decide on the treatment of the lateral malleolus and syndesmosis; treatment of medial malleolus fractures (when present) is most often ORIF

Specific injury patterns (four of them) can be recognized radiographically using the Lauge Hanson classification (see Fig. 21–25), and these patterns explain the position of the foot at the time of injury (first word) and the direction of the force causing the injury (second word); the injury patterns occur in stages based on the order that specific injuries occur; low-energy injuries may only go through stage I, and progressively higher energy injuries go through more of the stages; the four injury patterns (Lauge-Hansen) are as follows

Table 21–2
FRACTURES OF THE ADULT ANKLE

Fracture	Classification	Treatment	Most Common Complications of the Injury
Ankle fracture (see Figs. 21–25 through 21–29)	Lauge-Hansen (position of foot–direction of force) (see Fig. 21–25) Supination–adduction (see Figs. 21–25 and 21–26) Supination–external rotation (see Figs. 21–25 and 21–27) Pronation–abduction (see Figs. 21–25 and 21–28) Pronation–external rotation (see Figs. 21–25 and 21–29) Danis-Weber (A, B, C) (location of fibula fracture) (see Fig. 21–25) A. Fibula fracture is below ankle joint B. Fibula fracture begins at ankle joint and extends proximally C. High fibula fracture	Treatment of an ankle fracture is based on reduction of the mortise; most commonly medial malleolus fractures require ORIF A lateral malleolus fracture in an ankle with a medial malleolus fracture (bimalleolar fracture) is treated with ORIF Treatment of isolated lateral malleolus fractures depends on type A. Long leg cast B. Long leg cast vs. ORIF C. ORIF Posterior malleolar fragment is treated nonoperatively unless it involves more than one third of the articular surface of the distal tibia	Nonunion, malunion, post-traumatic arthritis, reflex sympathetic dystrophy, vascular injury
Avulsion fracture	Anatomic location	Symptomatically	Differentiation from accessory ossicles

ORIF, open reduction with internal fixation.

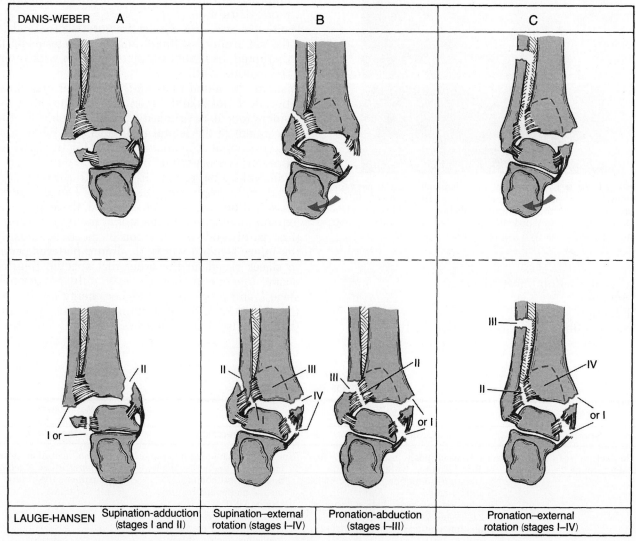

Figure 21-25 ■ Danis-Weber (AO/ASIF) and Lauge-Hansen classifications of ankle fractures. (From Trafton PG, Bray TJ, Simpson LA: Fractures and soft tissue injuries of the ankle. *In* Browner BD, Jupiter JB, Levine AM, et al [eds]: Skeletal Trauma. Philadelphia, WB Saunders, 1992, p 1891.)

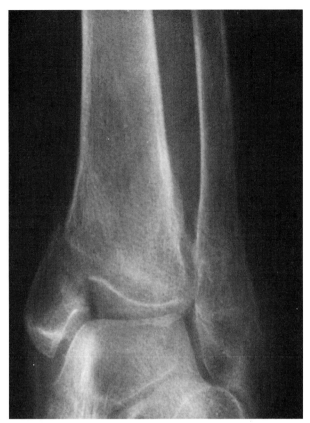

Figure 21–26 ■ AP radiograph of a supination-adduction (stage II) fracture. Note the transverse lateral malleolus fracture (Danis-Weber type A), which is nondisplaced, and the vertical medial malleolus fracture. (From Trafton PG, Bray TJ, Simpson LA: Fractures and soft tissue injuries of the ankle. *In* Browner BD, Jupiter JB, Levine AM, et al [eds]: Skeletal Trauma. Philadelphia, WB Saunders, 1992, p 1893.)

LATERAL   AP

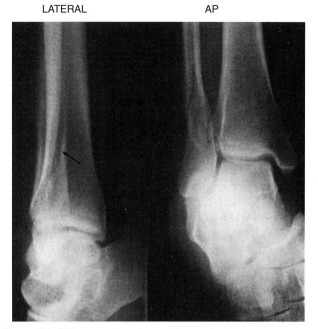

Figure 21–27 ■ Lateral and AP radiographs of a supination-external rotation (stage II) fracture. Note that the displacement of the distal fibular fracture (which runs obliquely from anterior inferior to posterior superior) is best seen on the lateral view (*arrow*). (From Trafton PG, Bray TJ, Simpson LA: Fractures and soft tissue injuries of the ankle. *In* Browner BD, Jupiter JB, Levine AM, et al [eds]: Skeletal Trauma. Philadelphia, WB Saunders, 1992, p 1893.)

Supination–adduction (see Fig. 21–25)
   Radiographic appearance—AP view shows a transverse lateral malleolus fracture (below the ankle mortise) with or without a vertical medial malleolus fracture (Fig. 21–26)
   Two stages
   I—lateral malleolus fracture
   II—medial malleolus fracture
Supination–external rotation (see Fig. 21–25)
   Radiographic appearance—AP view shows an oblique lateral malleolus fracture beginning at the ankle mortise and extending proximally, with or without a posterior malleolus fracture, with or without a transverse medial malleolus fracture; the lateral view best visualizes the lateral malleolus fracture (Fig. 21–27) because the fracture runs obliquely from anterior to posterior; this is in contrast to a pronation–abduction injury (Fig. 21–28), where the lateral malleolus fracture runs obliquely from medial to lateral and is best visualized on the AP view
   Four stages
   I—ATFL injury
   II—lateral malleolus fracture
   III—posterior malleolar fracture or injury to the PTFL
   IV—medial malleolus fracture
Pronation–abduction (see Fig. 21–25)
   Radiographic appearance—AP view shows a transverse medial malleolus fracture with or without an oblique lateral malleolus fracture that runs obliquely from medial to lateral; the oblique lateral malleolus fracture is best visualized on the AP view (see Fig. 21–28), in contrast

Table 21–3
DISLOCATIONS OF THE ADULT ANKLE

Dislocation	Classification	Treatment	Most Common Complications of the Injury
Tibiotalar (ankle) joint	Descriptive (anterior; posterior; medial; lateral)	Closed reduction via longitudinal traction Consider repair of ligamentous injuries Fracture-dislocations require operative stabilization	Missed associated fractures, vascular injuries, chronic ankle instability, post-traumatic arthritis

to the oblique lateral malleolus fracture of a supination–external rotation injury, which is best seen on the lateral view (see Fig. 21–27)

Three stages

I—medial malleolus fracture or deltoid ligament injury

II—syndesmotic ligament injury

III—lateral malleolus fracture

Pronation–external rotation (see Fig. 21–25)

Radiographic appearance—AP view shows evidence of a deltoid ligament injury (widened medial clear space) or a transverse medial malleolus fracture with a high short oblique fibula fracture with or without a posterior malleolus fracture (Fig. 21–29)

Four stages

I—medial malleolus fracture or deltoid ligament injury

II—ATFL injury

III—high fibular fracture

IV—posterior malleolus fracture

Most medial malleolar fractures require ORIF

High fibular ankle fractures and those with a syndesmotic injury require ORIF of the fibula and stabilization of the syndesmosis via a syndesmotic screw (Fig. 21–30)

Weber A fibula fractures and Weber B fibula fractures without syndesmotic disruption or displacement can be treated with casting

Deltoid ligament injuries are treated nonoperatively unless the ligament is interposed in the medial side of the joint, blocking reduction of the ankle mortise

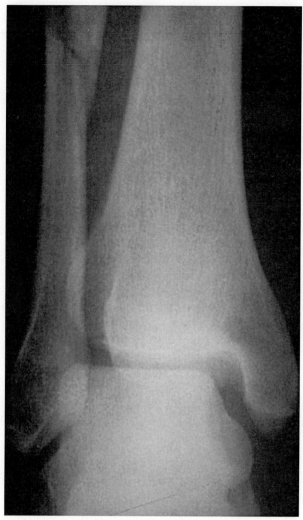

Figure 21–29 ■ AP radiograph of a pronation-external rotation (stage IV) fracture. Note the widened medial clear space (of a ruptured deltoid ligament), the laterally displaced fibula (indicating complete disruption of the syndesmosis), and the high fibula fracture. (From Trafton PG, Bray TJ, Simpson LA: Fractures and soft tissue injuries of the ankle. *In* Browner BD, Jupiter JB, Levine AM, et al [eds]: Skeletal Trauma. Philadelphia, WB Saunders, 1992, p 1898.)

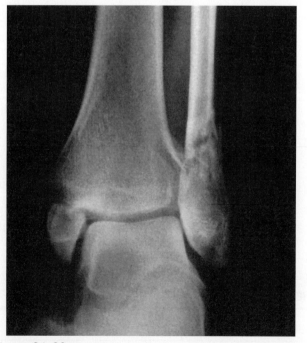

Figure 21–28 ■ AP radiograph of a pronation-abduction (stage III) fracture. Note the transverse medial malleolus fracture. The lateral malleolus fracture of a pronation-abduction injury is best visualized on the AP view. (From Trafton PG, Bray TJ, Simpson LA: Fractures and soft tissue injuries of the ankle. *In* Browner BD, Jupiter JB, Levine AM, et al [eds]: Skeletal Trauma. Philadelphia, WB Saunders, 1992, p 1895.)

Ankle dislocations (see Fig. 4–21C) (Table 21–3)

High-energy injuries that may be associated with an ankle fracture

Emergent closed reduction (via traction/manipulation) of the dislocation restores compromised arterial flow

Definitive treatment of a fracture-dislocation is usually ORIF (or external fixation with or without open reduction, with or without limited internal fixation)

TUMORS OF THE ANKLE

Soft Tissue

Clear cell sarcoma

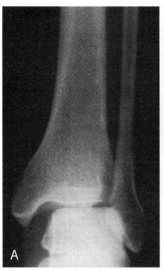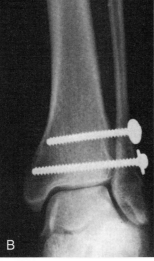

Figure 21–30 ■ *A*, AP radiograph of the ankle demonstrates widening of the medial clear space and lateral displacement of the talus, suggesting a syndesmotic ligament injury. *B*, Fixation of the syndesmosis with two screws after reduction of the syndesmosis. (From Trafton PG, Bray TJ, Simpson LA: Fractures and soft tissue injuries of the ankle. *In* Browner BD, Jupiter JB, Levine AM, et al [eds]. Skeletal Trauma. Philadelphia, WB Saunders, 1992, p 1916.)

DIFFERENTIAL DIAGNOSIS OF COMMON ANKLE COMPLAINTS

Pain

Tendon problems
Ankle sprain
Arthritis
Rheumatologic conditions
Osteochondral injuries of the talus
Nerve entrapments
Fractures
Dislocations

Instability

Ankle sprain
Charcot's ankle
Fractures
Dislocations

Weakness

Tendon problems
Nerve entrapments
Proximal condition causing myelopathy or radiculopathy

Tingling/Loss of Sensation

Charcot's ankle
Nerve entrapments
Proximal condition causing myelopathy or radiculopathy

Deformity

Tendon problems
Ankle sprains (swelling)
Arthritis
Rheumatologic conditions
Charcot's ankle
Fractures
Dislocations

Catching/Locking

Peroneal tendon subluxation/dislocation
Osteochondral injuries of the talus

Loss of Motion

Tendon problems
Arthritis
Rheumatologic conditions
Charcot's ankle
Fractures
Dislocations

PEARLS AND PITFALLS

Rotational injuries of the ankle causing a sprain or fracture can also result in a high fibula (Maisonneuve's) fracture (see Fig. 21–20); this fracture should not be missed! When in doubt, obtain x-rays of the entire length of the tibia and fibula

CHAPTER 22

The Adult Foot

FOOT ANATOMY

Bones (Fig. 22–1)

Seven tarsal bones
  Talus
  Calcaneus
  Navicular
  Cuboid
  Lateral cuneiform
  Middle cuneiform
  Medial cuneiform
Five metatarsal bones (one to five, medial to lateral)

Fourteen phalanges (proximal, middle, distal)
  Only two phalanges for the great toe (like the thumb)
Two sesamoid bones

Joints

Intertarsal joints
  Supporting ligaments are referred to by their common names (the bones that they connect) (Table 22–1)
Tarsometatarsal (Lisfranc's) joints (Fig. 22–2; see Fig. 22–1)

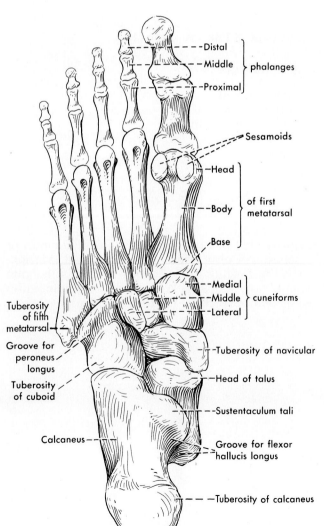

Figure 22–1 ■ Bones of the foot (as viewed from the plantar surface). (From Jenkins DB: Hollinshead's Functional Anatomy of the Limbs and Back, 6th ed. Philadelphia, WB Saunders, 1991, p 308.)

Table 22–1
LIGAMENTS OF THE INTERTARSAL JOINTS

Ligament	Common Name	Origin	Insertion
Interosseous talocalcaneal	Cervical	Talus	Calcaneus
Calcaneocuboid/calcaneonavicular	Bifurcate	Calcaneus	Cuboid and navicular
Calcaneocuboid-metatarsal	Long plantar	Calcaneus	Cuboid and first to fifth metatarsals
Plantar calcaneocuboid	Short plantar	Calcaneus	Cuboid
Plantar calcaneonavicular	Spring	Sustentaculum tali	Navicular
Tarsometatarsal	Lisfranc's	Medial cuneiform	Second metatarsal base

Gliding joints

These joints are very stable because of their bony architecture and supporting ligaments (see Fig. 22–2)

Intrinsic bony stability results because the second metatarsal base is recessed ("keystone effect") between the medial and lateral cuneiform and also because all the metatarsal bases are trapezoid shaped ("Roman arch")

Ligamentous stability is provided by

Strong transverse metatarsal ligaments—connect the lateral four metatarsal heads (in the first web space, the transverse metatarsal ligament runs from the second metatarsal head to the fibular [lateral] sesamoid) and the four lateral metatarsal bases (see Fig. 22–2)

Lisfranc's ligament—a strong ligament connecting the second metatarsal base to the medial cuneiform (see Fig. 22–2)

Metatarsophalangeal (MTP) joints (see Fig. 22–1)

Interphalangeal (IP) joints (see Fig. 22–1)

Muscles (Fig. 22–3)

There are **19 intrinsic muscles of the foot** (Table 22–2)

There is only one dorsal intrinsic muscle of the foot (extensor digitorum brevis—innervated by the deep peroneal nerve)

The 18 plantar intrinsic muscles of the foot are best considered in four layers

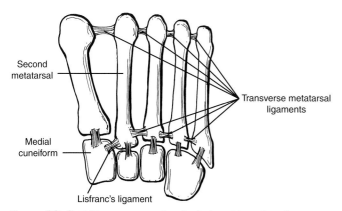

Figure 22–2 ■ Tarsometatarsal articulation. Note the "keystone effect" at the base of the 2nd metatarsal. (From Renstrom PAFH, Kannus P: Injuries of the foot and ankle. *In* DeLee JC, Drez D Jr [eds]: Orthopaedic Sports Medicine: Principles and Practice. Philadelphia, WB Saunders, 1994, p 1753.)

Nerves (Figs. 22–4 and 22–5)

Tibial nerve—divides into the medial and lateral plantar nerves and the medial calcaneal branches (as it courses deep to the flexor retinaculum); the medial and lateral plantar nerves provide motor innervation to all plantar intrinsics of the foot; the medial calcaneal branches are purely sensory

Medial plantar nerve

Like the median nerve of the hand

Runs close to the intersection of the flexor digitorum longus (FDL) and the flexor hallucis longus (FHL) (knot of Henry)

Provides plantar sensation to the medial 3½ digits

Provides motor innervation to

Flexor hallucis brevis (FHB)

Abductor hallucis

Flexor digitorum brevis (FDB)

First lumbrical

Lateral plantar nerve

Like the ulnar nerve of the hand

Provides plantar sensation to the lateral 1½ digits

Provides motor innervation to

Abductor digiti minimi

Quadratus plantae

Second to fourth lumbricals

Adductor hallucis

Flexor digiti minimi brevis (FDMB)

All seven interossei (four dorsal, three plantar)

The first branch of the lateral plantar nerve (to the abductor digiti minimi) runs between the deep fascia of the abductor hallucis longus and the quadratus plantae

Medial calcaneal branches

Provide sensation to the plantar heel

Deep peroneal nerve

Provides sensory innervations to the dorsal first web space

Provides motor innervation to the extensor digitorum brevis (EDB)

Sural nerve (dorsal lateral cutaneous nerve of the foot)

Provides sensory innervation to the lateral border of the foot

Superficial peroneal nerve (dorsal digital nerves)

Provides sensory innervation to the dorsum of the foot with the exception of the first web space

Saphenous nerve (terminal branches)

Provides sensory innervation to the medial border of the foot

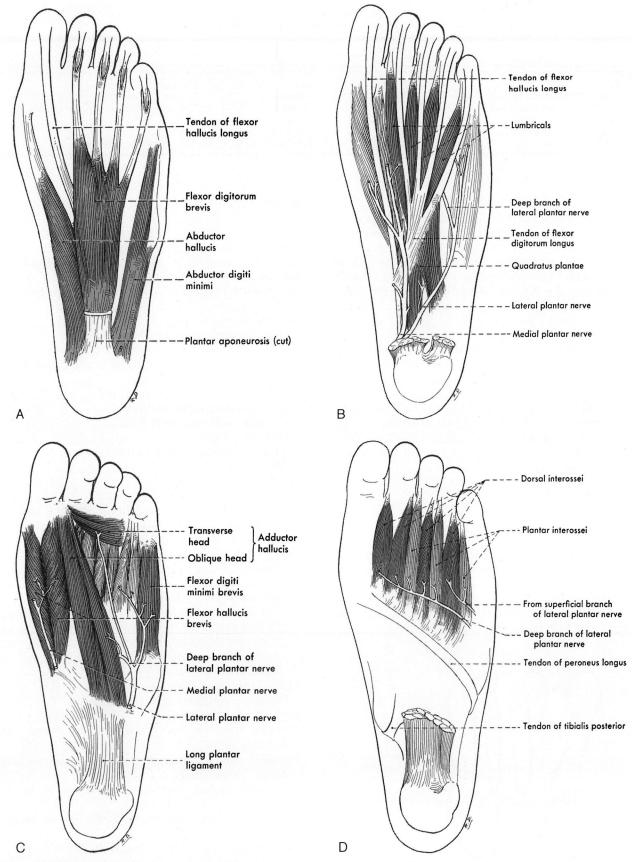

Tendon of flexor
hallucis longus

Flexor digitorum
brevis

Abductor
hallucis

Abductor digiti
minimi

Plantar aponeurosis (cut)

A

Tendon of flexor
hallucis longus

Lumbricals

Deep branch of
lateral plantar nerve

Tendon of flexor
digitorum longus

Quadratus plantae

Lateral plantar nerve

Medial plantar nerve

B

Transverse
head   } Adductor
Oblique head } hallucis

Flexor digiti
minimi brevis

Flexor hallucis
brevis

Deep branch of
lateral plantar nerve

Medial plantar nerve

Lateral plantar nerve

Long plantar
ligament

C

Dorsal interossei

Plantar interossei

From superficial branch
of lateral plantar nerve

Deep branch of lateral
plantar nerve

Tendon of peroneus longus

Tendon of tibialis posterior

D

Figure 22–3 ■ Plantar muscles of the foot and related anatomy. *A,* First (superficial) layer. *B,* Second layer. *C,* Third layer. *D,* Fourth layer. (From Jenkins DB: Hollinshead's Functional Anatomy of the Limbs and Back, 6th ed. Philadelphia, WB Saunders, 1991, pp 317–319.)

Table 22–2
INTRINSIC MUSCLES OF THE FOOT

Layer	Muscle	Origin	Insertion	Action	Innervation
Dorsal	Extensor digitorum brevis	Superolateral calcaneus	Base of the proximal phalanges	Extends the four lesser toes at the MTP and IP joints	Deep peroneal nerve
First plantar (most superficial)	Abductor hallucis	Calcaneal tuberosity	Base of the great toe proximal phalanx	Abducts the great toe	Medial plantar nerve
	Flexor digitorum brevis	Calcaneal tuberosity	Distal phalanges of the four lesser toes	Flexes the four lesser toes at the PIP joint	Medial plantar nerve
	Abductor digiti minimi	Calcaneal tuberosity	Base of the fifth toe	Abducts the small toe	Lateral plantar nerve
Second plantar	Quadratus plantae	Medial and lateral calcaneus	Tendon of flexor digitorum longus	Helps flex the distal phalanges	Lateral plantar nerve
	Lumbricals (four of them)	Flexor digitorum longus tendon	Base of the proximal phalanges	Flexes the MTP joint, extends the IP joint	Medial and lateral plantar nerves
Third plantar	Flexor hallucis brevis	Cuboid/lateral cuneiform	Proximal phalanx of the great toe	Flexes the great toe	Medial plantar nerve
	Adductor hallucis	Oblique head: peroneus longus tendon sheath Transverse head: deep transverse metatarsal ligament	Proximal phalanx of the great toe	Adducts the great toe	Lateral plantar nerve
	Flexor digiti minimi brevis	Base of the fifth metatarsal head	Proximal phalanx of the small toe	Flexes the small toe	Lateral plantar nerve
Fourth plantar (deepest)	Dorsal interossei (four of them)	Metatarsals	Base of proximal phalanges	Abducts the toes	Lateral plantar nerve
	Plantar interossei (three of them)	Metatarsals	Medial side of the proximal phalanges	Adducts the toes	Lateral plantar nerve

MTP, metatarsophalangeal; IP, interphalangeal; PIP, proximal interphalangeal.
Note: The second toe serves as a reference point for abduction and adduction of the toes.

Vessels (Fig. 22–6)

Dorsalis pedis artery
   The anterior tibial artery becomes the dorsalis pedis artery as it courses deep to the extensor retinaculum
   Deep plantar branch runs between the first and second metatarsals

   Supplies the plantar arch of the foot (the foot has only one arterial arch, whereas the hand has two arterial arches)
Posterior tibial artery
   Bifurcates to become the medial and lateral plantar arteries as it courses posterior and distal to the medial malleolus
   Lateral plantar artery is the main contributor to the plantar (arterial) arch

SURGICAL APPROACHES TO THE FOOT

Approaches to the Foot

Direct

HISTORY AND PHYSICAL EXAMINATION OF THE FOOT

History

Traumatic (injury) versus acquired condition
Referred pain
Chronicity
Age of the patient

Physical Examination

Observation
   Gait

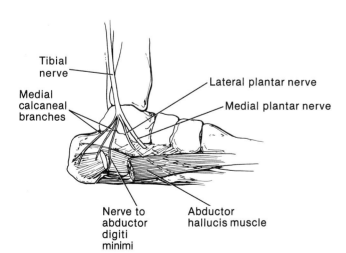

Figure 22–4 ■ Tibial nerve and its branches. (From Mann RA: Entrapment neuropathies of the foot. In DeLee JC, Drez D Jr [eds]: Orthopaedic Sports Medicine: Principles and Practice. Philadelphia, WB Saunders, 1994, p 1892.)

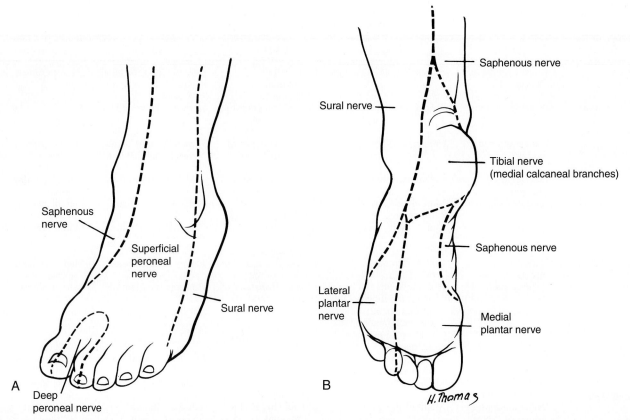

Figure 22–5 ■ *A,* Dorsal and *B,* plantar sensory innervation of the foot. (From Jaffe WL, Gannon PJ, Laitman JT: Paleontology, embryology, and anatomy of the foot. *In* Jahss MH [ed]: Disorders of the Foot and Ankle, 2nd ed. Philadelphia, WB Saunders, 1991, p 28.)

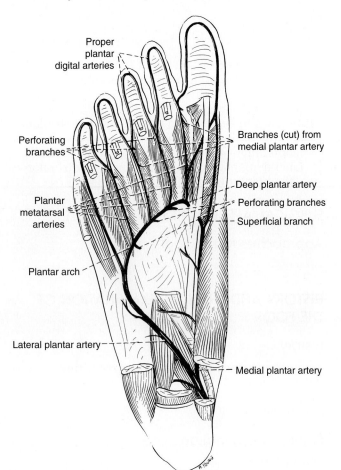

Figure 22–6 ■ Plantar arteries. (From Jenkins DB: Hollinshead's Functional Anatomy of the Limbs and Back, 6th ed. Philadelphia, WB Saunders, 1991, p 321.)

Shoe wear
Toes
Resting position of the foot
Skin changes
Swelling
Palpation
  Bones (see Fig. 22–1)
    First MTP joint (bunion)
    Navicular
    Fifth metatarsal base and head
    Calcaneus
    Sinus tarsi
    Metatarsal heads
    Toes
  Soft tissues
    Callosities
    Bursa (calcaneus, first MTP joint)
    Tibialis posterior tendon
    Dorsal extensor tendons
    Sinus tarsi
    Plantar fascia
    Toes
Motion (Fig. 22–7)
  Subtalar inversion/eversion (normal, 5 degrees each)
  Forefoot adduction (normal, 20 degrees)
  Forefoot abduction (normal, 10 degrees)
  First MTP joint flexion (normal, 45 degrees)
  First MTP joint extension (normal, 70–90 degrees)

Motions of the toes
Neurovascular exam
  Sensory (see Fig. 22–5)
  Strength testing (Table 22–3)
    Extrinsic toe dorsiflexors (extensor hallucis longus [EHL], extensor digitorum longus [EDL])
    Extrinsic toe plantar flexors (FHL, FDL)
    Intrinsic toe dorsiflexors (EDB)
    Intrinsic toe plantar flexors (FDB, FHB, FDMB, quadratus plantae, lumbricales)

DIAGNOSTIC TESTS FOR THE FOOT

Plain Radiographs

Anteroposterior (AP)
Lateral
Obliques (such as Broden's views)
Standing AP

Computed Tomography

Condition specific

Magnetic Resonance Imaging

Condition specific

Table 22–3
MUSCLES OF THE FOOT: THEIR ACTION, INNERVATION, AND NERVE ROOT DERIVATION

Action	Muscles Involved	Innervation	Nerve Root Derivation
Inversion	1. Tibialis posterior	Tibial	L4-5
	2. Flexor digitorum longus	Tibial	S2-3
	3. Flexor hallucis longus	Tibial	S2-3
	4. Tibialis anterior	Deep peroneal	L4-5
	5. Extensor hallucis longus	Deep peroneal	L5, S1
Eversion	1. Peroneus longus	Superficial peroneal	L5, S1-2
	2. Peroneus brevis	Superficial peroneal	L5, S1-2
	3. Peroneus tertius	Deep peroneal	L5, S1
	4. Extensor digitorum longus	Deep peroneal	L5, S1
Flexion of toes	1. Flexor digitorum longus	Tibial	S2-3
	2. Flexor hallucis longus	Tibial	S2-3
	3. Flexor digitorum brevis	Tibial (medial plantar nerve)	S2-3
	4. Flexor hallucis brevis	Tibial (medial plantar nerve)	S2-3
	5. Quadratus plantae (flexor accessorius)	Tibial (lateral plantar nerve)	S2-3
	6. Interossei	Tibial (lateral plantar nerve)	S2-3
	7. Flexor digiti minimi brevis	Tibial (lateral plantar nerve)	S2-3
	8. Lumbricales (metatarsophalangeal joints)	Tibial (1st by medial plantar nerve; 2nd through 4th by lateral plantar nerve)	S2-3
Extension of toes	1. Extensor digitorum longus	Deep peroneal	S5, S1
	2. Extensor hallucis longus	Deep peroneal	L5, S1
	3. Extensor digitorum brevis	Deep peroneal (lateral terminal branch)	S1-2
	4. Lumbricales (interphalangeal joints)	Tibial (1st by medial plantar nerve; 2nd through 4th by lateral plantar nerve)	S2-3
Abduction of toes	1. Abductor hallucis	Tibial (medial plantar nerve)	S2-3
	2. Abductor digiti minimi	Tibial (lateral plantar nerve)	S2-3
	3. Dorsal interossei	Tibial (lateral plantar nerve)	S2-3
Adduction of toes	1. Adductor hallucis	Tibial (lateral plantar nerve)	S2-3
	2. Plantar interossei	Tibial (lateral plantar nerve)	S2-3

Modified from Magee DJ: Orthopaedic Physical Assessment. Philadelphia, WB Saunders, 1992, p 475.

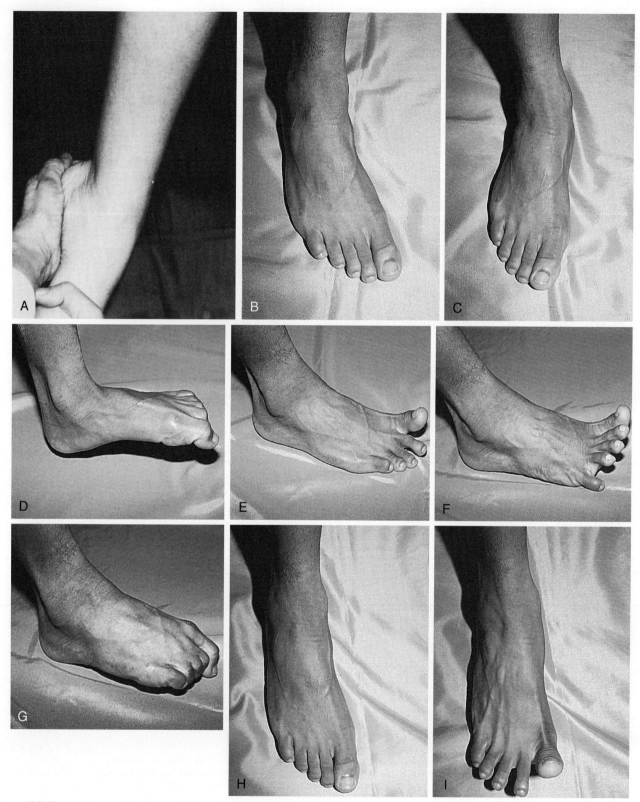

Figure 22–7 ■ Motions of the foot. *A*, Subtalar motion (inversion and eversion) is tested by holding and cupping the left heel in the left hand. The forefoot is grasped with the right hand and the arc of motion is recorded. *B*, Forefoot adduction. *C*, Forefoot abduction. *D*, First metatarsophalangeal (MTP) joint flexion. *E*, First MTP joint extension. *F*, Toe extension. *G*, Toe flexion. *H*, Toe adduction. *I*, Toe abduction. (*A* from Jahss MH: Disorders of the Foot. Philadelphia, WB Saunders, 1982, p 91.)

COMMON ADULT CONDITIONS OF THE FOOT

Foot conditions are most easily discussed by
Anatomic location (forefoot—metatarsals and distal; midfoot—the tarsal bones; and the hindfoot—talus and calcaneus)
Type of tissue involved (soft tissue, nail, bone)

Conditions of the Forefoot

Soft tissue conditions
Morton's neuroma
Etiology—degeneration and proliferation of the plantar digital nerve producing a painful mass near the metatarsal heads
Presentation—shooting pain radiating distally to the affected digits; most commonly painful when wearing shoes with a narrow toe box
Diagnosis—palpation between the metatarsal heads elicits painful symptoms; most common site is between the third and fourth metatarsals
Treatment—accommodative padding in the shoes, cortisone injections, surgical excision for cases refractory to conservative treatment
Hyperkeratotic disorders (corns)
Bony prominences are usually the cause
Treatment—supportive/shoe modification; surgical removal of offending bone
Intractable plantar keratoses
Plantar skin reaction from excess pressure (such as from a prominent metatarsal head, a long metatarsal, a hypermobile first ray, or forefoot varus or valgus)
Treatment—shoe modification/orthoses
Pathologic conditions of the nail (Table 22–4)
Bone problems
Hallux valgus (bunion) (Figs. 22–8 and 22–9)
Etiology—hereditary, may arise secondary to pes planus (flatfoot), or a long first metatarsal
Presentation—deformity at the first MTP joint

Table 22–4
TERMS FOR PATHOLOGIC CONDITIONS OF THE NAIL

Anonychia—Anonychia is the absence of nails. When the absence is congenital, it usually involves all of the nails, and the condition is permanent. This condition may also occur temporarily following trauma or as a result of systemic or local disease. It is also seen in the nail-patella syndrome.

Beau's lines—Beau's lines are transverse lines or ridges that mark repeated disturbances of nail growth. They may be associated with trauma or a systemic disease process.

Clubbing—Clubbing of the nail is associated with chronic pulmonary disease as well as cardiac disease.

Hapalonychia—Hapalonychia refers to extremely soft nails that may be prone to splitting. This is associated with endocrine disturbances and malnutrition as well as contact with strong alkali solutions.

Hemorrhage—Hemorrhage beneath the toenail may be associated with vitamin C deficiency, subacute bacterial endocarditis, and dermatologic disorders. Subungual hematoma follows trauma to the toenail bed.

Hyperkeratosis subungualis—Hypertrophy of the nail bed that may be associated with onychomycosis, psoriasis, and other dermatologic disorders.

Koilonychia—Concavity of the nail plate in both the longitudinal and transverse axes that is associated with nutritional disorders, iron deficiency anemia, and endocrine disorders.

Leukonychia—White spots or striations in the nail resulting from trauma or systemic diseases such as nutritional and endocrine deficiencies.

Onychauxis—A greatly thickened nail plate caused by persistent mild trauma and/or onychomycosis.

Onychia—Inflammation of the nail matrix causing deformity of the nail plate. Trauma, infection, and systemic diseases such as exanthemas are causes.

Onychitis—Inflammation of the nail.

Onychoclasis—Breakage or fracture of the nail plate.

Onychocryptosis—Ingrowing of the nails or more specifically hypertrophy of the nail lip. Also referred to as hypertrophied ungualabia, it is one of the most frequent pathologic conditions of the toenail.

Onychogryphosis—Claw nail or ram's horn nail. Extreme hypertrophy of the nail gives the appearance of a claw or horn. The condition may be congenital or a symptom of many chronic systemic diseases such as tinea infections. See onychauxis (synonym).

Onycholysis—Loosening of the nail plate beginning along the distal or free edge when trauma, injury by chemical agents, or diseases loosen the nail plate. This condition is associated with psoriasis, onychomycosis, acute fevers, and syphilis.

Onychoma—A tumor of the nail unit.

Onychomadesis—Complete loss of the nail plate.

Onychomalacia—Softening of the nail.

Onychomycosis—Fungal infection of the nail associated with fungal disease of the foot.

Onychorrhexis—Longitudinal ridging and splitting of the nails caused by dermatoses, nail infections, systemic diseases, senility, or injury by chemical agents.

Onychoschizia—Lamination and scaling away of the nails in thin layers caused by dermatoses, syphilis, or injury by chemical agents.

Onychosis—Disease or deformity of the nail plate.

Onychotrophia—Atrophy or failure of development of a nail caused by trauma, infection, endocrine dysfunction, or systemic disease.

Pachyonychia—Extreme thickening of all the nails. In this condition, the nails are more solid and more regular than in onychogryphosis. Usually this is a congenital condition associated with hyperkeratosis of the palms and soles.

Paronychia—Inflammation of the soft tissues around the nail margin. It may occur following infection or trauma. The infectious agent may be either bacterial or fungal.

Pterygium—The cuticle appears to grow distal to the nail plate and splits the nail into two or more portions that gradually reduce in size as the pterygium widens. This may result from trauma or poor circulation in the toes.

Modified from Coughlin MJ: Toe nail abnormalities. *In* Mann RA, Coughlin MJ: Surgery of the Foot and Ankle, 6th ed. St Louis, Mosby–Year Book, 1992, p 1036.

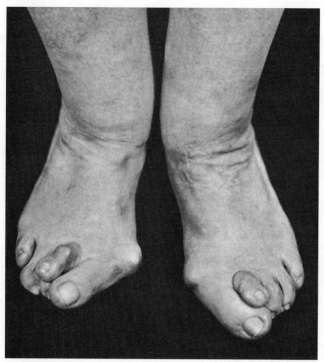

Figure 22–8 ■ Clinical example of a patient with severe bilateral bunions (hallux valgus). This patient also has bilateral overlapping second toes. (From Gartland J: Fundamentals of Orthopedics. Philadelphia, WB Saunders, 1987, p 401.)

with lateral deviation of the great toe and a large medial prominence at the first metatarsal head (see Fig. 22–8)

Diagnosis—radiographs (see Fig. 22–9) show

An increased hallux valgus angle (normal, ≤15 degrees)

An increased intermetatarsal angle (normal, ≤9 degrees)

Treatment options

Nonoperative—shoe modification to relieve pressure over the medial prominence

Operative—many types of operative corrections depending on the severity of the deformity

Hallux rigidus (Fig. 22–10)

Etiology—degenerative arthritis of the first MTP joint causing stiffness (at the joint); this may arise secondary to repetitive trauma or a metabolic disease, or after surgery

Presentation—pain and restricted motion of the first MTP joint; palpable bone spur on the dorsal aspect of the first metatarsal head

Diagnosis—palpable dorsal bone spur recreates painful symptoms on MTP joint range of motion; x-rays reveal MTP joint narrowing and osteophytes (bone spurs)

Treatment options

Nonoperative—nonsteroidal anti-inflammatory drugs (NSAIDs), orthoses

Operative—excision of the bone spur plus a portion of the joint surface

Hallux varus (Fig. 22–11)

Etiology—congenital or iatrogenic (such as after operative treatment of a hallux valgus deformity)

Presentation—discomfort in shoes, pain along the medial side of the great toe

Diagnosis—adducted position of the great toe

Treatment options

Nonoperative—valgus strapping and splinting

Operative—operative correction of the deformity

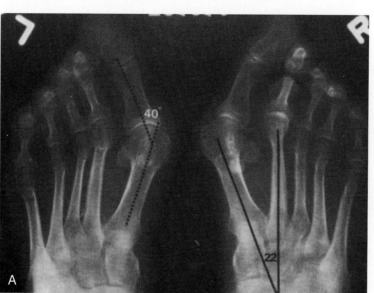
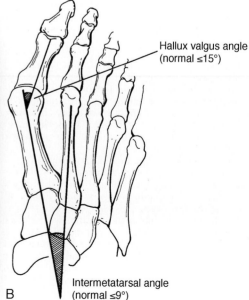

Figure 22–9 ■ *A,* Measurement of the hallux valgus angle (left) and the intermetatarsal angle (right). Note that both measurements in this example are abnormal. *B,* Drawing demonstrating angles. (*A* from Weissman BNW, Sledge CB: Orthopedic Radiology. Philadelphia, WB Saunders, 1986, p 657. *B* from Coughlin MJ: Conditions of the forefoot. *In* DeLee JC, Drez D Jr [eds]: Orthopaedic Sports Medicine: Principles and Practice. Philadelphia, WB Saunders, 1994, p 1847.)

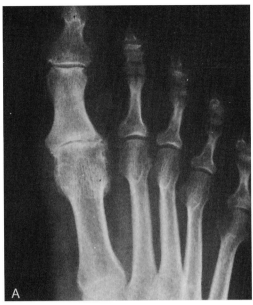
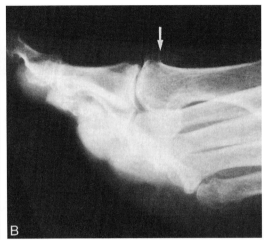

Figure 22–10 ■ Hallux rigidus. Note the loss of joint space at the great toe metatarsophalangeal joint seen on the AP view (*A*) and the dorsal osteophyte (*arrow*) seen on the lateral view (*B*). (From Weissman BNW, Sledge CB: Orthopedic Radiology. Philadelphia, WB Saunders, 1986, p 663.)

Sesamoiditis
  Etiology—repetitive trauma
  Presentation—pain in the area of the sesamoids (plantar surface of the great toe metatarsal head)
  Diagnosis—exclusion of a sesamoid fracture
  Treatment—relief of pressure on the sesamoids (pads, hard-soled shoes)

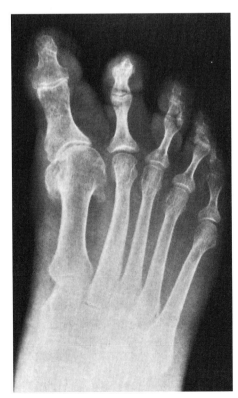

Figure 22–11 ■ AP radiograph demonstrating hallux varus. In this example, the varus deformity has resulted from overcorrection (surgically) of a hallux valgus. (From Weissman BNW, Sledge CB: Orthopedic Radiology. Philadelphia, WB Saunders, 1986, p 661.)

Sesamoid fractures (Fig. 22–12)
  Etiology—direct trauma or indirect trauma (hyperextension of the proximal phalanx on the metatarsal head, such as in runners)
  Presentation—pain in the area of the sesamoid bones (plantar surface of the great toe metatarsal head); the pain is aggravated with walking and subsides with rest
  Diagnosis—x-rays show the fracture (irregular borders); pain reproduced by dorsiflexion of the MTP joint of the great toe
  Treatment options
    Nonoperative—rest, immobilization
    Operative—excision of the involved sesamoid
Hammer toe (Fig. 22–13)
  Etiology—poorly fitting shoes lead to progressive "buckling" of the toes; characterized by a **contracture of the FDL tendon;** may also result from muscle imbalance in association with neuromuscular disorders
  Presentation—**plantar flexion of the proximal interphalangeal (PIP) joint** with dorsiflexion of the MTP joint; longer digits typically are affected more often; pain and discomfort in shoes
  Diagnosis—x-rays reveal dorsiflexion of the proximal phalanx with plantar flexion of the middle and/or distal phalanges
  Treatment—operative correction
Claw toe (Fig. 22–14)
  Etiology—often unclear, but may be associated with neuromuscular disorders, arthritic deformities, or metabolic disorders that cause the deformity; characterized by a **simultaneous contracture of the long extensors and long flexors of the toe** (and an imbalance between the intrinsic and extrinsic muscles of the foot)
  Presentation—usually affects multiple toes and

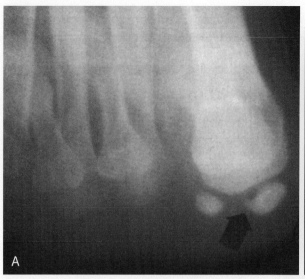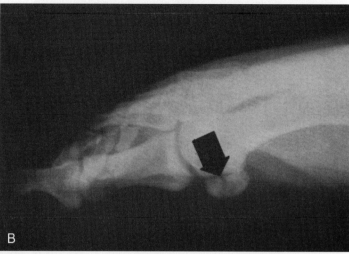

Figure 22–12 ■ *A,* Sesamoid view demonstrating a compression fracture of one of the sesamoids (*arrow*). *B,* Lateral view showing a fracture of one of the sesamoids (*arrow*). Note in both *A* and *B* that the tibial (medial) sesamoid is fractured and the fibular (lateral) sesamoid is uninjured. (From Jahss MH: Disorders of the Foot. Philadelphia, WB Saunders, 1982, p 1656.)

typically presents as a bilateral condition; the patient presents with **plantar flexion of the distal interphalangeal (DIP) joint and the PIP joint with dorsiflexion of the MTP joint** (see Fig. 22–14); **differentiated from a hammer toe by the hyperextension of the MTP joint**

Diagnosis—x-rays reveal a dorsiflexed position of the proximal phalanges and a plantarflexed position of the middle and distal phalanges

Treatment—operative correction of the deformity

Mallet toe (Fig. 22–15)

Etiology—poorly fitting shoes cause the toe to plantarflex at the DIP joint (with tightness of the FDL tendon)

Presentation—**plantar flexion of the DIP joint**

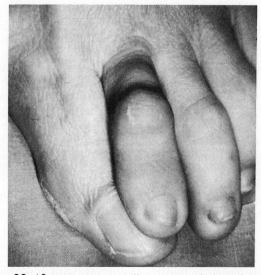

Figure 22–13 ■ Hammer toe. Illustration and clinical example. (From Jahss MH: Disorders of the Foot. Philadelphia, WB Saunders, 1982, p 639.)

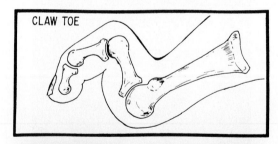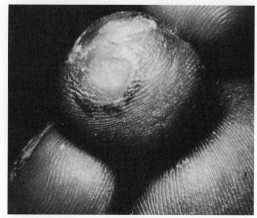

Figure 22–14 ■ Claw toe. Illustration and clinical example. (From Jahss MH: Disorders of the Foot. Philadelphia, WB Saunders, 1982, p 639.)

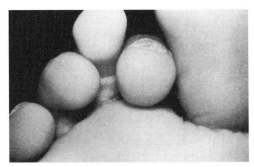

Figure 22–15 ■ Clinical example of a mallet toe. (From Jahss MH: Disorders of the Foot. Philadelphia, WB Saunders, 1982, p 625.)

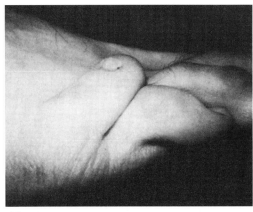

Figure 22–16 ■ Overlapping fifth toe. (From Jahss MH: Disorders of the Foot. Philadelphia, WB Saunders, 1982, p 646.)

(most common in the second toe); pain when the tip of the toe strikes the ground

Diagnosis—x-rays show a flexion contracture at the DIP joint

Treatment options

Nonoperative—padding to prevent the tip of the toe from striking the ground

Operative—release of the FDL tendon

Overlapping fifth toe (Fig. 22–16)

Etiology—usually congenital

Presentation—pain resulting from pressure from shoes on the toe; the fifth toe is externally rotated and compressed in the transverse plane

Treatment—operative correction varies according to the severity of the deformity

Underlapping fifth toe

Etiology—usually congenital

Presentation—the fifth toe is externally rotated and rides under ("underlaps") the fourth toe

Treatment—operative correction

Cock-up deformity of the fifth toe (Fig. 22–17)

Etiology—associated with a hammer toe deformity

Presentation—the proximal phalanx of the fifth

toe is at nearly a right angle in relation to the fifth metatarsal shaft

Treatment—operative correction

Tailor's bunion (bunionette) (Fig. 22–18)

Etiology—abnormal alignment of the metatarsal leads to lateral bowing of the diaphysis of the fifth metatarsal and a painful prominence of the lateral condyle of the fifth metatarsal head

Presentation—lateral or plantar keratosis; painful prominence

Diagnosis—x-rays reveal lateral bowing of the fifth metatarsal

Treatment options

Nonoperative—shoe modification

Operative—reconstruction

Subluxation of the second MTP joint

Etiology—the second ray is the longest in the foot and can result in pressure at the end of the toe that causes the toe to buckle and the proximal phalanx to ride up onto the dorsal aspect of the second metatarsal head

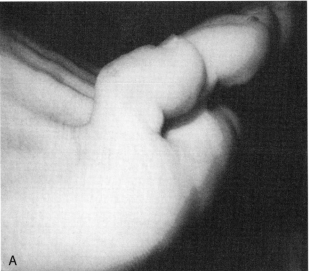
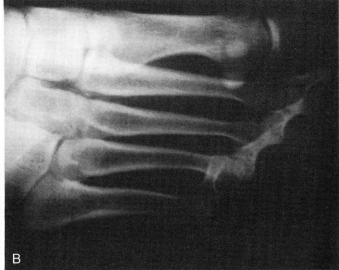

Figure 22–17 ■ *A*, Clinical photo and *B*, radiograph of a cock-up deformity of the fifth toe. (From Mann RA, Coughlin MJ: Lesser toe deformities. *In* Jahss MH [ed]: Disorders of the Foot and Ankle, 2nd ed. Philadelphia, WB Saunders, 1991, p 1226.)

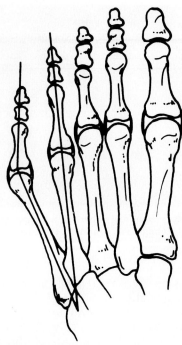

Figure 22–18 ■ Tailor's bunionette deformity showing the characteristic increase in the 4–5 intermetatarsal angle that results from lateral bowing of the fifth metatarsal. (From Cracchiolo A III: Surgical procedures of the lateral metatarsals. *In* Jahss MH [ed]: Disorders of the Foot and Ankle, 2nd ed. Philadelphia, WB Saunders, 1991, p 1270.)

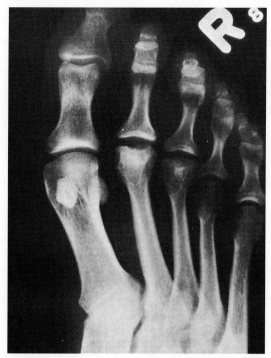

Figure 22–19 ■ Freiberg's infraction of the second and perhaps the third metatarsal heads. Note flattening, sclerosis, and irregularity of the second metatarsal head. (From Weissman BNW, Sledge CB: Orthopedic Radiology. Philadelphia, WB Saunders, 1986, p 668.)

Presentation—swelling of the second MTP joint with tenderness to palpation over the joint; pain on ambulation

Diagnosis—manipulation of the MTP joint elicits characteristic pain (differential diagnosis: MTP joint synovitis, capsular degeneration, Freiberg's infraction, arthritis)

Treatment options

Nonoperative—metatarsal pad, NSAIDs, shoe modification

Operative—when progressive deformity is present, correction of the deformity is indicated

Freiberg's infraction (Fig. 22–19)

Etiology—collapse of the subchondral area of the metatarsal head caused by avascular necrosis

Presentation—pain and limitation of motion of the affected joint; pain worsens with increased activity and is relieved by rest; most commonly affects the second metatarsal head

Diagnosis—x-rays confirm the diagnosis by demonstrating sclerotic changes in the early stages and osteolysis with collapse in the later stages

Treatment options

Nonoperative—alleviating discomfort by decreasing stress at the involved joint, short-leg walking cast, postoperative shoe

Operative—in later stages of the disease

Conditions of the Midfoot

Soft tissue problems
Plantar fibroma

Etiology—locally aggressive idiopathic proliferative fasciitis of the plantar aponeurosis; one of the most common benign soft tissue lesions seen in the foot; may be seen at any age but most commonly in the early decades; bilateral involvement is common

Presentation—tender nodules on the plantar fascia that produce discomfort with weight bearing

Treatment—operative excision (there is a high rate of recurrence)

Plantar warts (Fig. 22–20)

Etiology—papovavirus

Presentation—solitary, multiple, or a mosaic pattern; warts are painful

Diagnosis—pinpoint bleeding after trimming

Treatment—multiple methods (curettage and electrosurgery, carbon dioxide laser, salicylic acid, others)

Ganglion cyst

Etiology—continued stress on structures (joint capsule, tendon sheath) causes collagen tissue to undergo mucoid degeneration with the formation of amorphous gelatinous material

Presentation—most common area of the foot is in the tarsal area and over the tendon of the peroneus tertius; painful because of shoe pressure

Treatment—needle aspiration versus operative excision

Conditions of the Hindfoot

Soft tissue problems
Plantar fasciitis (Fig. 22–21)

Etiology—caused by overpull of the plantar fascia associated with microtrauma to the plantar fascia at its attachment (leading to chronic inflammation); a flatfoot (pes planus) deformity will place increased stress on the origin of the plantar fascia; a cavus foot may lead to increased stress on the heel caused by a lack of heel eversion necessary to absorb shock; also associated with nerve entrapments (irritation of the medial calcaneal nerve or entrapment of the nerve to the abductor digiti minimi)

Presentation—acute tenderness at the medial tubercle of the calcaneus and over the course of the plantar fascia

Diagnosis—x-rays may show a flatfoot or cavus foot deformity; a heel spur may also be present; lab studies are usually normal but one should rule out the seronegative spondyloarthropathies (HLA-B27)

Treatment

Nonoperative—NSAIDs, orthoses, corticosteroid injection, physical therapy, decrease in activity; conservative therapy should continue for 9 to 12 months before considering operative intervention

Operative—release of the plantar fascia is rarely required

Retrocalcaneal bursitis (Fig. 22–22)

Etiology—most common cause is overuse with the bursa compressed between the calcaneus and

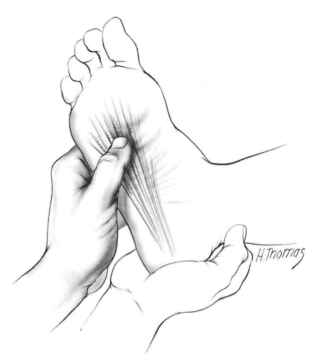

Figure 22–21 ■ Palpation of the plantar fascia reveals severe pain in patients with plantar fasciitis. (From Jahss MH: Disorders of the Foot. Philadelphia, WB Saunders, 1982, p 109.)

the Achilles tendon during dorsiflexion of the foot; may also be a new manifestation of other conditions such as gout, rheumatoid arthritis, or one of the seronegative spondyloarthropathies

Presentation—may see a prominence on the posterior aspect of the heel; edema; erythema

Diagnosis—hallmark is medial and lateral pain just anterior to the Achilles tendon at the level of the posterior superior calcaneal tuberosity;

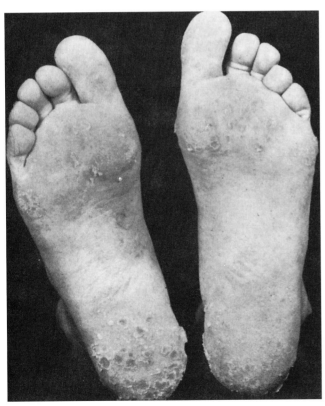

Figure 22–20 ■ Mosaic appearance of plantar warts. (From Jahss MH: Disorders of the Foot. Philadelphia, WB Saunders, 1982, p907.)

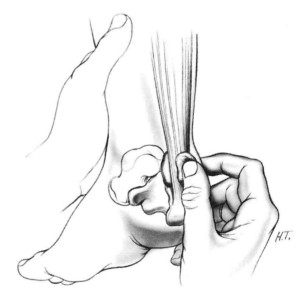

Figure 22–22 ■ Palpation of the retrocalcaneal bursa. Irritation is often caused by a tight shoe (pump bump). (From Jahss MH: Disorders of the Foot. Philadelphia, WB Saunders, 1982, p 105.)

MRI demonstrates the retrocalcaneal bursa clearly

Treatment

Nonoperative—NSAIDs, steroid injection, heel elevation (heel lift)

Operative—excision of the bursa alone is usually not helpful in relieving symptoms

Haglund's deformity (Fig. 22–23)

Etiology—similar to retrocalcaneal bursitis

Presentation—similar to retrocalcaneal bursitis

Diagnosis—x-rays may reveal a prominence of the posterior superior tuberosity of the calcaneus

Treatment

Nonoperative—heel lift

Operative—resection of the prominence of the posterior superior tuberosity of the calcaneus

Tarsal tunnel syndrome (see Chapter 21)

Entrapment of the first branch of the lateral plantar nerve

Etiology—entrapment occurs between the deep fascia of the abductor hallucis muscle and the medial aspect of the quadratus plantae muscle

Presentation—chronic heel pain, increased by running; pain radiates from the medial aspect of the heel into the medial ankle area and can radiate laterally across the foot

Diagnosis—tenderness over the first branch of the lateral plantar nerve deep to the abductor hallucis muscle; pressure at this point will reproduce symptoms

Treatment—surgical decompression of the nerve

Sinus tarsi syndrome (see Fig. 22–23)

Etiology

Trauma—prior inversion ankle sprain, fibula fracture, calcaneal or talar neck fracture

Biomechanical—pes cavus or pes planus foot structure

Arthritides—rheumatoid arthritis, gout, seronegative spondyloarthropathies

Presentation—pain on the lateral side of the foot aggravated by walking

Diagnosis—sharp pain when palpating the sinus tarsi; complete resolution of symptoms after an injection of local anesthetic into the sinus tarsi

Treatment

Nonoperative—series of injections of local anesthetic/steroid, NSAIDs, immobilization, physical therapy

Operative—sinus tarsi decompression

Other Foot Conditions

Rheumatoid foot (Fig. 22–24)

Etiology—rheumatoid arthritis

Presentation

Forefoot changes

Synovitis of the MTP joints—the lateral aspect of the MTP joints is often the first to be affected; progressive deformity leads to subluxation and dislocation; at the end stages of the disease the metatarsal head herniates through the plantar capsule and the base of the proximal phalanx comes to lie on the dorsal aspect of the metatarsal neck

Splaying of the forefoot—caused by chronic synovitis and ligamentous laxity

Claw toes—secondary to MTP involvement

Hallux valgus—with progression, may override or underride the lateral toes

Midfoot (tarsal and tarsometatarsal joints) changes—typically are not severely involved in the rheumatoid foot

May develop chronic synovitis and loss of the joint space leading to fibrosis and bony ankylosis

May develop a hypermobile metatarsocuneiform joint leading to transferred pressure to the lesser metatarsals and/or a hallux valgus deformity

Loss of the longitudinal arch caused by sagging of the metatarsocuneiform or naviculocuneiform joints

Hindfoot changes—occur much later in the process; related to destruction of the tissues surrounding the subtalar joint and occur as a result of changes in the tarsal joints

Ankylosis

Loss of the longitudinal arch

Diagnosis—based on clinical, laboratory, and radiographic findings

Rheumatoid arthritis begins in the feet in approximately 15% to 20% of cases; there is usually symmetric involvement

Intra-articular swelling with effusion is sometimes present, as is periarticular soft tissue swelling

There can be pain and erythema over the involved joint, with involvement of the PIP and MTP joints

In the early stages of the disease, x-rays may show only soft tissue swelling

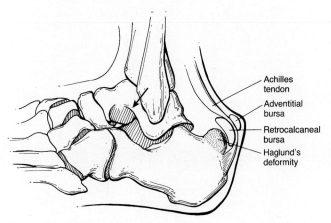

Figure 22–23 ■ This drawing illustrates the anatomic sites of involvement for Haglund's deformity and sinus tarsi syndrome. Sinus tarsi syndrome is caused by synovitis in the sinus tarsi (*arrow*). (From Bordelon RL: Heel pain. *In* DeLee JC, Drez D Jr [eds]: Orthopaedic Sports Medicine: Principles and Practice. Philadelphia, WB Saunders, 1994, p 1807.)

Achilles tendon

Adventitial bursa

Retrocalcaneal bursa

Haglund's deformity

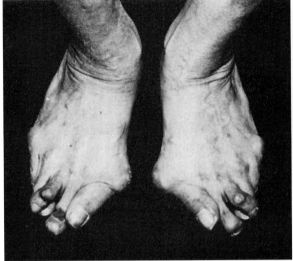
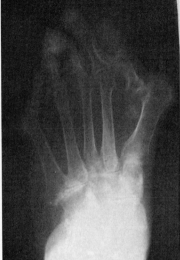
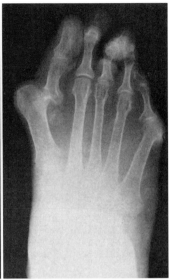
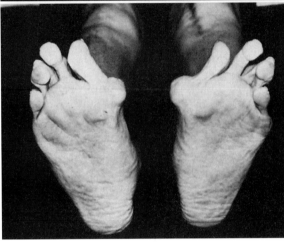

Figure 22–24 ■ Clinical and radiographic features of rheumatoid arthritis of the foot. Note the hallux valgus and lesser (2–5) toe deformities, the splaying of the forefoot, and the joint subluxations and dislocations. (From Jahss MH: Disorders of the Foot. Philadelphia, WB Saunders, 1982, p 1026.)

Treatment
　Nonoperative—drug therapy, physical therapy, orthotic devices
　Operative—each area affected (forefoot, midfoot, hindfoot) must be addressed; the operative procedure is based on an extensive clinical evaluation
Foot disorders in other arthritides (see Chapter 3)
　Crystal-induced arthritis of the foot (such as gout)
　The seronegative spondyloarthropathies (such as ankylosing spondylitis)
　Others
The diabetic foot
　Pathophysiology
　　Neuropathy—sensory neuropathy is the main source of almost all variations and most infections
　　　There is a loss of protective sensation combined with acute recurrent trauma or microtrauma; mechanical breakdown may lead to plantar ulcers, spontaneous fractures, and osteomyelitis
　　　Plantar ulcerations are almost always associated with areas of underlying bony prominences in the foot

Ulcerations on the dorsal, lateral, or medial aspects of the foot are usually caused by constant shoe pressure
Autonomic neuropathy—causes a loss of normal sweating of the skin of the foot, which leads to dry, scaly skin and possibly cracks and fissures that become potential areas for infection
Motor neuropathy—a loss of function and contracture of the intrinsic muscles of the foot; this is demonstrated by claw toe deformities that lead to a predisposition for ulcers on the dorsal aspect of the digit as well as on the plantar aspect of the metatarsal head caused by excess pressure
Mononeuropathy—usually affects the peroneal nerve, which can cause footdrop
Angiopathy
Presentation
　Must carefully evaluate patient's gait, structural deformities, bony prominences
　Must evaluate neurologic status—light touch, pinprick, vibratory status, temperature testing
　Must evaluate vascular status—Doppler pressures, examination of palpable pulses, warmth, and hair growth

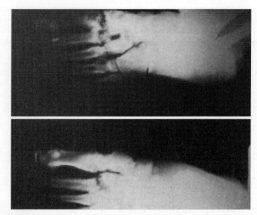

Figure 22–25 ■ Typical radiographic findings of Charcot's joints of the foot. In this example, there are advanced changes in Lisfranc's joint. (From Jahss MH: Disorders of the Foot. Philadelphia, WB Saunders, 1982, p 1379.)

Diagnosis—diagnostic studies include
  X-rays—to diagnose bony disorders
  Bone scans—sensitive in detecting early bone changes of osteomyelitis and Charcot's joints (more sensitive than plain radiographs)
  CT—useful in imaging bony changes
  MRI—useful for delineating the soft tissues and in imaging infections
Treatment

Ulcers
  Nonoperative—extra-depth shoes, total contact casting, prefabricated walking brace, wound care with dressing changes
  Operative—warranted for chronic and recurrent ulcerations
  Infections/abscesses—intravenous (IV) antibiotics, glucose control, operative débridement
  Osteomyelitis—resection of infected bone, IV antibiotics, amputation for uncontrollable infection
Charcot's joints (Fig. 22–25)
  Etiology—diabetes is the leading cause of a Charcot's joint of the lower extremity
    Theory no. 1—neurotraumatic: joint destruction, fractures, and collapse of the foot are caused by continued mechanical trauma in a joint that is pain insensitive
    Theory no. 2—neurovascular: joint destruction is caused by a neurally stimulated vascular reflex ("autosympathectomy") causing bone resorption and ligamentous changes
  Epidemiology
    Affects men and women equally
    Average duration of diabetes is 10 years before the occurrence of a Charcot's joint
    Occurs bilaterally in approximately 30% of cases
  Presentation

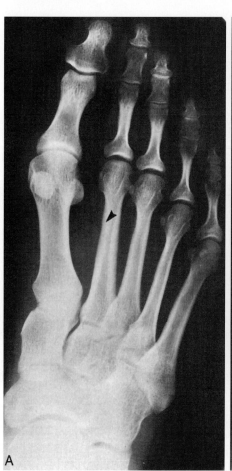
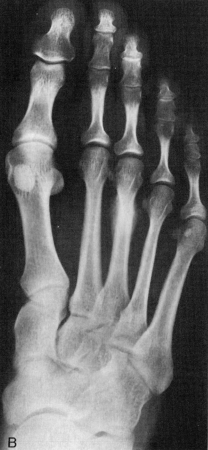

Figure 22–26 ■ Stress fracture of the third metatarsal. A, Early radiograph demonstrating a mild periosteal reaction along the third metatarsal shaft (the arrowhead demonstrates a normal vascular canal in the second metatarsal). B, 2 weeks later, the periosteal reaction is obvious. (From Weissman BNW, Sledge CB: Orthopedic Radiology. Philadelphia, WB Saunders, 1986, p 53.)

A

B

Pain can be a symptom even though the patient has a Charcot's joint

Acute—swelling of the ankle and foot with increased warmth and erythema; x-ray changes may be negative in early stages; differential diagnosis includes cellulitis or abscess

Subacute—less intense inflammatory changes with radiographic changes noted (i.e., "rocker-bottom foot," splayfoot, bony prominences)

Diagnosis—if differentiation between Charcot's foot and osteomyelitis cannot be made with noninvasive studies (bone scan, CT, MRI), a bone biopsy may be helpful

Treatment

Bracing

Avoid operative procedures

Infections of the Foot

Bacterial infections

Puncture wounds (through the rubber sole of a tennis shoe)—early manifestations include cellulitis and abscess formation; late complications include osteomyelitis and septic arthritis; treatment is irrigation and débridement (removal of any foreign bodies), and antibiotics (must cover for *Pseudomonas*)

Trauma creating open wounds—wound cleansing, débridement of devitalized tissue, and antibiotics are an essential part of the treatment; antibiotic coverage should be aimed to cover *Staphylococcus* and *Streptococcus*

Deep infections—penetrating wounds may lead to abscess formation and later osteomyelitis

Joint infections—can be spread by adjacent infection, by direct inoculation, or from septicemic illness (the most common organism is *Staphylococcus aureus*)

Bone infections—acute and chronic osteomyelitis (see Chapter 3)

Fungal infections

Tinea pedis—common infection of the skin and nails of the foot; symptoms include itching, cracking, and blisters; most common organisms are *Trichophyton rubrum* and *Trichophyton mentagrophytes*

FRACTURES AND DISLOCATIONS OF THE FOOT (Figs. 22–26 to 22–30)

Overview

The foot is made up of a large number of bones (seven tarsals, five metatarsals, 14 phalanges, and two sesamoids); the specific treatment of fractures and dislocations of the foot depends on the anatomic location and extent of injury (Tables 22–5 and 22–6)

Lawnmower injuries represent open fractures that are grossly contaminated and mandate operative débridement

The talus has a tenuous blood supply and is predisposed to avascular necrosis and fracture nonunion

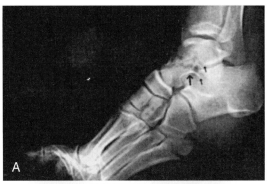
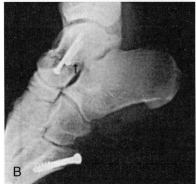

Figure 22–27 ■ *A*, Presentation and *B*, operative treatment of a talar neck fracture (also note the displaced fracture of the base of the fifth metatarsal). (From Hansen ST: Foot injuries. *In* Browner BD, Jupiter JB, Levine AM, et al [eds]: Skeletal Trauma. Philadelphia, WB Saunders, 1994, p 1962.)

TUMORS OF THE FOOT

Bone

Enchondroma

Soft Tissue

Plantar fibroma
Ganglion cyst
Glomus tumor
Giant cell tumor of tendon sheath
Kaposi's sarcoma
Clear cell sarcoma

DIFFERENTIAL DIAGNOSIS OF COMMON FOOT COMPLAINTS

Pain

Soft tissue problems
Tendon injuries
Ligamentous injuries
Bony conditions (such as metatarsalgia, tarsal coalition, bunions, other deformities)
Fractures
Stress fractures
Dislocations
Nerve injuries/disorders (such as neuromas)
Arthritis

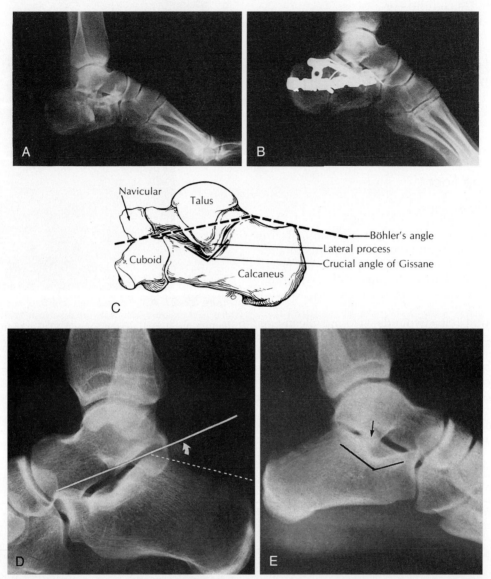

Figure 22–28 ■ *A*, Presentation and *B*, operative treatment of a calcaneus fracture. *C*, Two important radiographic measurements that should be made from the lateral radiograph when assessing an intra-articular calcaneus fracture. **Böhler's angle** is constructed by the intersection of two lines: (1) a line connecting the highest point of the anterior facet of the calcaneus and the highest point of the posterior facet of the calcaneus, and (2) a line connecting the highest point of the posterior facet of the calcaneus and the highest point on the posterior aspect of the calcaneus. Böhler's angle normally measures 25 to 40 degrees; depression of the subtalar joint from an intra-articular fracture results in an abnormal decrease in Böhler's angle. The **crucial angle of Gissane** represents an outline of the subtalar joint with the wedge-shaped lateral process of the talus pointed directly at the "crucial angle." The crucial angle of Gissane normally measures 120 to 145 degrees; this angle will be disrupted with a high-energy intra-articular calcaneus fracture. *D*, Radiographic measurement of Böhler's angle. *E,* Radiographic measurement of the crucial angle of Gissane. (*A* and *B* from Hansen ST: Foot injuries. *In* Browner BD, Jupiter JB, Levine AM, et al [eds]: Skeletal Trauma. Philadelphia, WB Saunders, 1994, p 1971; *C* and *E* from Heckman JD: Fractures and dislocations of the foot. *In* Rockwood CA, Green DP [eds]: Fractures in Adults, 2nd ed. Philadelphia, JB Lippincott, 1984, pp 1761 and 1771; *D* from Weissman BNW, Sledge CB: Orthopedic Radiology. Philadelphia, WB Saunders, 1986, p 645.)

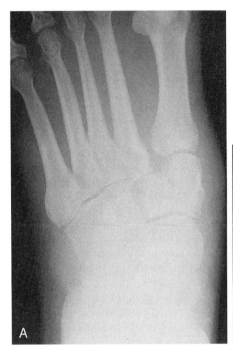

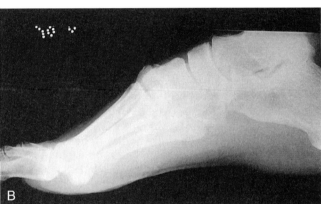

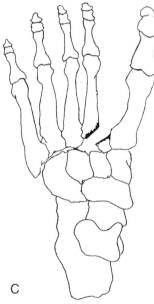

Figure 22–29 ■ Lisfranc's (tarsal metatarsal) fracture dislocation. *A,* AP radiograph showing a widened space between the first and second metatarsal base. *B,* Lateral radiograph showing dorsal displacement of the base of the second metatarsal. *C,* Schematic of the injury. (From Masear VR: Primary Care Orthopaedics. Philadelphia, WB Saunders, 1996, p 134.)

Table 22–5
FRACTURES OF THE ADULT FOOT

Fracture	Eponym or Other Name	Classification	Treatment	Most Common Complications of the Injury
Stress fracture (most common in the second metatarsal and calcaneus) (see Fig. 22–26)	March		Symptomatic (may require short leg cast)	
Talar neck (see Fig. 22–27)	Aviator's astragalus	Hawkins and Canale (I–IV) I. Nondisplaced	Short leg cast for 12 weeks (non–weight bearing for first 6 weeks)	Delayed union, nonunion, post-traumatic arthritis, avascular necrosis (Hawkins' sign is a radiolucency in the subchondral area of the talar dome; this is a *good* prognostic sign indicating remodeling and an adequate blood supply to the talus)
		II. Displaced with subtalar dislocation	Closed reduction; ORIF if reduction is not anatomic	
		III. Displaced with talar body dislocation	ORIF	
		IV. Displaced with talar head dislocation	ORIF	
Talar body			ORIF	Avascular necrosis, malunion, post-traumatic arthritis
Talar head			ORIF	Post-traumatic arthritis
Talar process		Lateral process	Short leg cast for 6 weeks	Nonunion
		Posterior process	Short leg cast for 6 weeks	
Calcaneus (see Fig. 22–28)		Essex-Lopresti (extra-articular, intra-articular) Sanders (I–IV)	Closed vs. operative treatment	Chronic heel pain and widening, peroneal tendinitis, post-traumatic arthritis, malunion, missed associated fractures (spine, lower extremity)
Midtarsal			ORIF	
Navicular		Descriptive	Operative treatment	Nonunion, avascular necrosis
Cuboid	Nutcracker		ORIF	
Tarsal metatarsal fracture dislocation	Lisfranc's (see Fig. 22–29)	Homolateral, isolated, divergent	Operative stabilization almost always required	Chronic pain, missed diagnosis
Metatarsal shaft			Closed reduction, operative stabilization may be required, short leg cast for 4 weeks	
Metatarsal head			Closed reduction vs. ORIF	
Fifth metatarsal, transverse fracture at base (junction of metaphysis and diaphysis)	Jones (see Fig. 22–30)		Non–weight-bearing short leg cast for 6 weeks, may require ORIF	Nonunion
Fifth metatarsal base avulsion fracture	Pseudo-Jones		Short leg walking cast for 3 weeks	

ORIF, open reduction with internal fixation.

Table 22–6
DISLOCATIONS OF THE ADULT FOOT

Dislocation	Eponym or Other Name	Treatment	Most Common Complications of the Injury
Subtalar	Basketball foot	Closed reduction and casting for 4 weeks; open reduction if irreducible by closed methods	Entrapment of the tibialis posterior tendon
Total talar		Open reduction	Avascular necrosis
Metatarsophalangeal		Closed reduction	
Phalangeal		Closed reduction	

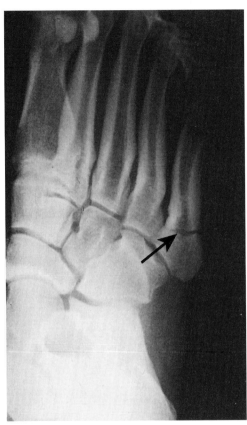

Figure 22–30 ■ Jones fracture (*arrow*). (From Masear VR: Primary Care Orthopaedics. Philadelphia, WB Saunders, 1996, p 135.)

Avascular necrosis (such as Freiberg's infraction)
Inflammatory conditions (such as synovitis, sesamoiditis, plantar fasciitis)
Rheumatologic conditions
Infections
Nail disorders
Tumors
Vaso-occlusive disorders

Instability

Ligamentous injuries
Fractures
Dislocations

Rheumatologic conditions
Neuropathic conditions

Weakness

Tendon injuries
Nerve injuries/disorders

Tingling/Loss of Sensation

Traumatic nerve injuries
Nerve entrapments (such as tarsal tunnel syndrome)
Lumbar radiculopathy
Neuromas
Tumors
Vaso-occlusive disorders
Neuropathic conditions (such as diabetes)

Deformity

Bony conditions (such as tarsal coalition, bunions, other deformities)
Fractures
Dislocations
Nerve injuries/disorders (atrophy, clawing)
Late effects of trauma
Rheumatologic conditions
Infections
Tumors

Loss of Motion

Tendon injuries
Ligamentous injuries
Bony conditions
Fractures
Dislocations
Late effects of trauma
Arthritis
Rheumatologic conditions
Infections
Tumors

PEARLS AND PITFALLS

A puncture wound through the rubber sole of a tennis shoe can lead to a serious infection

Glossary of Abbreviations

ABC	aneurysmal bone cyst
ABG	arterial blood gas
AC	acromioclavicular
ACL	anterior cruciate ligament
AD	autosomal dominant
ADI	atlantodens interval
ADM	abductor digiti minimi
AFO	ankle-foot orthosis
AIDS	acquired immunodeficiency syndrome
AIIS	anterior inferior iliac spine
ANA	antinuclear antibody
ANS	autonomic nervous system
AO	Arbeitgemeinschaft für Osteosynthese-fragen
AP	anteroposterior
APB	abductor pollicis brevis
APL	abductor pollicis longus
AR	autosomal recessive
ARDS	acute respiratory distress syndrome
AS	ankylosing spondylitis
ASIF	Association for the Study of Internal Fixation
ASIS	anterior superior iliac spine
ASO	antistreptolysin O
ATFL	anterior talofibular ligament
AVN	avascular necrosis
BMD	bone mineral density
BMP	bone morphogenic protein
BR	brachioradialis
CDH	congenital dislocation of the hip
CFL	calcaneofibular ligament
CMC	carpometacarpal
CMF	chondromyxoid fibroma
CNS	central nervous system
CP	cerebral palsy
CPK	creatine phosphokinase
CPM	continuous passive motion
CPPD	calcium pyrophosphate deposition disease
CT	computed tomography
CTLSO	cervicothoracolumbosacral orthosis
D/C	discharge
DCP	dynamic compression plating
DDH	developmental dysplasia of the hip
DEXA	dual energy x-ray absorptiometry
DIP	distal interphalangeal
DISH	diffuse idiopathic skeletal hyperostosis
DISI	dorsal intercalated segmental instability
DJD	degenerative joint disease
DP	dorsalis pedis
DVT	deep venous thrombosis
ECG	electrocardiograph
ECRB	extensor carpi radialis brevis
ECRL	extensor carpi radialis longus
ECU	extensor carpi ulnaris
EDC	extensor digitorum communis
EDL	extensor digitorum longus
EDM	extensor digiti minimi (same as EDQ [extensor digiti quinti])
EG	eosinophilic granuloma
EHL	extensor hallucis longus
EIP	extensor indicis proprius
ELISA	enzyme-linked immunosorbent assay
EMG	electromyography
EMS	emergency medical services
EPB	extensor pollicis brevis
EPL	extensor pollicis longus
ESR	erythrocyte sedimentation rate
FCR	flexor carpi radialis
FCU	flexor carpi ulnaris
FDL	flexor digitorum longus
FDM	flexor digiti minimi
FDP	flexor digitorum profundus
FDS	flexor digitorum superficialis
b-FGF	fibroblast growth factor (basic)
FHB	flexor hallucis brevis
FHL	flexor hallucis longus
FPB	flexor pollicis brevis
FPL	flexor pollicis longus
FTH	follow to healing
FWB(AT)	full weight bearing (as tolerated)
GAG	glycosaminoglycan
GC	gonococcal
GCT	giant cell tumor
HDL	high-density lipoproteins
HIV	human immunodeficiency virus
HKAFO	hip-knee-ankle-foot orthosis
HLA	human leukocyte antigen
HNP	herniated nucleus pulposus
HO	heterotopic ossification
HTO	high tibial osteotomy (same as PTO)
I & D	irrigation and débridement; incision and drainage
IGF-I	insulin-like growth factor I
IGF-II	insulin-like growth factor II
IL-I	interleukin I
IP	interphalangeal
IT	iliotibial
IV	intravenous
JRA	juvenile rheumatoid arthritis
KAFO	knee-ankle-foot orthosis

LCL	lateral collateral ligament
LDL	low-density lipoproteins
LLD	leg length discrepancy
MCL	medial collateral ligament
MCP	metacarpophalangeal
MED	multiple epiphyseal dysplasias
MEN	multiple endocrine neoplasias
MFH	malignant fibrous histiocytoma
MI	myocardial infarction
MO	myositis ossificans
MRI	magnetic resonance imaging
MSU	monosodium urate
MTA	metatarsus adductus
NCS	nerve conduction study
NOF	nonossifying fibroma (also known as a fibrous cortical defect)
NSAIDs	nonsteroidal anti-inflammatory drugs
OA	osteoarthritis
OCD	osteochondritis dissecans
ODM	opponens digiti minimi
OI	osteogenesis imperfecta
ON	osteonecrosis
OP	opponens pollicis
ORIF	open reduction with internal fixation
PA	posteroanterior
PB	peroneus brevis
PCL	posterior cruciate ligament
PDGF	platelet-derived growth factor
PE	pulmonary embolism
PEEP	positive end-expiratory pressure
Pen G	penicillin G
PFFD	proximal femoral focal deficiency
PGA	polyglycolic acid
PIN	posterior interosseous nerve
PIP	proximal interphalangeal
PL	peroneus longus; palmaris longus
PLA	polylactic acid
PMMA	polymethylmethacrylate
PMNs	polymorphonuclear leukocytes
POD	postoperative day (number)
PPD	purified protein derivative
PQ	pronator quadratus
PSIS	posterior superior iliac spine
PT	physical therapy; prothrombin time; pronator teres

PTFL	posterior talofibular ligament
PTH	parathyroid hormone
PTO	proximal tibial osteotomy (same as HTO)
PTT	partial thromboplastin time
PVNS	pigmented villonodular synovitis
PWB(AT)	partial weight bearing (as tolerated)
RA	rheumatoid arthritis
RBC	red blood cell
RF	rheumatoid factor
ROM	range of motion
RSD	reflex sympathetic dystrophy
SAC	space available for the (spinal) cord
SC	sternoclavicular
SCFE	slipped capital femoral epiphysis
SCIWORA	spinal cord injury without radiographic abnormality
SED	spondyloepiphyseal dysplasias
SH	Salter-Harris
SI	sacroiliac
SIADH	syndrome of inappropriate antidiuretic hormone secretion
SLAC	scapholunate advanced collapse
SLAP	superior glenoid labral tear in the anterior to posterior direction
SLE	systemic lupus erythematosus
TA	tibialis anterior
TB	tuberculosis
TDWB(AT)	touch-down weight bearing (as tolerated)
TENS	transcutaneous electrical nerve stimulation
TFCC	triangular fibrocartilage complex
TGF-β	transforming growth factor beta
THA	total hip arthroplasty
TJA	total joint arthroplasty
TKA	total knee arthroplasty
TLSO	thoracolumbosacral orthosis
TP	tibialis posterior
UCL	ulnar collateral ligament
UHMWPE	ultra–high molecular weight polyethylene
VISI	volar intercalated segmental instability
VMO	vastus medialis obliquus
WBAT	weight bearing as tolerated
WBC	white blood cell (count)

Suggested Readings

Orthopaedic Terminology
Hoppenfeld S, Zeide M: Orthopaedic Dictionary. Philadelphia, JB Lippincott, 1994.

Basic Science
Brinker MR, Miller MD: Basic sciences. *In* Miller MD (ed): Review of Orthopaedics, 2nd ed. Philadelphia, WB Saunders, 1996, pp 1–122.

Simon SR: Orthopaedic Basic Science. Chicago, American Academy of Orthopaedic Surgeons, 1994.

Musculoskeletal Conditions of Adults
Favus MJ: Primer on the Metabolic Bone Diseases and Disorders of Mineral Metabolism, 2nd ed. New York, Raven, 1993.

Miller MD: Review of Orthopaedics, 2nd ed. Philadelphia, WB Saunders, 1996.

Anatomy
Clemente CD: Anatomy: A Regional Atlas of the Human Body, 2nd ed. Baltimore, Urban & Schwarzenberg, 1981.

Gardner E, Gray DJ, O'Rahilly R: Anatomy: A Regional Study of Human Structure, 4th ed. Philadelphia, WB Saunders, 1975.

Gomez BA: Anatomy. *In* Miller MD (ed): Review of Orthopaedics, 2nd ed. Philadelphia, WB Saunders, 1996, pp 421–485.

Hollinshead WH: Anatomy for Surgeons: Volume 3: The Back and Limbs. New York, Hoeber-Harper, 1958.

Surgical Approaches
Gomez BA: Anatomy. *In* Miller MD (ed): Review of Orthopaedics, 2nd ed. Philadelphia, WB Saunders, 1996, pp 421–485.

Hoppenfeld S, de Boer P: Surgical Exposures in Orthopaedics: The Anatomic Approach. Philadelphia, JB Lippincott, 1984.

History and Physical Examination
Hoppenfeld S: Physical Examination of the Spine and Extremities. Norwalk, CT, Appleton-Century-Crofts, 1976.

Magee DJ: Orthopedic Physical Assessment, 3rd ed. Philadelphia, WB Saunders, 1997.

Pediatric Orthopedics
Lovell WW, Winter RB: Pediatric Orthopaedics. Philadelphia, JB Lippincott, 1978.

Stefko RM, Wenger DR: Pediatric orthopaedics. *In* Miller MD (ed): Review of Orthopaedics, 2nd ed, Philadelphia, WB Saunders, 1996, pp 123–167.

Tachdjian MO: Pediatric Orthopedics, 2nd ed. Philadelphia, WB Saunders, 1990.

Medical Considerations
Ewald GA, McKenzie CR: Manual of Medical Therapeutics, 28th ed. Boston, Little, Brown, 1995.

Fractures, Dislocations, and Traumatic Disorders
Browner BD, Jupiter JB, Levine AM, Trafton PG: Skeletal Trauma: Fractures, Dislocations, Ligamentous Injuries. Philadelphia, WB Saunders, 1992.

Charnley J: The Closed Treatment of Common Fractures, 3rd ed. New York, Churchill Livingstone, 1974.

Müller ME, Allgöwer M, Schneider R, Willenegger H: Manual of Internal Fixation, 3rd ed. Berlin, Springer-Verlag, 1991.

Rockwood Jr, CA, Green DP: Fractures in Adults, 2nd ed. Philadelphia, JB Lippincott, 1984.

Schatzker J, Tile M: The Rationale of Operative Fracture Care. Berlin, Springer-Verlag, 1987.

Operative Procedures (General Texts)
Chapman MW: Operative Orthopaedics. Philadelphia, JB Lippincott, 1988.

Crenshaw AH: Campbell's Operative Orthopaedics, 7th ed. St Louis, Mosby–Year Book, 1987.

Sports Medicine
Baker CL: The Hughston Clinic Sports Medicine Field Manual. Baltimore, Williams & Wilkins, 1996.

DeLee JC, Drez D Jr: Orthopaedic Sports Medicine: Principles and Practice. Philadelphia, WB Saunders, 1994.

Miller MD, Cooper DE, Warner JJP: Review of Sports Medicine and Arthroscopy. Philadelphia, WB Saunders, 1995.

Joint Arthroplasty
Krackow KA: The Technique of Total Knee Arthroplasty. St Louis, Mosby–Year Book, 1990.

Morrey BF, Chao EYS, Cooney WP III, Kavanagh BF, Kitaoka HB, Rand JA: Joint Replacement Arthroplasty. New York, Churchill Livingstone, 1991.

Shoulder
Miller MD, Cooper DE, Warner JJP: Review of Sports Medicine and Arthroscopy. Philadelphia, WB Saunders, 1995, pp 113–164.

Rockwood CA Jr, Matsen FA III: The Shoulder. Philadelphia, WB Saunders, 1990.

Elbow
Morrey BF: The Elbow and Its Disorders, 2nd ed. Philadelphia, WB Saunders, 1993.

Wrist
Lichtman DM, Alexander AH: The Wrist and Its Disorders, 2nd ed. Philadelphia, WB Saunders, 1998.

Taleisnik J: The Wrist. New York, Churchill Livingstone, 1985.

Hand
Green DP: Operative Hand Surgery, 2nd ed. New York, Churchill Livingstone, 1988.

The Hand: Primary Care of Common Problems. Aurora, American Society for Surgery of the Hand, 1985.

The Hand: Examination and Diagnosis. Aurora, American Society for Surgery of the Hand, 1978.

Spine
Frymoyer JW, Ducker TB, Hadler NM, Kostuik JP, Weinstein JN, Whitecloud TS III: The Adult Spine: Principles and Practice, 2nd ed. Philadelphia, Lippincott-Raven, 1997.

Herkowitz HN, et al (eds): Rothman-Simeone The Spine, 4th ed. Philadelphia, WB Saunders, 1998.

Knee
Miller MD, Cooper DE, Warner JJP: Review of Sports Medicine and Arthroscopy. Philadelphia, WB Saunders, 1995, pp 1–71.

Foot and Ankle
Jahss MH: Disorders of the Foot and Ankle, 2nd ed. Philadelphia, WB Saunders, 1991.

Mann RA, Coughlin MJ: Surgery of the Foot and Ankle, 6th ed. St Louis, Mosby–Year Book, 1992.

Commonly Used Medications in Musculoskeletal Medicine

Type of Medication	Brand Name (Company)	Generic Name	Sizes Available	Mechanism of Action	Adult Dosage	Maximum Daily Dosage	Comments
Anti-inflammatory (oral)	Clinoril (Merck)	Sulindac	150 mg, 200 mg	Inhibition of prostaglandin synthesis	150 to 200 mg bid	400 mg per day	
	Daypro (Searle)	Oxaprozin	250 mg, 500 mg	Inhibition of prostaglandin synthesis	600 mg bid	1800 mg per day or 26 mg/kg (whichever is lower)	
	Dolobid (Merck)	Diflunisal	250 mg, 500 mg	Inhibition of prostaglandin synthesis	250 to 500 mg q 8 to 12 hours	1500 mg per day	
	Feldene (Pfizer)	Piroxicam	10 mg, 20 mg	Inhibition of prostaglandin synthesis	20 mg per day	20 mg per day	
	Indocin (Merck)	Indomethacin	25 mg, 50 mg, 75 mg (SR)	Inhibition of prostaglandin synthesis	25 to 50 mg bid to tid	150 to 200 mg per day	
	Lodine (Wyeth-Ayerst)	Etodolac	200 mg, 300 mg, 400 mg, 500 mg, 600 mg	Inhibition of prostaglandin synthesis	400 to 1000 mg per day	1000 mg per day	
	Motrin (McNeil)	Ibuprofen	400 mg, 600 mg, 800 mg	Inhibition of arachidonic acid	400 to 800 mg tid	2400 mg per day	
	Naprosyn/Anaprox (Roche)	Naproxen	250 mg, 375 mg, 500 mg	Inhibition of prostaglandin synthesis	250 to 500 mg bid	1000 mg per day	
	Orudis (Wyeth-Ayerst)	Ketoprofen	25 mg, 50 mg, 75 mg	Inhibition of prostaglandin and leukotriene synthesis	75 mg tid or 50 mg q.d	300 mg per day	
	Relafen (SmithKline-Beecham)	Nabumetone	500 mg, 750 mg	Inhibition of prostaglandin synthesis	1000 to 2000 mg per day in single or divided dosages	2000 mg per day	
	Tolectin (Ortho-McNeil)	Tolmetin	200 mg, 400 mg, 600 mg	Inhibition of prostaglandin synthesis	300 mg tid	1800 mg per day	
	Toradol (Roche)	Ketorolac tromethamine	10 mg oral (also available in IV or IM 30 to 60 mg)	Inhibition of prostaglandin synthesis	20 to 40 mg orally for a maximum of 5 days or 60 to 120 mg IV/IM	40 mg orally and 120 mg IV/IM	
	Voltaren (Novartis)	Diclofenac	25 mg, 50 mg, 75 mg, 100 mg	Inhibition of prostaglandin synthesis	100 to 150 mg bid or tid	225 mg per day	

Type of Medication	Brand Name (Company)	Generic Name	Sizes Available	Mechanism of Action	Adult Dosage	Maximum Daily Dosage	Comments
Analgesic (oral)	Aspirin (Many manufacturers)	Acetylsalicylic acid	325 mg, 500 mg	Inhibition of prostaglandin synthesis and inhibition of platelet function	325 to 1000 mg q 4 to 6 hours (dosage for platelet effects for TIAs is 325 mg bid)	4000 mg per day	
	Tylenol (McNeil)	Acetaminophen	325 mg, 500 mg	Regulation of the hypothalamus	650 to 1000 mg q 4 to 6 hours as needed	4000 mg per day	
	Ultram (Ortho-McNeil)	Tramadol hydrochloride	50 mg	Central blockage of opioid receptors	50 to 100 mg q 6 hours	400 mg per day	
	Talwin Compound (Sanofi)	12.5 mg of pentazocine hydrochloride & 325 mg aspirin	—	Narcotic antagonist	2 tablets tid or qid	8 tablets per day	Schedule IV drug
	Darvocet/Darvon (Eli Lilly)	50 mg propoxyphene napsylate & 325 mg acetaminophen	—	Centrally acting narcotic	2 tablets q 4 hours as needed for pain	600 mg per day	Schedule IV drug
	Demerol (Sanofi)	Meperidine	50 mg, 100 mg	Opioid agonist	50 to 150 mg q 4 hours	600 mg per day	Schedule II drug
	Dilaudid (Knoll)	Hydromorphone hydrochloride	8 mg	Opioid agonist	8 mg q 3 to 4 hours as needed	48 mg per day	Schedule II drug
	Fiorinal with codeine (Novartis)	50 mg butalbital, 325 mg aspirin, 40 mg caffeine, & 30 mg codeine	—	Barbiturate and narcotic opioid agonist	1 or 2 tablets q 4 hours	6 tablets per day	Schedule III drug
	Lortab (UCB Pharma)	Hydrocodone bitartrate & acetaminophen	2.5/500 mg or 5/500 mg	Opioid analgesic and anticonvulsant	2.5 to 5 mg q 4 to 6 hours	8 tablets per day	Schedule III drug
	MS Contin (Purdue Frederick)	Morphine sulfate	15 mg, 30 mg, 60 mg, 100 mg, 200 mg	Opioid receptors	15 to 20 mg q 4 to 6 hours as needed for severe pain	Based on tolerance	Schedule II drug
	Oramorph (Roxane)	Morphine sulfate	15 mg, 30 mg, 60 mg, 100 mg	Opioid receptors	15 to 200 mg q 4 to 6 hours as needed for severe pain	Based on tolerance	Schedule II drug
	OxyContin (Purdue Pharma)	Oxycodone hydrochloride	10 mg, 20 mg, 40 mg, 80 mg	Opioid agonist	10 to 80 mg q 4 to 6 hours as needed	Based on tolerance	Schedule II drug

Percocet (Endo Labs)	5 mg oxycodone & 325 mg acetaminophen	—	Opioid agonist	1 to 2 tablets q 4 to 6 hours	8 to 10 tablets per day	Schedule II drug
Tylenol with codeine (Ortho-McNeil)	30 mg codeine & 300 mg acetaminophen	—	Opioid agonist	1 to 2 tablets q 4 to 6 hours as needed for pain	8 tablets per day	Schedule III drug
Tylox (Ortho-McNeil)	5 mg oxycodone hydrochloride & 500 mg acetaminophen	—	Opioid agonist	1 to 2 tablets q 4 to 6 hours as needed for pain	8 tablets per day	Schedule II drug
Vicodin (Knoll Labs)	10 mg hydrocodone bitartrate & 660 mg acetaminophen	5/500 mg	—	1 to 2 tablets q 4 to 6 hours as needed for pain	8 tablets per day	Schedule III drug
Wygesic (Wyeth-Ayerst)	65 mg proproxyphene hydrochloride & 650 mg acetaminophen	—	Centrally acting narcotic analgesic agent	1 to 2 tablets q 4 to 6 hours as needed for pain	390 mg per day or 6 tablets per day	Schedule IV drug

Type of Medication	Brand Name (Company)	Generic Name	Sizes Available	Mechanism of Action	Adult Dosage	Maximum Daily Dosage	Comments
Antibiotics (oral)—first-generation cephalosporins	Keflex (Many manufacturers)	Cephalexin monohydrate	250 mg, 500 mg	Inhibition of cell wall synthesis	250 to 500 mg q 6 hours	2000 mg per day	Gram-positive coverage
	Velosef (Lederle Standard)	Cephradine	250 mg, 500 mg	Inhibition of cell wall synthesis	250 mg, 500 mg q 6 hours	2000 mg per day	Gram-positive coverage
	Duricef (Bristol-Myers Squibb)	Cefadroxil monohydrate	500 mg, 1000 mg	Inhibition of cell wall synthesis	250 to 500 mg q 6 hours	2000 mg per day	Gram-positive coverage
Antibiotics (oral)—second-generation cephalosporins	Ceclor (Dura, Mylan, Eli Lilly)	Cefaclor	375 mg, 500 mg	Inhibition of cell wall synthesis	500 mg bid	4000 mg per day	Gram-positive coverage
	Ceftin (Glaxo Wellcome)	Cefuroxime axetil	125 mg, 250 mg, 500 mg	Inhibition of cell wall synthesis	125 to 500 mg q 12 hours	1000 mg per day	
Antibiotics (oral)—macrolides	Biaxin (Abbott)	Clarithromycin	250 mg	Inhibition of protein synthesis	500 mg q 8 to 12 hours	1500 mg per day	Aerobic and anaerobic gram-positive and gram-negative coverage and *Mycobacterium avium* coverage
	Erythromycin (Abbott/Mylan)	Erythromycin	250 mg, 500 mg	Inhibition of protein synthesis	250 mg q 6 hours or 500 mg q 12 hours	1000 mg per day	Gram-positive coverage for penicillin-insensitive organisms and patients who do not tolerate penicillin
	Zithromax (Pfizer)	Azithromycin	250 mg, 500 mg	Inhibition of protein synthesis	500 mg per day for 5 days of treatment	500 mg per day	Used primarily for respiratory infections
	Clecocin (Pharmacia, Upjohn)	Clindamycin hydrochloride	75 mg, 150 mg, 300 mg	Inhibition of protein synthesis	150 to 300 mg q 6 hours; 300 to 450 mg q 6 hours for severe infections	1800 mg per day	Used for anaerobic infections

Category	Brand (Manufacturer)	Generic	Strength	Mechanism	Dosing	Daily dose	Coverage
Antibiotics (oral)—penicillins	Amoxil (SmithKline-Beecham)	Amoxicillin	125 mg, 500 mg	Inhibition of cell wall synthesis	250 mg q 8 hours	1000 mg per day	Good coverage against gram-positive organisms that are not penicillinase resistant
	Augmentin (SmithKline-Beecham)	Amoxicillin/clavulanate	250 mg, 500 mg, 875 mg	Inhibition of cell wall synthesis	250 to 500 mg q 12 hours	1000 mg per day	Good coverage for respiratory infections and skin infections, especially animal bites
	Omnipen (Wyeth-Ayerst)	Ampicillin trihydrate	250 mg, 500 mg	Inhibition of cell wall synthesis	500 mg qid	2000 mg per day	Good coverage for gram-positive infections that are penicillinase sensitive
	Penicillin-VK (Wyeth-Ayerst)	Penicillin V potassium	250 mg, 500 mg	Inhibition of cell wall synthesis	250 to 500 mg q 6 to 8 hours	2000 mg per day	Good coverage for gram-positive nonpenicillinase resistant organisms
Antibiotics (oral)—tetracycline	Achromycin, Helidac, Tetracycline (Procter & Gamble, Lederle)	Tetracycline hydrochloride	500 mg	Inhibition of protein synthesis	500 mg bid to qid	2000 mg per day	Good coverage for various microbacteria, *Pasteurella*, *Brucella*, others
	Vibramycin (Pfizer)	Doxycycline hyclate	50 mg, 100 mg	Inhibition of protein synthesis	100 mg q 12 hours for the first day and then 100 mg qid for the following days treatment	200 mg per day	

Type of Medication	Brand Name (Company)	Generic Name	Sizes Available	Mechanism of Action	Adult Dosage	Maximum Daily Dosage	Comments
Antibiotics (oral)—quinolones	Cipro (Bayer)	Ciprofloxacin	100 mg, 250 mg, 500 mg, 750 mg	Inhibition of DNA gyrase enzymes	500 to 750 mg q 12 hours	1500 mg per day	Good coverage for aerobic gram-negative organisms and other difficult infections including chlamydia and microbacteria infections
	Floxin (Ortho-McNeil)	Ofloxacin	200 mg, 300 mg, 400 mg	Inhibition of DNA gyrase enzymes	200 to 400 mg q 12 hours	800 mg per day	Good coverage for gram-negative aerobes
Antibiotics (oral)—sulfonamides	Bactrim (Roche)	Trimethoprim-sulfamethoxazole	160 mg of trimethoprim, 100 mg of sulfamethoxazole	Sulfamethoxazole inhibits dihydrofolic acid synthesis and trimethoprim blocks dihydrofolic acid formations	1 double-strength to 2 double-strength tablets q 12 hours	4 tablets per day	Good coverage in urinary tract infection, bronchitis, and other problems
Antifungals (oral)	Fulvicin (Schering)	Griseofulvin	165 mg, 330 mg	Inhibition of cell wall synthesis	330 mg	330 mg per day	Good coverage for tinea, *Trichophyton*, *Microsporum* species
	Grifulvin V (Ortho Pharmaceutical)	Griseofulvin	250 mg, 500 mg	Keratin exfoliation	500 mg	500 mg per day	
	Flagyl (Searle)	Metronidazole	375 mg	Free-radical mechanism	750 mg tid	2250 mg per day	Good coverage for amebiasis and anaerobic infections

Category	Brand (Manufacturer)	Generic	Supply	Mechanism	Depends on effect (oral)	Effect to INR 2-3
DVT prophylaxis	Coumadin (DuPont)	Warfarin	1 mg, 2 mg, 2.5 mg, 4 mg, 5 mg, 7.5 mg, 10 mg	Inhibits vitamin K–dependent clotting factors	Depends on effect (oral)	Effect to INR 2-3
	Heparin (Wyeth-Ayerst)	Heparin	1000 to 20,000 U/mL	Inhibits factor X	Depends on effect (IV)	PTT to 1.5 to 2 times normal
	Lovenox (Rhone-Poulenc Rorer)	Enoxaparin sodium	30 mg/0.3 mL 40 mg/0.4 mL	Forms complexes between antithrombin III and factors IIa and Xa	15 to 40 mg (SC injection)	15 to 40 mg bid
	Ecotrin (SmithKline-Beecham)	Enteric-coated aspirin	325 mg	Antiplatelet	650 mg bid (oral)	—
Injectables—analgesics	Xylocaine (Astra)	Lidocaine	0.5%, 1%, 2%	Stabilizes neuronal membranes	1 to 5 mL	500 mg
	Marcaine (Abbott)	Bupivacaine hydrochloride	0.25%, 0.5%, 0.75% (10, 30, 50 mL vials)	Increases threshold for nerve stimulation	1 to 5 mL	200 mg
Injectables—steroids	Celestone (Schering)	Betamethasone	6 mg/mL (5-mL vials)	Anti-inflammatory	0.5 to 2.0 mL	3 or 4 doses
	Decadron (Merck)	Dexamethasone	4 mg/mL (5-mL vials)	Anti-inflammatory	2 to 4 mg (1 mL)	3 or 4 doses
	Hydrocortone (Merck)	Hydrocortisone	50 mg/mL (5-mL vials)	Anti-inflammatory	25 to 50 mg (1 mL)	3 or 4 doses
	Solu-Medrol (Pharmacia, Upjohn)	Methylprednisolone	125 mg/2 mL (2-mL vials)	Anti-inflammatory	125 mg/1 vial	125 mg (1 vial)
Injectables—hyaluronic acids	Hyalgan (Wyeth-Ayerst)	Hyaluronic acid	Prepackaged	Binds receptors and increases hyaluronic acid production	1 dose 4 to 5 times over 4 to 6 weeks (intra-articular)	—
	Synvisc (Orthologic)	Hylan fluid-gel mixture	Prepackaged	Binds receptors and increases hyaluronic acid production	1 dose 4 to 5 times over 4 to 6 weeks (intra-articular)	—

bid, twice a day; IM, intramuscular; INR, international normalized ratio; IV, intravenous; PTT, partial thromboplastin time; q, every; qid, four times a day; SC, subcutaneous; SR, substained release; TIA, transient ischemic attack; tid, three times a day.

Index

Note: Page numbers in *italics* refer to illustrations; page numbers followed by t refer to tables.

A

Aa (alveolar-arterial) gradient, 98
Abduction, of fingers, 184t, 205t
  of hip, 273, *274*, 275t
  of shoulder, 119, *124*, 126t
  of thumb, 184t, 205t
  of toes, 347, 347t, *348*
Abduction external rotation stress test, 328, *330*
Abductor(s), hip, 270, *271*
Abductor digiti minimi (ADM), *200*, 201, 345t
  strength testing of, 203, 205t
Abductor hallucis, 345t
Abductor pollicis brevis (APB), 184t, 200, *200*
  strength testing of, 203, 205t
Abductor pollicis longus (APL), forearm and, 165, *168*
  hand and, 200, *200*
  strength testing of, 203, 205t
  wrist and, 179, 179t, *181*, 184t
ABGs (arterial blood gases), 98
AC joint. See *Acromioclavicular (AC) joint.*
Acceleration, 16
Acetabulum, 269, *269*. See also *Pelvis.*
  fractures of, 264t, *267*, 267–268
Acetylsalicylic acid (aspirin), 370
Achilles tendon injury, 330, *330*, 333
Achondroplasia, 6t
Achromycin (tetracyline hydrochloride), 373
ACL. See *Anterior cruciate ligament (ACL).*
Acromioclavicular (AC) joint, 118, *122*
  degenerative disease of, 139
  diagnostic injection of, 135
  ligamentous injuries and, 143, 144t, *146*
  radiographic evaluation of, 135
  separation of, 139
  testing of, 128, *130*
Acromion, *131–132*
Acromioplasty, 118–119
Actin, of skeletal muscle, *10*, 11, 11t
Action potential, of neuron, 12
Acute tubular necrosis, 100
AD (autosomal dominant) disorders, 15
Adduction, of fingers, 184t, 205t
  of hip, 273, *274*
  of shoulder, 126t
  of thumb, 184t, 205t
  of toes, 347, 347t, *348*
Adductor(s), hip, 270, *271*
  thigh, 287, *287*
Adductor brevis, 270, *271*, 287, *287*
Adductor hallucis, 345t
Adductor longus, 270, *271*, 287, *287*
Adductor magnus, 270, *271*, 287, *287*
Adductor pollicis, hand and, 200, *200*
  strength testing of, 203, 205t
  wrist and, 179, 184t
Adhesive capsulitis, 140

ADM. See *Abductor digiti minimi (ADM).*
Adson's maneuver, 128, *130*
Adult respiratory distress syndrome (ARDS), 99
Aerobic conditioning, 11
Afferent nerve fibers, 12, *13*
Aging, articular cartilage changes with, 8
  dietary calcium requirement in, 6
Allen's test, digital, 205, *206*
  in wrist disorders, 184, *186*
Allergic reaction, to transfusion, 101
Allis reduction maneuver, 283, *283*
Allis' sign, 85, *85*
Allograft, *7*, *7*t
Alveolar-arterial (Aa) gradient, 98
Amoxicillin (Amoxil, Augmentin), 373
Ampicillin (Omnipen), 373
Amputation, of hand, 214, 214t
Anabolic steroids, 11
Analgesics, 370–371
  injectable, 375
Anconeus muscle, 157, 157t, *158*, 165, *167*
Ankle, 323–341
  anatomy of, 323–325, *323–327*
  conditions of, 332, 332–336, *334–336*
    diagnostic tests for, 330, 330–332, *331*
    differential diagnosis of, 341
    pediatric, 94, *94*, *95*
  fractures and dislocations of, 336–340, 337t, *338–341*, 339t
  history and physical examination of, 326–330, 328–330, 329t
  instability of, differential diagnosis of, 341
    testing for, 328, *329*
  surgical approaches to, 325–326
  tumors of, 340
Ankylosing spondylitis (AS), 27, *28*, 65–66, 255
Annular ligament, 154, *154*
Annular pulleys, 199, *199*
Anonychia, 349t
Anorexia, 6
Anterior circumflex humeral artery, 118, *123*
Anterior cord syndrome, 236, *236*
Anterior cruciate ligament (ACL), 294, *295*
  injury to, 307–308
  laxity of, 300–301, *301*
Anterior draw test, for ACL laxity, 300–301, *301*
  for ankle instability, 328, *329*
  for glenohumeral instability, *125*, 127
Anterior fat pad syndrome, 309
Anterior interosseous nerve, 165, *169*
Anterior interosseous syndrome, 171, *171*
Anterior longitudinal ligament, 240, *242*
Anterior talofibular ligament (ATFL), 324, *324*
Anterior tibial artery, 325, *326*
Antibiotics, 372–374

Antibiotics *(Continued)*
  indications for and side effects of, 36, 41t
Antifungals, 374
Anti-inflammatory medication, 369
Antimicrobial agents, 36, 40t
Aorta, 240
APB. See *Abductor pollicis brevis (APB).*
Ape hand deformity, 172t, *173*
APL. See *Abductor pollicis longus (APL).*
Apophyseal joint, 221, *222*, 240, *242*
Apprehension test, 119–127, *125*
AR (autosomal recessive) disorders, 15
ARDS (adult respiratory distress syndrome), 99
Areflexia, 6
Arm, 149–152
  anatomy of, 149–151, *149–151*
  conditions of, 151–152
    diagnostic tests for, 151
    pediatric, 73, 73t
  fractures and dislocations of, 152, *152*, 152t
  history and physical examination of, 151
  surgical approaches to, 151
  tumors of, 152
Arterial blood gases (ABGs), 98
Arteriography, 24
Arterioles, 4, *4*
Artery of Adamkiewicz, 240
Arthritis, 25t, 25–30, 26t. See also *Osteoarthritis (OA); Rheumatoid arthritis (RA).*
  hemorrhagic, 30, *31*
  infectious, 29–30
  inflammatory, 26–29, 27t, *27–30*
  noninflammatory, 25, 25–26, *26*
  of ankle, 335, *335*, *336*
  of elbow, 158–159, *159*
  of hand, *211*, 211–212, *212*
  of hip, *278*, 278–279
  of wrist, 188
  patellofemoral, 310
  pediatric, 65–66
  tibiofemoral, 310
Arthrography, 24
  of shoulder, 135, *135*
  of wrist, 185, *187*
Arthropathy(ies). See specific type.
Arthroplasty, in tibiofemoral arthritis, 310–311, *311*
  joint replacement, 107–109, *108–110*
  shoulder, 118
Arthroscopy, in tibiofemoral arthritis, 310
  of ankle, 332
  of hip, 277
  of knee, 305, *306*
  of shoulder, 135, *136*
Articular cartilage, 7–8, 8t, *9*
  as orthopaedic material, 17
  injury to, 307